THE COMPLETE BOOK OF

NATURAL & MEDICINAL CURES

THE COMPLETE BOOK OF

NATURAL & MEDICINAL CURES

HOW TO CHOOSE THE MOST POTENT
HEALING AGENTS FOR OVER 300
CONDITIONS AND DISEASES

By the Editors of **PREVENTION** Magazine Health Books

Rodale Press, Emmaus, Pennsylvania

Library of Congress Cataloging-in-Publication Data

The Complete book of natural and medicinal cures : how to choose the most potent
   healing agents for over 300 conditions and diseases / by the editors of Prevention
  Magazine Health Books.
       p.   cm.
     Includes index.
     ISBN 0–87596–190–8 hardcover
      1. Therapeutics—Popular works.   2. Naturopathy—Popular works.
    I. Prevention Magazine Health Books. II. Title: Natural and medicinal cures.
   RM122.5.C65   1994
   615.5—dc20   94–4888
                                                     CIP

Distributed in the book trade by St. Martin's Press

      18   20   19   17   hardcover

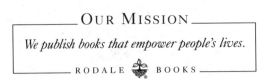

OUR MISSION

We publish books that empower people's lives.

RODALE ⚘ BOOKS

The Complete Book of Natural and Medicinal Cures
Editorial and Design Staff

Editor: Russell Wild

Authors:
HEALING FOODS: Ellen Michaud
VITAMINS, MINERALS AND OTHER SUPPLEMENTS: Sara J. Henry
HERBAL REMEDIES: Brenda Becker, Michael Castleman
MEDICATIONS: Matthew Hoffman

Contributing Writers: Brian Paul Kaufman, Sid Kirchheimer, Gale Maleskey, Elisabeth Torg

Contributing Editor: Alice Feinstein

Researchers and Fact Checkers: Susan E. Burdick, Carlotta Cuerdon, Christine Dreisbach, Valerie Edwards-Paulik, Jan Eickmeier, Theresa Fogarty, Sandra Salera-Lloyd, Deborah Pedron, Sally A. Reith, Anita Small, Bernadette Sukley, Michelle M. Szulborski

Book and Cover Designer: Vic Mazurkiewicz

Copy Editor: Jane Sherman

Office Manager: Roberta Mulliner

Office Staff: Julie Kehs, Mary Lou Stephen

Prevention Magazine Health Books

Editor-in-Chief, Rodale Books: Bill Gottlieb

Executive Editor: Debora A. Tkac

Research Manager: Ann Gossy Yermish

Copy Manager: Lisa D. Andruscavage

Advisers for *The Complete Book of Natural and Medicinal Cures*

HEALING FOODS

Kristi A. Steinmetz, R.D., Ph.D., consulting nutritional epidemiologist in the Division of Epidemiology at the University of Minnesota in Minneapolis.

VITAMINS, MINERALS AND OTHER SUPPLEMENTS

Howerde E. Sauberlich, Ph.D., professor of nutrition in the Department of Nutrition Sciences at the University of Alabama at Birmingham.

HERBAL REMEDIES

James A. Duke, Ph.D., a botanist retired from the U.S. Department of Agriculture and author of *The CRC Handbook of Medicinal Herbs*.

Norman R. Farnsworth, Ph.D., director of the Program for Collaborative Research in the Pharmaceutical Sciences at the University of Illinois at Chicago.

William J. Keller, Ph.D., professor and head of the Division of Medicinal Chemistry and Pharmaceutics at Northeast Louisiana University School of Pharmacy in Monroe.

Daniel B. Mowrey, Ph.D., director of the American Phytotherapy Research Laboratory in Salt Lake City, Utah, and author of *The Scientific Validation of Herbal Medicine*.

Varro E. Tyler, Ph.D., professor of pharmacognosy at Purdue University School of Pharmacy in West Lafayette, Indiana, and author of *The Honest Herbal*.

MEDICATIONS

E. Don Nelson, Pharm.D., professor of clinical pharmacology at the University of Cincinnati and director of the Ohio Prevention and Education Resource Center in Cincinnati.

Contents

CONTENTS

PART II

CONTENTS

PART III

CONTENTS

CONTENTS

PART IV

CONTENTS

CONTENTS

Healing Wisdom at Your Fingertips

Back pain. Headache. Stiff and achy joints. It hardly matters what's troubling you—you're likely to be showered with health advice.

"Constipated?" asks your husband—thrusting a generous bowl of bran cereal your way—"Here, eat this." Mother recommends you try one of her trusted suppositories. Margaret, your best friend, swears that nothing works better than a steaming cup of herbal tea. Whom do you listen to? What do you take?

The answer: Take a few minutes to sit down with *The Complete Book of Natural and Medicinal Cures.* No offense to your well-meaning family and friends, but what you really need is the advice of bona fide medical experts—the kind of advice featured on every page of this book.

My colleagues at *Prevention* Magazine Health Books spent months interviewing medical authorities to find the most recent and accurate information on a multitude of healing agents. What they've come up with is a revealing and practical guide to the curative power of hundreds of foods, vitamins and minerals, herbs and medications.

You might start your exciting journey to greater health with The Cure Finder, a comprehensive guide to finding just the right remedy for any of over 300 conditions. Or you can turn directly to one of the four big sections in this book to find the healing agents listed alphabetically. And if you have any question about where to locate something, there's a large index in the back of the book.

Before you know it, you'll not only find yourself healthier and happier, but *you* will be the one everyone turns to for health advice!

Russell Wild

Russell Wild
Editor

The Cure Finder

Finding Just the Right Remedies

Concerned about allergies? Arthritis? Want to find out quickly which chapters to turn to? Use this convenient listing of more than 300 health problems as a ready guide.

ANEMIA
Copper, 161
Folic Acid, 183
Iron, 194
Male Hormones, 530
Meats and Poultry, 64
Pumpkin, 89
Vitamin B_{12}, 131

ANGINA
Angina Medications, 367
Hawthorn, 309
Pineapple, 83

ANXIETY
Amino Acids, 124
Gotu Kola, 306
Sedatives, 580
Selenium, 234
Sleeping Pills, 588

APPETITE, EXCESSIVE
Amino Acids, 124
Fiber, 174

APPETITE LOSS
Folic Acid, 183
Thiamin, 240
Zinc, 243

ARRHYTHMIAS
Copper, 161
Hawthorn, 309
Heart Rhythm Drugs, 504

ARTHRITIS
Angelica, 259
Arthritis Drugs, 427
Astragalus, 262
Berries, 42
Boron, 144

Cayenne, 275
Cilantro and Coriander, 281
Copper, 161
Feverfew, 297
Fish, 55
Fish Oil, 178
Ginger, 298
Gout Drugs, 500
Immune System
  Suppressants, 508
Meadowsweet, 319
Painkillers, 557
Pantothenic Acid, 221
Potatoes, 84
Primrose Oil, 228
Selenium, 234
Turmeric, 339
Vervain, 342

ASTHMA
Asthma Drugs, 433
Astragalus, 262
Berries, 42
Coffee, 285
Fish, 55
Ginkgo, 300
Potatoes, 84

ATHEROSCLEROSIS
Beta-Carotene, 135
Chromium, 159
Copper, 161
Fish Oil, 178
Magnesium, 205
Potassium, 224
Silicon, 238
Vitamin C, 149

ATHLETE'S FOOT
Antifungal Drugs, 393
Black Walnut, 266

ATOPIC DERMATITIS
Primrose Oil, 228

ATTENTION PROBLEMS
Stimulants, 596
Zinc, 243

AUTISM
Vitamin B_6, 128

AUTOIMMUNE DISORDERS
Immune System
Suppressants, 508
Thyroid Drugs, 605

B

BACKACHE
Calcium, 154

BACK STRAIN
Painkillers, 557

BACTERIAL INFECTIONS
Antibiotics, 377
Antiseptics and Antibiotic
Creams, 418
Buckthorn, 267
Clove, 284
Dill, 288
Ear Drugs, 482
Eucalyptus, 292
Eye Drugs, 486
Thyme, 338

BALDNESS
Baldness Drugs, 438
Biotin, 142

BIRTH DEFECTS
Beans, 39
Folic Acid, 183
Okra, 76

BLADDER CANCER
Apricots, 35
Beta-Carotene, 135
Greens, 60
Selenium, 234

BLEEDING PROBLEMS
Bioflavonoids, 139
Iron, 194
Vitamin K, 199

BLISTERS
Antibiotics, 377
Antiseptics and Antibiotic
Creams, 418

BLOATING
Enzymes, 171

BLOOD CLOTS
Garlic, 58
Garlic Tablets, 186
Meadowsweet, 319
Pineapple, 83
Vitamin E, 168

BRAIN DISORDERS
Muscle Relaxants, 544

BREAST CANCER
Beta-Carotene, 135
Cancer Drugs, 452
Carrots, 45
Citrus Fruits, 49
Cruciferous Vegetables, 52
Greens, 60

Potassium, 224
Potatoes, 84
Primrose Oil, 228
Prunes, 88
Pumpkin, 89
Radishes, 90
Riboflavin, 231
Rosemary, 326
Sea Vegetables, 93
Selenium, 234
Soy, 96
Squash, 98
Sweet Potatoes, 99
Tarragon, 335
Tea, 336
Tomatoes, 102
Tropical Fruits, 103
Turmeric, 339
Vitamin A, 119
Vitamin B$_6$, 128
Vitamin C, 149
Vitamin D, 164
Vitamin E, 168
Wheat, 105
White Willow, 344
Yogurt, 107

CANDIDIASIS
Antifungal Drugs, 393

CAPILLARY PROBLEMS
Bioflavonoids, 139

CARDIOVASCULAR DISEASE
See **Atherosclerosis;**
Heart Disease

CARPAL TUNNEL SYNDROME
Vitamin B$_6$, 128

CATARACTS
Cherries, 47
Inositol, 189
Iron, 194
Riboflavin, 231
Vitamin C, 149
Vitamin E, 168

CELIAC DISEASE
Buckwheat, 44

CERVICAL CANCER
Apricots, 35
Beans, 39
Beta-Carotene, 135
Cherries, 47
Citrus Fruits, 49
Folic Acid, 183
Greens, 60
Milk, 69
Peppers, 82
Selenium, 234
Squash, 98
Sweet Potatoes, 99
Tomatoes, 102
Tropical Fruits, 103
Vitamin C, 149

CHEST CONGESTION
Anise, 261
Coffee, 285
Ephedra, 291
Eucalyptus, 292
Horehound, 310
Hyssop, 312
Mullein, 322
Oregano, 323
Peppermint, 324
Tea, 336
Thyme, 338
Wild Cherry, 346

CHOLESTEROL PROBLEMS

CHRONIC FATIGUE SYNDROME

CIRCULATION PROBLEMS

CIRRHOSIS

COLDS

COLD SORES

COLIC
Anise, 261
Chamomile, 278
Dill, 288
Fennel, 293

COLITIS
See **Inflammatory Bowel Disease**

COLON CANCER
Apples, 33
Beta-Carotene, 135
Calcium, 154
Carrots, 45
Corn, 51
Fiber, 174
Figs, 54
Folic Acid, 183
Melons, 68
Okra, 76
Onions, 78
Peppers, 82
Rice, 91
Rosemary, 326
Sea Vegetables, 93
Selenium, 234
Soy, 96
Wheat, 105
White Willow, 344
Yogurt, 107

CONCENTRATION DIFFICULTY
Iron, 194
Magnesium, 205

CONFUSION
Potassium, 224
Thiamin, 240
Vitamin B$_{12}$, 131

CONGESTION
See **Chest Congestion; Nasal Congestion**

CONJUNCTIVITIS
Eye Drugs, 486

CONSTIPATION
Apricots, 35
Buckthorn, 267
Cascara Sagrada, 273
Corn, 51
Fenugreek, 295
Fiber, 174
Figs, 54
Laxatives, 522
Magnesium, 205
Okra, 76
Prunes, 88
Pumpkin, 89
Rice, 91
Sea Vegetables, 93
Senna, 333
Squash, 98
Sweet Potatoes, 99
Vervain, 342

CONVULSIONS
Gotu Kola, 306
Seizure Drugs, 584

COORDINATION DIFFICULTY
Thiamin, 240
Vitamin B$_{12}$, 131

COUGHING
Camphor, 272
Cold Remedies, 463
Cough Medicines, 467
Fenugreek, 295

ENDOMETRIOSIS
Female Hormones, 491

EPILEPSY
Gotu Kola, 306
Seizure Drugs, 584

ESOPHAGEAL CANCER
Citrus Fruits, 49
Peppers, 82
Riboflavin, 231
Selenium, 234
Tropical Fruits, 103
Vitamin C, 149
White Willow, 344

ESOPHAGEAL REFLUX
Antacids, 372

EYE DISEASE, IN DIABETES
Citrus Fruits, 49

EYE DRYNESS
Eye Drugs, 486

EYE INFECTIONS
Antiviral Drugs, 422

**EYE REDNESS
AND IRRITATIONS**
Eye Drugs, 486
Goldenseal, 304

F

FACIAL HAIR, EXCESSIVE
Female Hormones, 491

FATIGUE
Angelica, 259
Astragalus, 262
Coffee, 285
Folic Acid, 183
Iron, 194
Magnesium, 205
Pantothenic Acid, 221
Selenium, 234
Stimulants, 596
Thiamin, 240
Vitamin B_{12}, 131

**FEET, BURNING
AND TICKLING IN**
Pantothenic Acid, 221

**FEET AND HANDS,
TINGLING IN**
Vitamin B_{12}, 131

FEVER
Balm, 263
Meadowsweet, 319
Oregano, 323
White Willow, 344

FINGERNAIL PROBLEMS
Biotin, 142
Silicon, 238

FLATULENCE
See Gas

FLEAS
Brewer's Yeast, 147
Thiamin, 240

FLU
    Antiviral Drugs, 422
    Bioflavonoids, 139
    Echinacea, 289
    Ginger, 298
    Meadowsweet, 319
    Tarragon, 335
    Tea, 336
    Vaccines, 617

FOOT PAIN, IN DIABETES
    Cayenne, 275

FORGETFULNESS
    See **Memory Loss**

FRACTURES
    Calcium, 154
    Manganese, 209
    Vitamin D, 164

FROSTBITE
    Aloe, 257

FUNGAL INFECTIONS
    Antifungal Drugs, 393
    Black Walnut, 266
    Cinnamon, 282
    Ear Drugs, 482
    Thyme, 338

G

GAIT PROBLEMS
    Vitamin B_{12}, 131

GALLSTONES
    Apples, 33
    Fiber, 174
    Gallstone Medications, 498
    Lecithin, 202

GAS
    Allspice, 256
    Anise, 261
    Anti-gas Drugs, 397
    Dill, 288
    Enzymes, 171
    Fennel, 293
    Ginger, 298
    Peppermint, 324

GASTRITIS
    Meadowsweet, 319

GASTROINTESTINAL CANCER
    Acidophilus, 121
    Vitamin C, 149

GIARDIASIS
    Parasite Drugs, 564

GLAUCOMA
    Eye Drugs, 486

GLUCOSE INTOLERANCE
    Copper, 161

GOITER
    Iodine, 191

GOUT
    Cherries, 47
    Gout Drugs, 500

GRAVES' DISEASE
    Thyroid Drugs, 605

GROWTH PROBLEMS
    Pituitary Drugs, 571
    Riboflavin, 231
    Zinc, 243

Vitamin E, 168
Wheat, 105
White Willow, 344

HEMORRHOIDS
Anal and Rectal Drugs, 363
Bioflavonoids, 139
Butcher's Broom, 270
Corn, 51
Fiber, 174
Iron, 194
Sea Vegetables, 93
Witch Hazel, 347

HEPATITIS
Milk Thistle, 320

HERPES
Antiviral Drugs, 422
Balm, 263
Bioflavonoids, 139
Cascara Sagrada, 273
Tarragon, 335
Vitamin B_6, 128

HIGH BLOOD PRESSURE
Bananas, 36
Black Walnut, 266
Blood Pressure
   Medications, 445
Calcium, 154
Celery Seed, 277
Copper, 161
Fish, 55
Fish Oil, 178
Garlic, 58
Garlic Tablets, 186
Ginseng, 302
Hawthorn, 309
Kiwi, 63

Lecithin, 202
Magnesium, 205
Milk, 69
Oils, 72
Potassium, 224
Potatoes, 84
Pumpkin, 89
Tropical Fruits, 103
Vitamin C, 149
Yogurt, 107

HIGH BLOOD SUGAR
See **Diabetes**

HIGH CHOLESTEROL
See **Cholesterol Problems**

HIGH TRIGLYCERIDES
Beans, 39
Citrus Fruits, 49
Fish, 55
Fish Oil, 178
Garlic, 58
Niacin, 218
Pantothenic Acid, 221
Tropical Fruits, 103

HIP FRACTURES
Calcium, 154

HISTOPLASMOSIS
Antifungal Drugs, 393

HIVES
Antihistamines, 400

HODGKIN'S DISEASE
Cancer Drugs, 452

INFECTION
Antibiotics, 377
Antifungal Drugs, 393
Antiseptics and Antibiotic
  Creams, 418
Antiviral Drugs, 422
Cilantro and Coriander, 281
Cold Remedies, 463
Ear Drugs, 482
Echinacea, 289
Eye Drugs, 486
Goldenseal, 304
Parasite Drugs, 564
Selenium, 234
Vaccines, 617

INFERTILITY
Fertility Drugs, 495
Pituitary Drugs, 571

INFLAMMATION
Anti-inflammatory Drugs, 405
Arthritis Drugs, 427
Berries, 42
Bioflavonoids, 139
Chamomile, 278
Cilantro and Coriander, 281
Enzymes, 171
Feverfew, 297
Ginkgo, 300
Gotu Kola, 306
Gout Drugs, 500
Painkillers, 557
Peppermint, 324
Pineapple, 83
Potatoes, 84
Primrose Oil, 228
Selenium, 234
Turmeric, 339
Vervain, 342
White Willow, 344

INFLAMMATORY BOWEL DISEASE
Inflammatory Bowel Disease
  Drugs, 518

INSECT BITES AND STINGS
Balm, 263
Clove, 284
Mullein, 322

INSOMNIA
Amino Acids, 124
Antihistamines, 400
Balm, 263
Chamomile, 278
Gotu Kola, 306
Pantothenic Acid, 221
Sleeping Pills, 588
Valerian, 341

INTESTINAL POLYPS
Wheat, 105

IRON-DEFICIENCY ANEMIA
Iron, 194
Meats and Poultry, 64

IRRITABILITY
Iron, 194
Thiamin, 240

IRRITABLE BOWEL SYNDROME
Antidepressants, 382
Fiber, 174
Okra, 76
Peppermint, 324

ITCHING
Antihistamines, 400
Anti-itch Drugs, 410
Oregano, 323

J

JAUNDICE
Oregano, 323

JOCK ITCH
Black Walnut, 266

JOINT PAIN
Allspice, 256

K

KAPOSI'S SARCOMA
Hyssop, 312

KASHIN-BECK DISEASE
Selenium, 234

KERATITIS
Eye Drugs, 486

KIDNEY PROBLEMS
Fish, 55
Potassium, 224
Potatoes, 84

KIDNEY STONES
Magnesium, 205
Vitamin B_6, 128

L

LACTOSE INTOLERANCE
Acidophilus, 121
Enzymes, 171

LARYNGEAL CANCER
Citrus Fruits, 49
Tropical Fruits, 103

LEARNING PROBLEMS
Lecithin, 202

LEG NUMBNESS
Gotu Kola, 306
Thiamin, 240

LEG VEIN PROBLEMS
Butcher's Broom, 270

LETHARGY
See Fatigue

LEUKEMIA
Cascara Sagrada, 273
Vitamin D, 164

LIP INFLAMMATION
Riboflavin, 231

LIVER CANCER
Lecithin, 202
Selenium, 234

LIVER PROBLEMS
Amino Acids, 124
Lecithin, 202
Milk Thistle, 320
Turmeric, 339

LOW BLOOD SUGAR
Brewer's Yeast, 147
Chromium, 159
Diabetes Drugs, 476

LUNG CANCER
Apricots, 35
Berries, 42
Beta-Carotene, 135
Carrots, 45
Cherries, 47

Citrus Fruits, 49
Folic Acid, 183
Greens, 60
Milk, 69
Peppers, 82
Pumpkin, 89
Rosemary, 326
Selenium, 234
Squash, 98
Sweet Potatoes, 99
Tomatoes, 102
Tropical Fruits, 103
Vitamin A, 119
Vitamin C, 149

M

MACULAR DEGENERATION
Vitamin A, 119
Zinc, 243

MALARIA
Malaria Drugs, 527

MEASLES
Vaccines, 617
Vitamin A, 119

MELANOMA, MALIGNANT
Sun Protectors, 600

MEMORY LOSS
Ginkgo, 300
Gotu Kola, 306
Lecithin, 202
Meats and Poultry, 64
Riboflavin, 231
Vitamin B$_{12}$, 131
Zinc, 243

MENINGITIS
Antibiotics, 377

MENKES' DISEASE
Copper, 161

MENOPAUSE SYMPTOMS
Angelica, 259
Female Hormones, 491
Fenugreek, 295

MENSTRUAL BLEEDING, HEAVY
Bioflavonoids, 139

MENSTRUAL CRAMPS
Allspice, 256
Balm, 263
Birth Control
    Medications, 440
Black Haw, 265
Calcium, 154
Chamomile, 278
Female Hormones, 491
Feverfew, 297
Menstrual-Problem
    Drugs, 534
Painkillers, 557
Peppermint, 324
Rosemary, 326
Valerian, 341

MENSTRUAL IRREGULARITIES
Birth Control
    Medications, 440
Menstrual-Problem
    Drugs, 534
Pituitary Drugs, 571

MENTAL FATIGUE
Boron, 144

MENTAL ILLNESS
Anti-psychotic Drugs, 415

MENTAL PROBLEMS
Zinc, 243

MENTAL SKILLS, REDUCED
Meats and Poultry, 64

METABOLIC DISORDERS
Thyroid Drugs, 605

MIGRAINES
Antidepressants, 382
Feverfew, 297
Migraine Drugs, 539
Painkillers, 557
White Willow, 344

MOOD CHANGES
Iron, 194
Lecithin, 202
Vitamin B$_{12}$, 131

MORNING SICKNESS
Ginger, 298
Nausea Drugs, 548

MOSQUITOES
Balm, 263
Brewer's Yeast, 147
Thiamin, 240

MOTION SICKNESS
Ginger, 298
Nausea Drugs, 548

MOUTH, CRACKS AT CORNERS OF
Riboflavin, 231

MOUTH CANCER
See **Oral Cancer**

MULTIPLE SCLEROSIS
Ginkgo, 300

MUMPS
Vaccines, 617

MUSCLE CRAMPS OR SPASMS
Calcium, 154
Muscle Relaxants, 544
Valerian, 341

MUSCLE SORENESS
Allspice, 256
Camphor, 272
Cayenne, 275
Eucalyptus, 292
Peppermint, 324
Witch Hazel, 347

MUSCLE SPRAIN
Painkillers, 557

MUSCLE WEAKNESS
Iron, 194
Magnesium, 205
Pantothenic Acid, 221
Potassium, 224
Vitamin B$_{12}$, 131

N

NAIL PROBLEMS
Biotin, 142
Silicon, 238

NARCOLEPSY
Stimulants, 596

NASAL CONGESTION
Cold Remedies, 463
Decongestants, 472
Peppermint, 324

NAUSEA
Antihistamines, 400
Ginger, 298
Nausea Drugs, 548
Thiamin, 240

NECK SWELLING
Iodine, 191

NERVOUSNESS
Astragalus, 262
Balm, 263
Chamomile, 278
Gotu Kola, 306
Valerian, 341

NEUROLOGICAL DISORDERS
Inositol, 189
Painkillers, 557
Shellfish, 95
Vitamin B_6, 128
Vitamin B_{12}, 131

NIGHT VISION IMPAIRMENT
Vitamin A, 119

NOSE, RUNNY
Antihistamines, 400
Cold Remedies, 463

NUMBNESS IN LEGS
Gotu Kola, 306
Thiamin, 240

O

ONYCHOMYCOSIS
Antifungal Drugs, 393

ORAL CANCER
Beta-Carotene, 135
Citrus Fruits, 49
Milk, 69
Peppers, 82
Tropical Fruits, 103
Vitamin C, 149
Vitamin E, 168

ORAL THRUSH
Antifungal Drugs, 393

OSTEOPOROSIS
Boron, 144
Calcium, 154
Magnesium, 205
Osteoporosis Drugs, 553
Vitamin D, 164
Yogurt, 107

OVARIAN CANCER
Milk, 69
Soy, 96

OVERWEIGHT
Beans, 39
Corn, 51
Ephedra, 291
Potatoes, 84
Prunes, 88
Sea Vegetables, 93
Shellfish, 95
Stimulants, 596

P

PAIN
Allspice, 256
Antidepressants, 382
Anti-inflammatory Drugs, 405
Arthritis Drugs, 427
Cayenne, 275
Clove, 284
Cold Remedies, 463
Ear Drugs, 482
Female Hormones, 491
Gout Drugs, 500
Painkillers, 557
Ulcer Medications, 612
Vervain, 342
White Willow, 344

PALENESS
Folic Acid, 183
Iron, 194

PANCREATIC CANCER
Citrus Fruits, 49
Peppers, 82
Tropical Fruits, 103
Vitamin C, 149

PANCREATITIS
Enzymes, 171

PANIC ATTACKS
Sedatives, 580

PARASITIC INFECTIONS
Parasite Drugs, 564

PARKINSON'S DISEASE
Parkinson's Disease
Drugs, 567

PEPTIC ULCERS
See Ulcers

PERIPHERAL NEUROPATHY
Inositol, 189

PERIPHERAL VASCULAR DISEASE
Ginkgo, 300

PERNICIOUS ANEMIA
Vitamin B_{12}, 131

PERTUSSIS
Vaccines, 617

PIMPLES
See Acne

PINKEYE
Eye Drugs, 486

PITUITARY PROBLEMS
Pituitary Drugs, 571

PNEUMONIA
Antibiotics, 377

POISON IVY
Anti-itch Drugs, 410

SPINAL CORD INJURY
Muscle Relaxants, 544

SPINAL FRACTURES
Osteoporosis Drugs, 553
Vitamin D, 164

STOMACH CANCER
Beta-Carotene, 135
Citrus Fruits, 49
Garlic Tablets, 186
Milk, 69
Onions, 78
Peppers, 82
Squash, 98
Sweet Potatoes, 99
Tropical Fruits, 103
Vitamin C, 149
White Willow, 344

STOMACH ULCERS
See **Ulcers**

STOMACH UPSET
Allspice, 256
Anise, 261
Balm, 263
Chamomile, 278
Cinnamon, 282
Peppermint, 324
Pineapple, 83

STRESS
Ginseng, 302
Pantothenic Acid, 221
Sedatives, 580
Sleeping Pills, 588

STROKE
Bananas, 36
Citrus Fruits, 49

Cruciferous Vegetables, 52
Fish, 55
Ginkgo, 300
Greens, 60
Muscle Relaxants, 544
Peppers, 82
Pineapple, 83
Potassium, 224
Potatoes, 84
Pumpkin, 89
Selenium, 234
Vitamin A, 119
White Willow, 344

SUDDEN INFANT DEATH SYNDROME
Biotin, 142

SUNBURN
Aloe, 257
Sun Protectors, 600

SWELLING
Anti-inflammatory Drugs, 405

SWIMMER'S EAR
Ear Drugs, 482

T

TARDIVE DYSKINESIA
Lecithin, 202

TASTE LOSS
Zinc, 243

TEETHING PAIN
Chamomile, 278

TETANUS
Vaccines, 617

THROAT CANCER
Beta-Carotene, 135
Citrus Fruits, 49

THYROID PROBLEMS
Iodine, 191
Thyroid Drugs, 605

TINNITUS
Ginkgo, 300

TIREDNESS
See **Fatigue**

TONGUE, RED
Riboflavin, 231

TOOTHACHE
Allspice, 256
Chamomile, 278
Clove, 284
White Willow, 344

TOOTH DECAY
Cinnamon, 282
Molybdenum, 211

TRAVELER'S DIARRHEA
Clove, 284

TUBERCULOSIS
Tuberculosis Drugs, 609

U

ULCERATIVE COLITIS
Fish, 55
Fish Oil, 178

Folic Acid, 183
Inflammatory Bowel Disease
Drugs, 518

ULCERS
Bananas, 36
Chamomile, 278
Cinnamon, 282
Fiber, 174
Ginger, 298
Iron, 194
Licorice, 316
Meadowsweet, 319
Slippery Elm, 334
Turmeric, 339
Ulcer Medications, 612

URINARY INCONTINENCE
Incontinence Drugs, 513

URINARY TRACT INFECTIONS
Antibiotics, 377
Berries, 42
Cinnamon, 282
Meadowsweet, 319

UTERINE CANCER
Selenium, 234

V

VAGINAL YEAST INFECTIONS
See **Yeast Infections**

VARICOSE VEINS
Bioflavonoids, 139

PART

I

HEALING
FOODS

Healing Foods

You Are What You Eat

The evidence is overwhelming that what we put in our mouths can either put us on the road to health or bottle us up with disease.

"Perhaps five of the ten leading causes of death in the United States are nutritionally caused," says Neil Stone, M.D., chairman of the American Heart Association's nutrition committee and associate professor of medicine at Northwestern University in Chicago. "And as such, diseases like heart disease, cancer and stroke can often be prevented."

In fact, scientists say that a little more attention to our diets might slash the death rates for these diseases by as much as 70 percent.

"There are four broad ways in which diet can produce disease," explains John Potter, M.D., Ph.D., professor of epidemiology at the University of Minnesota in Minneapolis. "We eat too much, we eat too much of the wrong things, we don't eat enough of the right things, and we eat things in our foods like preservatives and pesticide residues that the body doesn't handle well—

or at least not in the quantities we consume."

The result is clogged arteries, overburdened hearts, stone-filled gallbladders, ruined livers and a variety of chemical enemies running around our bodies that can deal out a dozen different types of cancer.

How do so many people get into such a predicament? "I think it's useful to think about the way our gatherer/hunter ancestors ate," says Dr. Potter. "And notice that I didn't say 'hunter/gatherer.' Most of the evidence is that we've always gathered much more than we've hunted."

The point is that our ancestors consumed mostly fruits, roots, leaves, nuts and seeds, with an occasional piece of meat if someone got lucky with a club. Their only milk came from the breast, eggs were a rare treat and potato chips and ice cream were unheard of.

"This is the diet to which humans are adapted," says Dr. Potter. "It contains not just low fat, high fiber and lots of vitamins and minerals but also other things we are only now discovering are essential to the maintenance of a disease-free human."

Great Discoveries

Ten years ago scientists began to develop highly sensitive tools for use in genetic engineering and molecular biology," explains Dick Huston, Ph.D., a nutritional bio-chemist who heads an interdisciplinary Functional Foods for Health program at the University of Illinois at Chicago. "And for the past few years those tools have been used to pry open the secrets of food."

The result has been discovery after discovery at the molecular level. Researchers have discovered that broccoli contains sulforaphane,

---

FOOD FOR A HEALTHY HEART

You already know that a healthy heart demands a low-fat, low-cholesterol diet. But other than holding off on double helpings of bacon, what else can you do to keep your heart on the job? "It's important to eat a balanced diet rich in fruits and vegetables," says Neil Stone, M.D., chairman of the American Heart Association's nutrition committee and associate professor of medicine at Northwestern University in Chicago.

The Heart Association's advice summarizes a smorgasbord of studies that indicate that a well-balanced diet, low in saturated fat, can protect your heart. Some foods may reduce cholesterol levels; others may reduce the amount of damage cholesterol can do. Other foods may reduce your body's ability to produce the blood clots that can jam arterial highways and trigger heart attacks.

However they work, research suggests that the following foods can help increase the likelihood that your heart will remain the healthy workhorse it was designed to be. But don't pick one food, eat it at every meal and think you're going to prevent a heart attack. The key, experts say, is balance.

Apricots	Garlic	Nuts	Pineapple
Beans	Grapefruit	Oil*	Prunes
Carrots	Greens	Okra	Pumpkin
Cherries	Kiwi	Onions	Squash
Fish	Mangoes	Oranges	Sweet potatoes

*Canola and olive oil may help prevent heart disease, but only when used as a *substitute* for other fats in the diet.

TOP CANCER FIGHTERS

Studies indicate that eating more than seven servings a week of fresh fruits and green and yellow vegetables may reduce your risk of various types of cancer by as much as 80 percent.

According to research from around the world, here are a few of the most potent cancer fighters available. Eat a wide variety to assure yourself maximum protection.

Apricots	Figs	Papaya
Berries	Garlic	Prunes
Bok choy	Grapefruit	Pumpkin
Broccoli	Guava	Radishes
Brussels sprouts	Honeydew	Romaine lettuce
Cabbage	Kale	Soy
Cantaloupe	Kiwi	Spinach
Carrots	Mangoes	Sweet potatoes
Casaba melons	Mustard greens	Swiss chard
Cherries	Okra	Tomatoes
Collards	Onions	Watercress
Endive	Oranges	Winter squash

a substance that may help prevent cancer. Brussels sprouts, rutabagas and mustard greens contain indoles, which may reduce the risk of breast and other cancers. Beans, soy products, grains, potatoes, spinach, broccoli and radishes contain protease inhibitors, which may also be potent cancer-fighting compounds. And garlic and onions contain organosulfides, which may be able to prevent tumors from growing and prevent the blood clots that trigger heart attacks.

The list of substances in plant foods that can help us fight disease is long. Lycopenes in tomatoes, beta-carotene in dark orange and leafy green vegetables, bromelain in pineapple and hesperidin, naringin, nobiletin, tangeretin and sinensetin in citrus—all may have the ability to prevent cancer. What's more, some may have the ability to fight heart disease and stroke as well.

As a result, "we've come to realize that it's no longer right to think of foods as only carbohydrates, proteins and fats," says Gary Fraser, M.D., Ph.D., professor of medicine and epidemiology at Loma Linda University in California and lead researcher of the Adventist Health Study, a landmark research effort in which the eating habits of some 34,000 people were analyzed. "There are literally hundreds of biochemically active substances in foods. And many are of value in fighting both heart disease and cancer."

Of course, along with the discoveries of new compounds in foods, scientists have also been confirming the long-known healing powers of our old allies—vitamins, minerals and fiber.

Studies have shown that vitamin C can reduce your risk of cancer, lower blood pressure, reduce blood sugar and increase levels of HDL cholesterol, the kind of cholesterol that protects your heart. Calcium not only helps prevent osteoporosis, it can reduce the risk of high blood pressure—and of colorectal cancer by 67 percent. Potassium can reduce the risk of stroke by 40 percent. And fiber is something of a nutritional wonder: Studies indicate it can help prevent high blood pressure, control blood sugar, lower cholesterol, alleviate constipation, soothe irritable bowels and help you lose weight.

Evidence from the Kitchen

While some scientists have been studying individual foods, others have been studying groups of foods and the way people eat them. What they've found is that people who eat a variety of foods that contain a mixture of protective vitamins, minerals and other substances do, in fact, have less disease.

It is possible, says Dr. Potter, that the reason cancer has become almost epidemic is that we are not consuming enough of these protective substances. A federal survey has found that on any given day, 45 percent of us have no fruit at all, while 22 percent have no vegetables.

In the Adventist Health Study conducted by Dr. Fraser and his colleagues—a study that included more than 34,000 men and women who are primarily vegetarians—researchers discovered that those who ate three to seven servings of fruit a week reduced their risk of lung cancer by 70 percent.

"We looked at heart disease and cancer," says Dr. Fraser. "And across the board we found that those who ate lots of produce enjoyed decreased risk from both diseases."

Other scientists have found similar results. Studies at the National Cancer Institute showed that male cigarette smokers who ate one serving of dark yellow or leafy green vegetables every other day cut their risk of lung cancer in half. Studies at the University of Hawaii showed that men who regularly ate tomatoes and dark green and cruciferous vegetables also cut their risk of lung cancer in half, while women cut their risk by even more.

Researchers abroad are reporting similar findings. Italian studies indicate that those who regularly eat melon have a 40 percent lower risk of colorectal cancer, while those who eat fresh fruit, green vegetables and fish reduce their risk of a heart attack anywhere from 40 to 60 percent. Studies in China have found that people who eat spinach, squash, eggplant and green beans reduce their risk of stomach cancer anywhere from 25 to 50 percent. And a study in Greece reveals that women who eat the most cucumbers, lettuce and raw carrots are five to eight times less likely to develop breast cancer than women who eat the least.

Back to Basics

What all these studies add up to is that people should tend toward a vegetarian diet," says Dr. Fraser. "We have found that vegetables, fruits and nuts are protective, while there's some preliminary evidence that people who eat three or more flesh foods a week are at increased risk of bladder and colon cancer. Also, men who eat the most meat have an increased risk of fatal heart disease."

Eating lots of meat, it seems, has a powerful correlation with disease.

The American Heart Association promotes a balanced diet rich in fruits, vegetables and whole grains. They suggest we get less than 30 percent of our calories from fat and less than 10 percent from saturated fat. We should consume less than 300 milligrams of cholesterol—roughly the amount found in three ounces of pot roast and one egg a day.

One way to attain such goals is to limit meat consumption. This *doesn't* mean we all have to become strict vegetarians—fish, skinless chicken and low-fat dairy products are all good foods. And even an occasional slab of roast beef shouldn't do anyone great harm. But the bulk of our calories should come from the garden, says Dr. Fraser.

"These recommendations match exactly the diet that I suspect we're naturally adapted to," says Dr. Potter. Not only did our ancestors' diet consist mostly of plant foods, but those foods weren't refined, nor did they contain dyes, preservatives or fillers. "The best direction we can take to reduce risk of chronic diseases is to eat a very wide variety of plant food, and to eat it as simply and as unprocessed as possible," says Dr. Potter.

A simple, plant-rich diet can lead to a life that is healthier *and* longer. Studies of thousands of people in the United States, Netherlands, Denmark, Britain and Germany have all demonstrated that a diet rich in fruits and vegetables may cut deaths from all causes in half.

On the following pages, you'll be introduced to a variety of nutritious foods. Use these pages as a tool to relearn the ways of the gatherer.

Apples

Crispy Cures

> **POTENTIAL HEALING POWER**
>
> May help:
> - Lower cholesterol
> - Prevent gallstones
> - Reduce risk of colorectal cancer

Crisp. Crunchy. Sweet. Sometimes tart. Biting into one of the more than 300 varieties of apples that are produced throughout the United States can evoke the sharp sweetness of a New England morning or the hazy peace of a Washington farm. But along with a touch of nostalgic Americana, that burst of juice spurting from a fresh apple also brings a mouthful of health-giving nutrients that may help prevent cancer, reduce cholesterol levels and possibly even lower your risk of developing gallstones.

How? Scientists really aren't sure. In the past a lot of discussion has centered around pectin and lignin, two types of fiber that abound in apples. But researchers are now beginning to suspect that the health-promoting effects granted by apples are somehow derived from eating the whole fruit rather than getting a dose of any one constituent.

In a Belgian study of 3,669 men and women, for example, researchers found that those who regularly ate a lot of apples had one-third the risk of developing colon cancer and 76 percent less risk of developing rectal cancer, as compared to those who never ate apples. Only whole, raw apples had a protective effect, reported the scientists. Canned or stewed fruit did not.

The real benefit of apples may be that they put foods that contain cancer-causing agents on a fast track, says Harris Clearfield, M.D., director of gastroenterology at Hahnemann University in Philadelphia. "Apples increase the stool's transit time through your colon," he explains. As a result, "the carcinogens in food have less contact time with your colon, which—in susceptible people—means less chance of getting cancer."

Drop Your Cholesterol by 15 Points

As if preventing cancer weren't more than enough to justify a visit to the closest orchard, researchers at Central Washington University have also discovered that apple fiber can reduce cholesterol levels by 15 points.

The researchers recruited 26 men with high cholesterol. Thirteen were fed three cookies a day for six weeks—cookies loaded with the equivalent of five apples' worth of fiber. The other 13 didn't get cookies. After the six weeks were up, the researchers compared the cholesterol levels of the two groups. The men who ate the apple cookies lowered their cholesterol levels an average of 7 percent—or 15 points.

Although the apple-rich cookies used in the study are not commercially available, other researchers have found similar results in people who ate two or three apples a day. It's also easy to get similar amounts of fiber by eating a variety of fruits, vegetables and whole grains each day.

As most people today know, however, there is both "good" and "bad" cholesterol. Too much of the bad (LDL) clogs up your arteries and sets the stage for heart attacks, while the good (HDL) actually wraps the bad stuff in a protein package and escorts it out of your arteries. But which kind of cholesterol is getting reduced on an apple-enriched diet?

To find out, another team of researchers fed hamsters a high-fat, high-cholesterol diet, which sent their cholesterol levels soaring. Then they put the hamsters on a diet, 10 percent of which consisted of dried apples. After six months, the researchers analyzed the hamsters' cholesterol levels and found that the "bad" cholesterol was cut in *half*, while the animals' levels of

"good" cholesterol had remained the same.

Cut Your Risk of Gallstones

Because hamsters have a digestive system very much like that of humans, researchers at Paul-Sabatier University in France also used hamsters to study how an apple-rich diet can affect the body's digestive organs and fluids.

They discovered two amazing things: One, that animals with a high cholesterol level had significantly damaged intestines. And, two, after the hamsters ate an apple-rich diet for a couple of months, the damaged intestines actually returned to normal.

But the researchers' discoveries were only beginning. In examining the hamsters' digestive fluids, they also found that an apple-rich diet alters the composition of bile, a digestive liquid from which gallstones are sometimes formed. In animals with high cholesterol levels, measurements of bile composition taken while the animals were on a regular diet indicated that their potential to form gallstones was high. After the animals had spent two months on an apple-rich diet, however, measurements indicated that their risk of gallstones was low.

Although the researchers caution that further studies are needed to confirm this effect, it may be that a diet rich in apples can actually prevent gallstones—in people as well as hamsters.

Fortunately for their health, Americans have fallen in love with apples. Between apples, applesauce and apple juice, we each eat around 40 pounds of apples a year.

Which is the most healthful product? "A fresh apple," answers apple expert Mark McLellan, Ph.D., professor of food science at Cornell University's Agriculture Experimental Station in Geneva, New York. "Everything's there.

When you make applesauce, you remove the skin, the core and the seeds, and that causes a loss of cellulose fiber. When you make juice, you usually remove not only the cellulose fiber in the skin but most of the pectin fiber that's found in the pulp as well. And that's a significant loss of dietary fiber," he says.

Anybody for a nice big Red Delicious?

Apricots

Tiny Protectors

Apricots are tiny, tart, sunshine-colored fruits packed with both fiber and beta-carotene, a form of vitamin A that is abundant in orange and yellow fruits and vegetables.

Although fiber is important in preventing constipation and lowering cholesterol, it's the beta-carotene that's knocking the socks off scientists. Results from a study at Harvard Medical School indicate that beta-carotene may well prevent the cholesterol in your blood from undergoing chemical changes that allow it to damage your arteries and set the stage for heart disease.

> **POTENTIAL HEALING POWER**
>
> May help:
> - Combat constipation
> - Prevent cholesterol from damaging your arteries
> - Protect against certain cancers

Moreover, in a review of beta-carotene research completed to date, scientists at the National Cancer Institute and the University of California, Los Angeles, have concluded that consuming more beta-carotene-rich foods like apricots may cut your risk of lung cancer—in *half*.

And in a joint study over a nine-year period by the University of Oxford in England and the University of Tampere in Finland, researchers compared 766 people who had cancer with 1,419 people who did not. Relying on new technology that uses a simple blood test to determine the amount of beta-carotene people have eaten, the researchers estimated that those who did *not* have cancer consumed 5 to 14 percent more beta-carotene from fruits and vegetables than those who had the disease—a key difference. The protective effect was particularly strong against lung and bladder cancers, two forms of the disease most related to smoking.

Fortunately, the sunny flavor of apricots makes it easy to add them around the edges of almost any meal or snack. Add dried apricot bits to a fresh green salad or slice a few fresh fruits over an icy sorbet. Try stewed apricots with cereal in the morning, apricot nectar with a cookie at night or dried apricots and almonds as an afternoon snack. The result will be a burst of fresh, sunny flavor—and a body armed against disease.

Bananas

Nature's Perfect Fast Food

Eating bananas ain't monkey business. We've known for some time that bananas can help give the slip to high blood pressure and reduce our risk of stroke. We're now finding out that bananas may also help cure ulcers, lower cholesterol and possibly more.

The magic ingredient, at least as far as your circulatory system is concerned, appears to be potassium. For example, in a study of 859 men and women conducted at the University of California, San Diego, in conjunction with the University of Cambridge School of Medicine in England, researchers discovered that those who ate a single daily serving of potassium-rich foods such as bananas had a 40 percent lower risk of stroke.

Other researchers have found that those who add potassium to their diets can not only help prevent stroke but reduce their blood pressures as well. The effect is so pow-

> **POTENTIAL HEALING POWER**
>
> May help:
> - Prevent high blood pressure
> - Heal ulcers
> - Relieve recurrent heartburn
> - Control cholesterol
> - Prevent strokes

erful, scientists say, that practically every time they add potassium to someone's diet, their blood pressure goes down. When they take the potassium *out* of someone's diet, blood pressure goes up.

In a study in India, for instance, researchers added potassium to the diets of 37 men with high blood pressures and watched their readings drop 16 points over the next eight weeks. Half a world away, researchers at Temple University in Philadelphia took potassium *out* of the diets of 12 people with high blood pressures and watched the pressures jump 7 points over the next ten days.

How many daily servings of potassium-rich foods does it take to lower blood pressure? Scientists aren't sure. But a study at the University of Naples in Italy found that 81 percent of those with high blood pressure who ate three to six servings a day of potassium-rich foods such as bananas could cut their medication in half. Some could even eliminate it entirely.

The All-Natural Ulcer Remedy

Research to date into the effects of bananas on ulcers indicates that bananas—rather than an expensive drug—may one day be just what the doctor ordered.

"There are laboratory and animal studies to suggest that bananas may have a protective effect on the stomach," says William Ruderman,

M.D., chairman of the Department of Gastroenterology at the Cleveland Clinic–Florida in Fort Lauderdale.

Although further research is necessary to demonstrate exactly what goes on when a banana slides through the digestive system, a study at the Kasturba Medical College in India offers a strong clue. Researchers concluded that a naturally occurring chemical found in bananas—protease inhibitor—actually may zap the bacteria that can cause stomach ulcers.

Another study, at the University of New England in Australia, found that bananas may also prevent the recurrence of ulcers as effectively as the high-priced drugs that are now used—and without any of the common side effects. The key in this animal study seemed to be that the bananas used were so ripe that they were almost brown. Bananas at this stage apparently produce a substance that armor-plates the stomach's protective lining, while at the same time reducing the body's secretion of stomach acid.

Body-Wide Benefits

While researchers continue to look at ulcers, they are also checking out other therapeutic effects of bananas. In studies with animals at the University of Kerala in India, for example, researchers have found that unripe dried bananas may lower LDL cholesterol—the "bad" kind of cholesterol that clogs your arteries—and prevent chemical changes within the heart that can cause cardiovascular disease.

Other researchers in New Delhi have found that dried banana powder may reduce or eliminate pain in those who have non-ulcer dyspepsia, a condition characterized by recurring heartburn.

Fortunately, bananas are the overwhelming favorite fruit snack of Americans. We've increased our consumption of the fruit by about 30 percent over the past couple of decades.

Barley

Breakfast of Gladiators

POTENTIAL HEALING POWER
May help: • Lower cholesterol   • Prevent heart disease

No wonder this grain has a reputation as the original power food. Several thousand years ago, Greek gladiators were eating barley for strength and stamina. In fact, the locals dubbed these warriors barley eaters.

Modern-day barley eaters are most likely to enjoy these chewy pearls in soups or stews. But barley more than holds its own stuffed into peppers or poultry or baked with mushrooms and beef broth. Any way you cook it, barley is good, healthy food, especially when it comes to battling high cholesterol.

Smart for the Heart

Like oats, barley contains soluble fiber—particularly beta-glucans—that can help reduce cholesterol. Cutting cholesterol, of course, is like sending roses to your heart.

"We think barley affects cholesterol by creating a gelatinous condition in the intestine that interferes with cholesterol and fat absorption into the body," explains Rosemary Newman, Ph.D., professor of foods and nutrition at Montana State University in Bozeman.

In tests, people with high cholesterol who ate barley as their main source of carbohydrates lowered their total cholesterol by 11 percent, while their "bad" LDL dropped 16 percent. "No, we weren't stuffing them with barley," Dr. Newman says. Each day, these people ate a breakfast cereal made with barley flakes and a flatbread and a muffin made with barley flour.

A ½-cup serving of cooked barley contains about 1.5 grams each of soluble and insoluble fiber, approximately the same amount as in oatmeal. "And geneticists are developing new strains of barley that may have as much as twice that amount of soluble fiber," according to Dr. Newman.

Beans

For Dream Cuisines

Red beans, black beans, pink beans, green beans—there's such a selection of beans scattered throughout markets today that it's almost impossible not to find at least one fresh, frozen, canned or dried variety that will tickle your taste buds.

Yet who would think that anything so colorful and tasty would also be potent enough to reduce cholesterol levels, stabilize blood sugar, reduce appetite and help fight off cancer?

"I think of beans as a broad-based nutrient-rich food," says Joanne Slavin, Ph.D., professor of nutrition at the University of Minnesota in St. Paul. "They just don't get eaten enough. They're a good source of protein, starch and particularly fiber, which can help lower cholesterol."

In a study at the University of Kentucky, for example, researchers asked 24 men with high cholesterol levels to eat between four and five ounces of canned beans with tomato sauce a day over a three-week period. The result? The men's cholesterol dropped anywhere from 9 to 12 percent, depending on how many beans they ate. And the more they ate, the lower their cholesterol tended to go.

What's more, triglyceride levels—levels of a particularly nasty blood fat that can frequently predict a propensity for heart attacks—dropped 6 percent for those who had normal levels before the study began and *13 percent* among those who had high levels.

As the researchers concluded, beans may very well lower cholesterol and triglyercides as effectively as many medications—*and* with fewer side effects.

Naturally, the results of a bean-intensive diet will vary from person to person according to individual factors such as your current cholesterol, says James W. Anderson, M.D., professor of medicine at the Veterans Administration Medical Center and at the University of Kentucky in Lexington. "People with readings over 250 show better results than those with levels in the low 200s."

Double Trouble for Cancer

Beans also contain two potentially effective cancer fighters— phytate and protease inhibitors— that can either help prevent or arrest cancer at the cellular level.

Protease inhibitors may block cancer-causing agents from gaining a foothold in your cells. Then,

should a tumor somehow begin to form in some unguarded cell, they seem to help keep the tumor from growing.

Phytate is a substance that had been considered something of a nuisance by nutritionists because it grabs hold of iron in foods and escorts it out of the body before it has a chance to do its job. But while phytate may grab iron as it cruises through your body, it may grab carcinogens on its way to the door as well, elevating its status considerably.

Protect Your DNA

As impressive as the cancer-fighting phytates and protease inhibitors may be, however, the folate contained in beans may be of even more importance to women. That's because a deficiency among pregnant women can cause life-threatening holes in the spine or skull of the baby, scientists suggest. And among all women, folate deficiency may set the stage for cervical cancer.

In a study at the University of Alabama, for example, researchers compared the diets of 294 women with a viral infection that can lead to cancer with the diets of 170 women who did not have the infection. The study showed that even a minor folate deficiency can apparently make the DNA in cervical cells vulnerable to the virus, which can set up housekeeping. And once inside the cell, the virus may sometimes transform the cells into a cancer-friendly habitat that doctors label cervical dysplasia.

A second study, this one at the University of Illinois, found similar results. "Women who had clear deficiencies in folate were approximately *three times* more likely to

---

AMERICA'S BEST-LOVED BEANS

Can't tell your lentils from your limas? Here's a quick primer on beans.

Black beans. These beans add chewiness to soups, casseroles and rice dishes. Originally found in South American and Caribbean dishes, they have now found their way into American kitchens. Half a cup of cooked beans has at least six grams of fiber, 64 percent of the Recommended Dietary Allowance (RDA) for folate and 18 percent of the RDA for iron.

Black-eyed beans. Sometimes known as black-eyed peas, cowpeas or even black-eyed suzies, black-eyed beans are tiny, cream-colored beans with a distinctive black mark. They are particularly popular served with rice in the South. Half a cup has more than eight grams of fiber, 89 percent of the RDA for folate and 22 percent of the RDA for iron.

Chick-peas. Sometimes called garbanzo beans, these round, pale yellow nuggets are frequently used in salads. Half a cup has seven grams of fiber, 40 percent of the RDA for folate and 16 percent of the RDA for iron.

Kidney beans. These beans are best known for their supporting role in Texas chili. Half a cup has nearly seven grams of fiber, 57 percent of the RDA for folate and 26 percent of the RDA for iron.

Lentils. Biblical beans that are used as a major protein source in the Middle East, lentils provide a rich-flavored base for soups and stews. Half a cup provides five grams of fiber, 89 percent of the RDA for folate and 33 percent of the RDA for iron.

Navy beans. These beans are usually found in canned pork 'n' beans, Boston baked beans and many of the bean-and-tomato-sauce recipes found in American cookbooks. Half a cup has nearly five grams of fiber, 64 percent of the RDA for folate and 23 percent of the RDA for iron.

have cervical dysplasia than women who did not," says Faith Davis, Ph.D., associate professor of epidemiology and one of the study's authors.

How can women protect their cervix from the cancer-friendly virus to begin with? By eating beans. Researchers report that a mild to moderate folate deficiency is relatively common, yet the Recommended Dietary Allowance for adults—between 180 and 200 micrograms per day—is an amount easily found in a little more than a half-cup of lentils or a little less than a full cup of kidney beans.

What kind of beans are *most* therapeutic? Well, a series of studies at the University of Kentucky indicates that one bean's pretty much as good as another. And Dr. Slavin agrees. So pick your favorite, toss a handful into a salad, boil them with rice, simmer them in soup or bake them with a rich and savory tomato sauce. The result will be a taste-tempting treat that's destined to reduce your chances of cancer—and give your cholesterol a good swift kick in the pants.

To reduce the gas-inducing properties of beans, try Beano, an over-the-counter natural enzyme available at most pharmacies and supermarkets. Or soak your beans for at least three hours, discard the soaking water and then cook them thoroughly in fresh water. That allows the gas-producing ingredients to break down in a pot rather than in your gut.

Berries

Brimming with Benefits

Strawberries, blueberries, raspberries, blackberries, cranberries—it seems as though much of our world is designed to have a berry within reach from the first warm days of spring to the last cool days before frost.

And a good thing, too. Berries may help protect your body from

POTENTIAL HEALING POWER
May help:
• Prevent certain cancers
• Ward off urinary tract infections
• Battle arthritis
• Reduce allergy symptoms
• Relieve asthma

cancer, urinary tract infections, viruses and inflammatory diseases such as arthritis. They may also help reduce your allergy symptoms. They might even help prevent eye and nerve damage in people who have diabetes.

All berries are packed with quercetin, a cousin of vitamin C that can help smother the inflammatory process that damages eyes and nerves as a result of diabetes and that causes the symptoms of allergies, bursitis, asthma and arthritis. Quercetin also may decrease the infectious power of such viruses as herpes, polio and Epstein-Barr. It may even be helpful in healing wounds.

Berry for berry, strawberries may be the most health-promoting because they are also the richest source of a cancer-fighting substance called ellagic acid. Also found in raspberries, blackberries and loganberries, ellagic acid can apparently help prevent cancer by partially neutralizing three different cancer-causing agents: nitrosamines, which are chemicals found in tobacco and processed foods;

aflatoxins, substances produced by mold found on certain foods; and polycyclic aromatic hydrocarbons, invisible by-products of combustion found in the atmosphere and tobacco smoke.

Strawberries are also a rich source of vitamin C, with one cup providing 141 percent of the Recommended Dietary Allowance. This vitamin richness, scientists think, gives strawberries a second powerful preventive weapon against lung cancer. In a study at the Louisiana State University Medical Center in New Orleans, an area known to have high cancer rates, researchers asked 1,253 area residents who had lung cancer about their diets, then questioned 1,274 people who did not have lung cancer. Researchers found that those who ate the most fruit were less likely to have lung cancer. In fact, they were able to conclude that eating a lot of strawberries reduced the chances of lung cancer in Louisiana by 30 percent.

Buckwheat

Oh! Susanna's Favorite Food

Mention buckwheat and what vision pops into your head? If it's a stack of steaming hot flapjacks, dripping with maple syrup, you're attuned to the collective consciousness of millions of Americans, past and present. Buckwheat pancakes fueled the pioneers. They even appear in one frontier song, which has poor Susanna crying with a buckwheat cake in her mouth, while her sweetheart searches for her with a banjo on his knee.

Because of its name, you might think buckwheat is a grain. In fact, it is from an entirely different plant family than wheat and most grains. It's closely related to rhubarb. But like wheat, buckwheat makes excellent breads and cereals. That makes it a possible selection for most (but not all) adults with celiac disease, an intestinal problem that can be controlled by avoiding gluten, a sticky protein found in wheat and other grains.

But those people with celiac disease who stand to benefit aren't the only ones who can enjoy buckwheat. This is one food that has a little something to offer everyone. To those with diabetes, buckwheat offers a very special package of nutritional benefits.

Diabetes Duelist

Buckwheat has a "stick-to-your-ribs" reputation. That's because its mix of amylose, a type of starch, and amylopectin, a water-soluble fiber, are absorbed very slowly in the intestines, explains Eunsook T. Koh, Ph.D., professor of nutrition at the University of Oklahoma in Oklahoma City.

That same slow absorption can improve glucose (sugar) tolerance in people with Type II (non-insulin-dependent) diabetes, suggests a study by Dr. Koh. Slow absorption helps keep blood sugar from roller-coastering and so helps keep blood insulin levels stable. This means there's less chance of damage to organs such as the eyes or kidneys by high glucose levels.

The people in Dr. Koh's study ate either buckwheat, rice, potatoes or a soybean-rice mixture as their main source of carbohydrate for three weeks. "They ate buckwheat three times a day, with meals, as a kind of pancake," Dr. Koh says. "In all cases the meals containing buckwheat produced the smallest increase in blood glucose and in insulin levels."

Besides in pancakes, you can enjoy buckwheat cooked as a hot cereal, steamed in a pilaf or stuffed in a chicken breast. "Many buckwheat recipes are of Eastern Euro-pean origin. Our best customers are Russian or Polish," says Clifford Orr, a director of the National Buckwheat Institute in Penn Yan, New York. One well-known recipe, *kasha varnitchkes*, is made with a combination of nutty-flavored roasted buckwheat (known as kasha) and bow-tie pasta.

Carrots

Nutrient-Rich Roots

If Bugs Bunny ever dies, it probably won't be from heart disease or cancer. That's because carrots, a rich source of both beta-carotene and fiber, have been found to help prevent cancer and reduce the risk of a heart attack.

In one of the first studies to reveal the therapeutic value of carrots, researchers at the Wolfson Gastrointestinal Laboratory in Edinburgh, Scotland, measured the cholesterol levels of five hospital employees between the ages of 25 and 41, fed them the equivalent of seven ounces of raw carrots a day for three weeks, then measured their cholesterol again. The result? The employees' cholesterol levels fell an average of 11 percent.

Since high cholesterol levels are a

POTENTIAL HEALING POWER
May help: • Lower cholesterol   • Prevent heart attacks   • Ward off certain cancers

major risk factor for heart disease, that was more than enough to put carrots on the "eat" list for many both here and abroad. But a group of Swedish scientists have recently given us an even better reason to munch: They've discovered that root vegetables such as carrots can actually reduce the chances of having a heart attack—independently of their effect on cholesterol.

These researchers have found that two key players are involved in the cellular repair squads that roam your arteries: the clot-*forming* plasminogen activator inhibitor (PAI-1) and the clot-*busting* tissue plasminogen activator (tPA). These two naturally occurring substances generally keep each other in check, but a few years ago researchers began to realize that people who had high levels of PAI-1—the clot former—were more likely to have heart attacks than those who didn't.

Thinking that there must be a way to tilt the clot-forming/busting ratio more in people's favor, Swedish researchers at Umea University Hospital in Norsjo—a community with a higher-than-average rate of heart disease—set out to see if there was some natural way, pos-

sibly through diet, to decrease PAI-1. On a hunch they questioned 260 men and women between the ages of 30 and 60 about what they ate, then ran blood tests to determine their levels of PAI-1 and tPA.

The results were nothing short of amazing: The more root vegetables such as carrots people ate, the more clot-busting tPA they had patrolling their arteries, and the less clot-forming PAI-1.

The bottom line, concluded the researchers, was that those who ate six or more servings of root vegeta-

ORANGE OVERLOAD

Are you eating too many carrots? Take a look at the palms of your hands, says Paul Lachance, Ph.D., chairman of the food science department at Rutgers University in New Brunswick, New Jersey.

If they're beginning to turn a yellowish-orange, then there's a good chance that you're eating more carrots than your body can use. That's because the same chemicals in yellow-orange vegetables that protect your body against heart disease and cancer—beta-carotene and other carotenoids—can actually turn your skin a rather odd shade of yellow-orange when you eat too many.

Most people need around five or six milligrams of beta-carotene a day to gain the beneficial effects of carotenoids, explains Dr. Lachance. That's the equivalent of a single carrot. More than that—say several carrots a day—and you may begin to turn yellow-orange within a couple of months.

First the palms of your hands change color, then the soles of your feet and the rest of your body. And eating a lot of dark green leafy vegetables, tomatoes or sweet potatoes—all of which are packed with carotenoid cousins—can create the same effect. Even a vegetable cocktail—whether it's canned or freshly made—can turn you into a walking carrot if it's downed three or more times a day for several months.

Too many carotenoids won't hurt you, adds Dr. Lachance, except, perhaps, socially.

bles a week—raw or cooked—were significantly less likely to have a heart attack than those who didn't.

What do they mean by "significantly less"? Scientists are always reluctant to give precise numbers, but a study conducted at the Mario Negri Institute of Pharmacological Research in Italy may give us a clue. Over a five-year period, researchers there compared the diets of 287 women between the ages of 22 and 69 who had had heart attacks with a similar group of women who had not. They found that a major difference between the two groups was that those who ate more carrots had one-third the risk of heart attack as compared with those who ate less carrots.

A Crunchy Life Preserver

Heart disease is the number-one killer of Americans, but cancer isn't far behind. A number of studies indicate that eating carrots can help protect against lung and other cancers.

In a study of 3,669 men and women in Belgium, for example, researchers found that eating almost any vegetable reduces the risk of colon cancer, but that eating fiber-rich carrots in particular reduced the risk by as much as 24 percent.

What's more, a joint study by the University of Athens in Greece and the Harvard School of Public Health found that women who ate raw carrots every day were *five to eight times* less likely to develop breast cancer than women who did not eat carrots. Given the fact that breast cancer rates are on the rise in the United States, it's fortunate that the consumption of fresh carrots is growing as well. Americans are now eating 33 percent more than they did two decades ago.

Cherries

Pucker Power

Sweet cherries, the kind of cherries most of us enjoy fresh from a roadside stand on hot summer days, are low in fat, high in fiber and—if you believe a common folk remedy—able to help cure gout.

Yet, it's actually the sweet cherry's

POTENTIAL HEALING POWER
May help:
• Prevent certain cancers
• Combat cataracts
• Protect against heart disease
• Cure gout

sour cousin—the sour cherry we usually bake into an all-American pie on the Fourth of July—that packs the most nutritional power.

Sour cherries are one of the few foods packed with three of the nutrients—beta-carotene, vitamin C and vitamin E—usually referred to as antioxidants.

Together, these three nutrients form a powerful defense against molecular mavericks called free radicals, which are released by your exposure to toxic chemicals, radiation and sunshine. Without that protection, scientists suspect, these free radicals can damage your cells and trigger cataracts, cancer and heart disease.

Notice how all those diseases are the ones we normally associate with aging? Some of the things we normally characterize as an "inevitable" part of old age may not be so inevitable. Eating antioxidant-packed fruits such as sour cherries may very well slow the hands of time.

In a U.S. Department of Agriculture study, for example, people who reported eating more than 1½ daily servings of antioxidant-rich foods were almost *four* times less likely to develop cataracts than those who said they ate less. There are basic ways that cataracts form, the researchers subsequently reported. And one or another of the antioxidants tends to counteract them all.

Antioxidant foods also seem to protect against cancer. In a 20-year study of more than 4,000 men conducted in Finland, researchers found that the more antioxidant fruits nonsmoking men ate, the less likely they were to develop lung cancer. And a study of women found that a diet rich in antioxidants apparently cut the women's risk of cervical cancer in *half*.

And in another Finnish study, scientists found that antioxidants were able to reduce factors that affect the way red blood cells clump together to form heart-stopping clots.

Unfortunately, while sour cherries are such a nutritional bargain, they are also a bit too tart to enjoy eating them raw. Cooking them, however, destroys some of the vitamin C.

Citrus Fruits

Sun-Kissed Disease Fighters

POTENTIAL HEALING POWER

May help:
- Lower cholesterol
- Defend against certain cancers
- Protect against heart attack
- Lower risk of stroke
- Prevent allergy symptoms
- Fight diabetes-related eye disease

Citrus County, Florida, may well be one of the healthiest places in the world to live. Oranges, grapefruits and tangerines all grow abundantly in this neck of the woods—basking in the fierce white sun, the intense humidity and the loving appreciation of thousands of winter residents who can step outside from December through March to pick one of nature's most therapeutic gifts.

"Citrus fruits are packed with natural substances that may prevent cancer, reduce allergy symptoms and help protect the heart," says John Attaway, Ph.D., director of scientific research for the Florida Department of Citrus in Lakeland.

Most notably, all citrus, from the odd little kumquat to the common lemon or lime, is loaded with vitamin C. This nutrient is known for its ability to neutralize potentially cancer-causing free radicals—those destructive oxygen molecules formed in the body by anything from normal metabolism and infections to cigarette smoke and pollution. More specifically, studies have shown that vitamin C may help protect against cancers of the esophagus, larynx, mouth, throat, pancreas, stomach, rectum, breast, cervix and lung.

Another cancer-fighting substance found in citrus is D-limonene, a natural constituent of citrus oils, which has been shown in laboratory studies to provide a defense against breast cancer. D-limonene may block the formation of a tumor by detoxifying the invading carcinogen. Failing that, it may halt the subsequent cancer's growth.

Other natural cancer fighters found in citrus are flavonoids, which, in the laboratory at least, have been found to stop an invading cancer in its tracks.

"There are at least six different flavonoids present in citrus," explains Dr. Attaway. The four major ones are naringin, hesperidin, nobiletin and tangeretin. Naringin is principally found in grapefruit, while hesperidin and nobiletin are found in oranges. Tangeretin is primarily found in tangerines. Two other flavonoids—sinensetin and quercetin—are present in most citrus in smaller quantities.

"Researchers working on tangeretin at Ghent University in Belgium have found the substance prevents the invasion of cancer into healthy cells," says Dr. Attaway. It imprisons the cancer in the cell where it initially starts, prevents its growth and, for all intents and purposes, neutralizes the disease.

But cancer is not the only disease citrus can fight, adds Dr. Attaway. Tangeretin may also—along with nobiletin and sinensetin—keep red blood cells from clumping together to form the clots that can trigger a heart attack. And hesperidin and quercetin block the release of histamine, thus reducing its ability to cause allergy symptoms.

Clear Your Arteries with Grapefruit

Naringin, the flavonoid in grapefruit, is of particular interest to scientists because it may slow the progression of heart disease as well as of a serious vision problem linked to diabetes.

One study at the University of Florida indicates that as little as half a grapefruit—pink, red or white—a day may be able to prevent the overly aggressive clumping together of red blood cells that may jam arteries and lead to heart attacks, strokes and blindness that comes from diabetes.

What's more, another study at the University of Florida revealed that the pectin found in white grapefruit reduced the risk of heart disease itself. The study, which involved 27 men and women with total cholesterol levels ranging from a borderline 208 to a mind-boggling 420, found that a daily half-ounce supplement of grapefruit pectin over a four-week period helped reduce cholesterol levels by 21 points—making grapefruit pectin as effective as some of the drugs doctors frequently prescribe to lower cholesterol.

As if that weren't enough, an added plus is that grapefruit pectin reduced only the "bad" kind of cholesterol (LDL) that clogs your arteries. Levels of the "good" kind (HDL)—the kind that actually helps transport bad cholesterol out of the body—did not change.

"The only problem is that it seems to take a significant amount of grapefruit to get a significant reduction in cholesterol levels," says Dick Matthews, Ph.D., professor of food science at the University of Florida in Gainesville. "To get the kinds of reductions made in the pectin study, for example, you'd need to eat a number of grapefruit a day."

But if a significant amount of grapefruit produces a significant reduction in cholesterol, will a small amount produce a small reduction? "My feeling is that even small intakes may have a positive effect on cholesterol levels," says Dr. Matthews.

Corn

Golden High-Fiber Goodness

POTENTIAL HEALING POWER
May help:
• Relieve constipation
• Prevent colon cancer
• Thwart hemorrhoids
• Reduce cholesterol
• Lower triglycerides

T he mainstay of Native American diets for thousands of years, corn remains a popular food for modern Americans. There's nothing corny about this succulent kernel, which provides an array of health benefits.

Corn is mostly a complex carbohydrate, the kind of starchy food the American Heart Association says should make up at least half our calories each day.

And even though it's a popular source of oil, sweet corn itself is low in fat. "Only about 10 percent of its calories come from fat, mostly the health-protective polyunsaturated and monounsaturated fats, which makes it a good choice for people who are trying to protect their hearts by reducing fat in the diet," says Felicia Busch, R.D., a dietitian in St. Paul, Minnesota, and a spokesperson for the American Dietetic Association. Corn is also great for people trying to lose weight. A single plain ear of corn (about a half-cup serving of kernels) has only about 80 calories.

Corn also provides about three grams of fiber per ear. "It has both soluble and insoluble fiber, so you get the benefits of both for the price of one," Busch says. The insoluble fiber may help to protect against constipation and hemorrhoids, not to mention colon cancer. And the soluble fiber may help reduce blood cholesterol levels.

A study by researchers at Georgetown University Hospital in Washington, D.C., showed that people who added 17 to 34 grams a day of fiber-rich corn bran to their daily diets had a 20 percent drop in cholesterol levels within 12 weeks. Not only that, but they also enjoyed a *31 percent* dive in triglycerides, another type of potentially harmful blood fat.

Try fresh, air-popped popcorn to fill up on corn fiber. One cup provides over a gram of fiber, with only 23 calories and a negligible amount of fat. Eschew the oil and salt and season your popcorn with garlic, curry or even cinnamon.

To keep fresh sweet corn a healthy food, don't slather it with salted butter, Busch cautions. "Try using reduced-fat liquid margarine or butter-flavored sprinkles," she suggests.

Even better, try eating it plain. That's no hardship if you can get your hands on some truly fresh sweet corn—corn that's picked after the kettle is boiling. "If you can, buy corn-on-the-cob the same day you intend to eat it," Busch says. "Fresh sweet corn has a delicate, sugary sweet taste that does not need garnishment."

Cruciferous Vegetables

The Ideal Anti-cancer Family

POTENTIAL HEALING POWER
May help:
• Prevent heart disease
• Protect against stroke
• Prevent certain cancers
• Stabilize diabetes
• Boost immunity
• Lower cholesterol

Cruciferous vegetables are the mushy things that smelled up the kitchens of our childhood. Cooked until pronounced dead, crucifers such as brussels sprouts and broccoli launched the resolution that, once liberated into the adult world, none of us would allow a single forkful to pass our lips again. Ever.

Fortunately, few of us have held to that childhood vow. Instead, most of us have gone on to discover that when lightly steamed and appropriately sauced, these members of the cabbage family are actually tender, occasionally crunchy, sources of fiber that contain chemicals that may boost your body's defenses against cancer.

All the crucifers—including broccoli, brussels sprouts, cabbage, cauliflower, kale, kohlrabi, rutabagas and turnips—contain glucobrassicin, a naturally occurring compound that, once in your body, may help form substances called indoles. Studies have shown that indoles may help prevent breast cancer.

They also contain dithiolthiones, interesting substances that may help protect you from an assorted variety of potentially cancer-causing compounds. Cruciferous vegetables also contain benzyl isothiocyanate, a substance that may also help prevent cancer, or—if the cancer's already present—may help suppress its growth.

Broccoli Power

But all of these protective substances pale when compared to a powerful compound found in broccoli, and probably in other crucifers as well.

"Most cancer-causing chemicals—carcinogens—are not in themselves toxic," explains Jeffrey Blumberg, Ph.D., associate director of the U.S. Department of Agriculture's Human Nutrition Research Center on Aging at Tufts University in Boston. "But when they enter the body, these chemicals may be activated by a family of enzymes known as Phase I enzymes." When this happens, they are converted into small, highly reactive molecules that may attack the DNA found in the body's cells and initiate the cancer process.

Fortunately the body produces a second family of enzymes—Phase II enzymes—that can neutralize the maverick molecules and render them harmless.

But no defense system is effective enough to block every carcinogen that invades the body, says Dr. Blumberg, who is also chief of the Antioxidants Research Laboratory at Tufts. That's why researchers from Johns Hopkins University School of Medicine have turned their microscopes on various foods to see if the anticancer activity of Phase II enzymes can be boosted, and what substances, if any, might do the job.

BROCCOFLOWER: THE NEW KID ON THE BLOCK

Look! Over in the produce section! It's a broccoli! It's a cauliflower! No—it's broccoflower, the neon green hybrid from California that combines the best qualities of both vegetables.

It's sweet and mild, without the cabbagey flavor that turns some people off from cauliflower. It's also softer than broccoli, which means it's easier to chew.

The new-fangled crucifer is also a nutritional wonder. Each half-cup serving contains hefty vitamin C levels—as much as 125 percent of the Recommended Dietary Allowance, which puts it on a par with broccoli—and more heart-helping beta-carotene than either broccoli *or* cauliflower. And as a cruciferous vegetable, it includes other compounds, most notably indoles, that researchers believe may help prevent some kinds of cancer.

The way to choose a fresh head of broccoflower is to check the jacket leaves. If they're wilted, yellow or limp, look for another. Cook and eat it just as you would broccoli or cauliflower.

The result of their work? After years of painstaking research they have discovered that sulforaphane, the substance found in broccoli, can indeed boost the activity of Phase II enzymes. "This lays the foundation for a revolution in preventive health, in which naturally occurring plant chemicals are used to lower the risk of disease," says Dr. Blumberg. It suggests that Mother was right telling you to finish your broccoli.

Tone Up Your Defenses

While you're finishing your broccoli, you may also want to gobble up other crucifers. They all have much to crow about.

A half-cup serving of brussels sprouts, for example, packs in 81 percent of the Recommended Dietary Allowance (RDA) of vitamin C and 11 percent of the RDA for folate, both of which are necessary to keep your immune system on the job. The same serving also has enough fiber to help control diabetes and lower cholesterol.

Cabbage, cauliflower and kale are all good sources of fiber, and a half-cup serving contains roughly half a day's supply of vitamin C. Kale is also a respectable source of beta-carotene, which may reduce the risk of heart attack and stroke. What's more, a single serving of kohlrabi provides 74 percent of your daily requirement of vitamin C.

Fortunately for most of us, our tastes have changed since we were kids. The American consumption of fresh broccoli has jumped more than 400 percent over the past 20 years.

Figs

Middle Eastern Jewels

POTENTIAL HEALING POWER
May help:
• Prevent constipation
• Lower cholesterol
• Prevent colon cancer

Figs are rich, honey-flavored delicacies that evoke images of an oasis amidst warm desert sands. They originated somewhere between southwest Asia and the eastern Mediterranean—not far from where the Garden of Eden is reputed to have been. They were so highly valued in ancient Greece that their export was forbidden.

But aside from their rich, full

flavor, dried figs—which is the way most of us eat these little gems—contain an impressive five grams of fiber per three-fig serving, enough to help prevent constipation, lower cholesterol and perhaps even reduce our chances of developing colon cancer.

When fiber goes through the digestive system, scientists explain, it mops up globs of cholesterol and carries them out of the body. It's thought that fiber may mop up and usher out cancer-causing substances as well.

Although, on average, Americans eat only three ounces of figs per person every year, fig consumption is on the rise, according to industry sources.

Fish

The Best Entrée on the Menu

From sea to shining sea, more Americans are visiting their fishmongers than ever before. Seafood restaurants are more popular than ever, fish counters in supermarkets everywhere have expanded their inventories, and cookbooks on grilling, baking, broiling and steaming fish are leaping off bookstore shelves. What's more, consumption of seafood has jumped 24 percent over the past two decades.

Why has the tide risen so much? "The most important reason we eat fish is because it's naturally low in fat and cholesterol," says Lynne W. Scott, R.D., director of the Diet Modification Clinic at Baylor College of Medicine in Houston. "It's a

POTENTIAL HEALING POWER

May help:
- Thwart heart disease
- Prevent stroke
- Reduce symptoms of psoriasis
- Treat Raynaud's disease
- Ease arthritis pain
- Lower blood pressure
- Reduce cholesterol

good source of protein, and any fat the fish has is polyunsaturated, which does not raise cholesterol."

Ah-huh. Fat. Cholesterol. In the wake of reports indicting saturated fat and cholesterol as major causes of clogged arteries, Americans have cut back on fatty red meat with a vengeance. The U.S. Department of Agriculture reports that consumption of beef has dropped 20 percent over the past two decades and—

isn't that a coincidence?—consumption of fish and seafood has jumped by nearly a quarter.

And why not? To a newly fat-conscious nation, fish for lunch or dinner presents a healthful alternative. It's lower in fat than most meats, and fish is generally a good source of omega-3 fatty acids, those super dietary compounds that seem to buoy up heart health.

A Friend on the Inside

Scientists started checking into the omega-3 fatty acids in fish when a few of them noted that Greenland Eskimos and Japanese fisherfolk seemed to have little heart disease—despite a high-fat, high-cholesterol diet. When the scientists began to investigate, it dawned on them that these northerners derived most of the fat in their diets from fish rather than meat. Could that explain their healthy hearts?

One of the first studies to examine this idea was conducted by researchers from the University of Leiden in the Netherlands. They asked 852 middle-aged men who were free of heart disease about their diets, then kept an eye on each of them for the next 20 years. During that time 80 of the men died from heart disease. When the scientists analyzed who lived and who died and who ate what, they found that death from heart disease was more than 50 percent lower among those who ate an average of at least an ounce of fish a day than among those who didn't.

Study after study followed, confirming the heart-healthy effects of fish and eventually suggesting that the therapeutic agents are the omega-3's in its oil. Scientists pointed out that when we ingest fish, the omega-3's partially replace other, more harmful fats that have been deposited in our cells. And once in residence, the omega-3's are

---

THE BEST SOURCES OF OMEGA-3'S

Which fish has the most heart-healthy omega-3's? "Generally, warm-water fish such as flounder and snapper are lower in omega-3's than cold-water fish such as salmon and mackerel," says Lynne W. Scott, R.D., director of the Diet Modification Clinic at Baylor College of Medicine in Houston.

A single, daily $2^1/_2$-ounce serving of almost any cold-water fish will convey the amount of omega-3's that most experts agree will help protect you from cardiovascular disease.

Aside from salmon and mackerel, other top choices are herring, sardines, anchovies, tuna, sablefish and whitefish.

able to decrease the body's production of substances that constrict arteries and thicken blood while simultaneously increasing production of other substances that relax arteries and thin blood. They also increase body activities that can dissolve blood clots.

All told, scientists have discovered that the omega-3's reduce or inhibit no fewer than 17 different factors suspected of putting you at risk for heart disease and increase no fewer than 7 different factors that may protect you.

The result is more open, flexible arteries throughout your body and blood that's not likely to gum up the works. And that means less chance of a heart attack—or a stroke.

A Fillet Full of Miracles

Continuing investigations have revealed that the oil found in fish not only has the potential to prevent and treat heart disease but may also help reduce the symptoms of psoriasis, ulcerative colitis, asthma, Raynaud's disease and rheumatoid arthritis; lower high blood pressure; prevent life-threatening disruption of normal heart rhythms; prevent skin cancer and other types of tumors from growing; extend life expectancy in those with severe kidney disease; and lower cholesterol and triglycerides.

How much fish should we be eating?

Nobody knows for sure. When researchers discovered that fish oil maintained its therapeutic effect whether it was packaged in a gelcap by a machine or packaged by nature in a fish, they started experimenting with high doses of the encapsulated oil to test its therapeutic limits. Although they at first thought that huge doses of omega-3's might be necessary for people to reap the benefits, now scientists are beginning to think otherwise. In fact, a government review of dozens of research studies on omega-3's concluded that regular, small amounts of fish in the diet may be enough to gain at least the cardiovascular protection of omega-3's.

The Canadian government has already developed a set of specific recommendations for various age groups. Men between the ages of 25 and 49 should eat enough fish to get 1.5 grams of omega-3's in their diet every day, suggest the Canadians. Women of that age need 1.1 gram. And men between the ages of 50 and 74 should get 1.3 grams of omega-3's, while women of the same age should get 1.1 gram.

In terms of fish consumption, this equals a single, $2^{1}/_{2}$-ounce serving of fatty fish once a day—an amount that the National Heart, Lung and Blood Institute reports could help reduce heart disease by 40 percent among those who are most at risk.

The bottom line on fish?

If it swims, eat it.

Garlic

An Aromatic Healer

"S*in ajo, no hay cocina*" is a Latin American folk saying that could be engraved over the doorposts of millions of kitchens throughout the world. Loosely translated, it means "without garlic there is no kitchen."

For much of the world, that phrase accurately expresses a central—almost mystical—relationship between garlic and cooking. Whether you're in Italy, France, Lebanon or China, the distinctive way in which garlic is used largely defines a country's cuisine. What's more, given the therapeutic value of garlic, how much is used may also influence the health of a nation.

"Garlic is now getting a tremendous amount of attention," says Barbara Klein, Ph.D., professor of food and nutrition at the University of Illinois in Urbana and associate editor of the *Journal of Food Science*. "We don't know a lot about it, but we do know that garlic contains sulfur compounds that fight cancer and foster cardiovascular health."

The Heart of the Matter

In a landmark study in India, researchers wanted to see what effect garlic might have on a fat-laden diet. So they added roughly 2 1/2 ounces of butter to the diets of 40 postgraduate students for several weeks. Half of these students were also given a garlic-oil supplement equivalent to seven cloves of garlic a day.

For students fed only butter, the results were predictable: Eating all that fat raised their cholesterol levels, triglyceride levels and the tendency of their blood to clot. In other words, they took several paces in the direction of having a heart attack. Students eating butter *plus* garlic, however, found that their cholesterol levels increased far less than those on the butter-only diet. What's more, the butter-plus-garlic group's triglycerides actually *dropped* by 16 percent, their platelets were 16 percent less likely to clump together and block arteries, and their body's clot-busting ability increased by 36 percent!

This study clearly demonstrated that garlic can offset some of the nastier health effects of a diet that's slathered in fat. But what happens when garlic is added to a more normal diet?

Apparently you get healthier. In a European study of people with elevated cholesterol levels, cholesterol dropped an average of 21 percent for those who took roughly a gram of garlic powder daily for 16 weeks. Levels of triglycerides—those particularly nasty blood fats—dropped 24 percent.

Other European studies have had similar results, and one even seems to indicate that garlic may also lower blood pressure. In that study, 47 people with high blood pressure were given 600 milligrams of garlic powder a day for 12 weeks. When their blood pressures were checked at the end of the study, scientists found that blood pressure had dropped right along with cholesterol and triglyceride levels: Diastolic blood pressure—the bottom number on a blood pressure reading and the one that is most likely to indicate cardiovascular stress—decreased an average of 11 percent.

The garlic powder used in these studies may be a little more convenient to use than garlic cloves. The amount used is equivalent to roughly 1½ to 2½ cloves of raw garlic.

The Cancer Connection

Another area of keen interest to garlic researchers is cancer prevention. At the University of California, Los Angeles, for example, researchers added aged garlic extract to test tubes containing cancer cells from humans and mice. A week later, they checked the tubes and found that the cancer cells had stopped growing.

KISS WITH CARE

People throughout the world may love the taste of fresh garlic, although not everyone loves the smell, particularly when it lingers on the breath.

But if you eliminate the smell, will you also eliminate garlic's therapeutic powers? The answer seems to be yes, says Barbara Klein, Ph.D., professor of food and nutrition at the University of Illinois in Urbana.

Although many companies are trying to grow odorless garlic, no one has yet proved that it's possible to have the health benefits without the aroma. Unfortunately, says Dr. Klein, it seems to be the same chemical compounds that give you bad breath that also help protect the heart and fight cancer.

What's more, in a study at Pennsylvania State University, laboratory animals were fed garlic and also subjected to a chemical that's known to turn normal mammary cells cancerous. "In some studies," says John Milner, Ph.D., head of the nutrition department, "we observed a 70 percent reduction in the number of tumors."

Why? Scientists really aren't sure. Dr. Milner's guess is that garlic might directly affect the DNA of a cell. But other researchers are now beginning to suspect that garlic may have the ability to actually inactivate cancer-causing substances that invade the body.

Greens

Prolong Your Salad Days

POTENTIAL HEALING POWER
May help:
• Prevent certain cancers
• Combat heart disease
• Protect against strokes

Crisp or wilted, smooth or crinkled, rounded or ruffled—it just doesn't matter. Because whether you prefer romaine or endive, collard greens or dandelion, chicory or watercress, there's probably not a green alive that isn't just bursting with heart-healthy, cancer-crunching nutrients.

"Leafy dark green vegetables are one of the best sources available for beta-carotene," explains Paul Lachance, Ph.D., chairman of the food science department at Rutgers University in New Brunswick, New Jersey. "You only need around five or six milligrams of beta-carotene a day to gain its preventive effects." This amount is easily obtained from a bowl of fresh spinach or a single serving of cooked dandelion or collard greens.

Why is beta-carotene so important? Preliminary studies from Harvard and elsewhere indicate that beta-carotene may well prevent the "bad" kind of cholesterol (LDL) from undergoing chemical changes that allow it to damage your arteries and set the stage for heart disease.

What's more, an ongoing study at Harvard may give doctors reason to prescribe greens to their patients who already have heart disease. For 12 years, every other day, researchers have been giving a 50-milligram supplement of beta-carotene—about the amount found in seven or eight servings of most cooked greens—to some of the study's 20,000 participants. So far, the number of heart attacks and strokes among the beta-carotene recipients is about half what you would normally expect to see.

GREEN GOLD

Most greens are rather arbitrarily separated into cooking greens—beet, collard, dandelion, lamb's-quarters and mustard—and salad greens—chicory, watercress, endive, lettuce and spinach.

But don't get hung up on classifications. Most people like to mix and match their greens anyway. And since most greens are equally at home either steaming on the dinner plate or perked up in a salad bowl, try experimenting with them both ways.

To give you an idea of how much protective value may be on your plate, here's a breakdown of greens based on beta-carotene content, arguably their most powerful health-giving nutrient. Scientists say you need five to six milligrams a day to gain the benefits of beta-carotene.

Green	How Served	Beta-Carotene (mg)
Mustard spinach	raw	8.91
Collards	boiled	6.10
Dandelion greens	raw	4.62
Spinach	boiled	4.42
Beet greens	boiled	4.41
Chicory	raw	4.32
Swiss chard	boiled	3.30
Garden cress	raw	2.79
Mustard greens	boiled	2.55
Spinach	raw	2.26
Watercress	raw	0.96
Romaine lettuce	raw	0.87
Swiss chard	raw	0.71
Loose-leaf lettuce	raw	0.64
Endive	raw	0.62

NOTE: All values are for a 1-cup serving.

The Cancer Squelcher

Scientists at the National Cancer Institute and the University of California, Los Angeles, have also suggested that the more beta-carotene-rich foods we consume, such as greens, the lower our risk of cancer. In particular, they suspect that eating beta-carotene-rich foods may actually cut our risk of lung cancer in *half*. The scientists further predicted that any community in which people ate five or more servings a day of foods rich in beta-carotene might experience a decline of 15 to 31 percent in lung cancer.

In a large study conducted by two European universities over a nine-year period, researchers compared 766 people who had cancer with 1,419 people who did not. The researchers found that those who did *not* have cancer had 5 to 14 percent *more* beta-carotene in their blood than those who had cancer. The protective effect was strongest against smoking-related cancers—particularly those of the lung and bladder.

Slashing Women's Cancer

Gathering momentum is the idea that vegetables rich in beta-carotene may be effective at helping to prevent certain cancers particular to women.

A joint study between the University of Athens and the Harvard School of Public Health found that women who ate lettuce every day were 40 percent less likely to develop breast cancer than women who did not.

What's more, a study of more than 2,000 women conducted among four Latin American nations indicates a similar relationship between beta-carotene-rich foods and cervical cancer. In that study, women who regularly ate beta-carotene-rich vegetables were 32 percent less likely to have cervical cancer.

At the University of Hawaii, researchers compared the diets of 404 men and women with lung cancer to those of 968 people who did not have the disease. Men who ate dark green vegetables such as watercress, spinach, bok choy, Swiss chard, dark lettuces and other green leaves were only *half* as likely to develop lung cancer as those who avoided them. Women who ate dark green vegetables were *four times* less likely to develop lung cancer than those who did not.

To capture the full nutritious benefit of any green, food experts recommend choosing fresh rather than packaged greens. When fresh greens are not readily available, frozen greens are preferable to canned.

Kiwi

A Wonder from Down Under

Kiwi is that tan, hairy-looking little fruit that you often see next to the pineapples or coconuts at your supermarket. Looking for all the world as though it's lost its mother—or at least its proper bin—the kiwi is nevertheless packed with even more disease-fighting power than many of its statelier neighbors.

Originally from China, kiwis contain hefty amounts of fiber—but where they really shine is in their incredibly high level of vitamin C. Consider that the tiny kiwi has 75 milligrams of vitamin C—that's 124 percent of the Recommended Dietary Allowance and more than either an orange or an eight-ounce glass of grapefruit juice! Vitamin C has been found to have a significant effect on cholesterol levels, high blood pressure and breast cancer.

In a study at Tufts University, in Boston, for example, researchers looked at the relationship between blood pressure, cholesterol levels and vitamin C. They found that the higher your intake of vitamin C, the

---

TAKE IT OFF—TAKE IT ALL OFF

You dropped the kiwi in your shopping basket, paid for it at the register and carted it all the way home. Now it sits, brown and hairy, on your counter. And now you stand, puzzled and uncertain, with your knife poised.

So how do you peel a kiwi?

Like a potato. Slice off both ends of the fruit and peel spirally from end to end. The ugly brown skin will fall away to reveal the luscious soft green fruit beneath.

Some people prefer to cut the kiwi in half and eat it with a spoon, much like a soft-boiled egg.

lower your blood pressure and LDL cholesterol—the kind that encourages heart disease. Moreover, the higher your intake of vitamin C, the higher your HDL cholesterol—the kind that actually helps get rid of the bad. As vitamin C levels increased, blood pressure generally dropped anywhere from 4 to 11 percent. The bad LDL cholesterol levels dropped about 4 percent, and the good HDL cholesterol levels increased from 4 to 9 percent.

And when researchers from cancer centers at major universities around the world reviewed the dietary records of more than 10,000 women, they concluded that a major factor in whether or not women develop breast cancer is the amount of vitamin C in the diet. If all women across North America would increase their consumption of vitamin C–rich foods such as kiwi until they were getting at least 380 milligrams of vitamin C per day, concluded the researchers, breast cancer in North America would be reduced by 16 percent.

Fortunately, more and more people are beginning to take advantage of the vitamin C kiwi has to offer. Barely known to Americans a decade ago, we now eat more fuzzy little fruit than we do cherries!

Meats and Poultry

They're Not All Created Equal

POTENTIAL HEALING POWER
May help:
• Prevent iron-deficiency anemia
• Prevent memory loss
• Bolster your immune system

You're walking along a buffet table loaded down with prime rib, turkey, roasted chicken and barbecued pork. And you'd really like to plunge your fork right in. But you've heard about how the saturated fat in meat can clog arteries and lead to heart disease and stroke.

What do you do? Bypass the prime rib? Turn your back on that magnificent barbecued pork? Or is there some way you can have your cake . . . er, meat . . . and eat it, too?

"If you go to a party and they're serving prime rib, go ahead and have some. Eating a higher-fat food on a special occasion is all right," says Susan Kleiner, R.D., Ph.D., former professor of nutrition at Case Western Reserve University in Cleveland, Ohio, who is now a high-performance nutrition consultant to clients such as the Cleveland Browns professional football team and the Cleveland Cavaliers professional basketball team. "The trick is to eat lean the rest of the day and to eat no more than a six-ounce portion," she says. And, of course, you should be following a low-fat lifestyle. But low fat doesn't mean you have to banish meat forever.

A Plateful of Iron and Zinc

Eating meat *is* tricky. Too much and the saturated fat makes your cholesterol levels go up and your arteries load up on plaque. Your brain and your heart begin to wonder if you really care about your health.

But eat too little—or none at all—and life can become a struggle to get an adequate supply of iron and zinc, especially for women.

Iron is necessary to make hemoglobin, the part of red blood cells that picks up oxygen in the lungs and transports it to muscles and organs all over your body, explains Dr. Kleiner. No iron, no oxygen. No oxygen, no energy. And the result is anemia—a malaise so debilitating that some people won't have the energy to get out of bed.

And because of blood losses during menstruation and the need for the body to keep churning out new red blood cells, women in particular are at risk for developing an iron deficiency.

Zinc is just as necessary, says Dr. Kleiner. It's the middleman directly responsible for jump-starting over 200 enzymes that will eventually be involved in metabolic processes that do everything from priming your reproductive pump to keeping your immune system on its toes to helping you remember where you put your keys.

In one study, for example, researchers measured the effect of low zinc intakes on the memories of 14 young, healthy people. Over a seven-month period, the study participants were placed on diets supplying very low amounts of zinc, followed by periods of adequate zinc intake. They periodically took a series of tests. The result? When they consumed low amounts of zinc, they scored poorly on 10 out of 15 tasks requiring short-term memory, spatial skills and attention. They also performed more slowly.

Although both iron and zinc are available from vegetables and grains, meat provides the best packaging and the richest source of these minerals, says Dr. Kleiner. A single serving of most meats will give you one-fifth to one-third of your body's Recommended Dietary Allowance (RDA) for both. And, unlike the iron and zinc in grains and vegetables, the iron and zinc in meat is in a form that your body can easily absorb and put to work.

THE LEANEST CUTS

Not all meats are created (or prepared) equal. Let the table below help you choose the leaner cuts. Your heart—and your waistline—will thank you.

Meat	Fat (g)	Calories	Calories from Fat (%)
Beef			
Top round steak	4.2	153	25
Eye round roast	4.2	143	26
Shank cross-cuts	5.4	171	28
Tip round steak	5.9	157	34
Bottom round roast	7.0	178	35
Arm pot roast	7.1	184	35
Lamb			
Foreshank	5.1	159	29
Shank	5.7	153	33
Leg	6.6	162	36
Sirloin	7.8	173	40
Pork			
Tenderloin	4.1	141	26
Ham, cured	6.5	140	42
Ham, fresh	9.4	187	45
Poultry			
Turkey white meat	2.7	133	18
Chicken breast	3.1	142	19
Turkey dark meat	6.1	159	35
Chicken leg	8.0	181	40
Veal			
Leg	2.9	128	20
Arm roast	4.9	139	32
Sirloin	5.3	143	33
Blade roast	5.9	145	36
Loin	5.9	149	36

NOTE: All values are for 3 ounces, cooked.

What's more, says Dr. Kleiner, meat also contains all the amino acids your body needs to build sound, healthy tissue—and, once again, unlike other foods, it makes every one of them available in a single, convenient package. Meat also contains the full range of energy-boosting B vitamins. In addition, pork is an excellent source of thiamin—a single serving of tenderloin contains half the RDA. And most cuts of poultry contain roughly one-third the RDA for niacin.

Cut the Meat, Not the Minerals

So how do you tap the rich reservoir of vitamins, minerals and amino acids meat has to offer without falling into the trap of saturated fat?

"Leaner cuts and smaller portions are really the trick," says Dr. Kleiner. "For beef, the round cuts—round tip, top round, eye of round—are the leanest, followed by the loins—sirloin, tenderloin and top loin." The cut labeled "select" will have the least fat. And if you have a yen for burgers one night, just ask your supermarket's meat-cutter to grind a "select" cut—top round, perhaps—specifically for that purpose.

For pork, the loins are the leanest cuts; for poultry, the breast. All visible fat should be trimmed from meat, and the skin should be removed from poultry.

"Portions for both red meat and poultry should range between four and six ounces each, eaten no more than once a day," says Dr. Kleiner. "Beef and pork should be eaten no more than three times a week. Poultry—generally the leanest of meats—can be eaten every day if you like."

The one problem leaner cuts of meat present is that they may not have quite the flavor and moisture of their fattier counterparts. "That's why we've learned to change our cooking techniques," says Dr. Kleiner. "We've learned to marinate foods before they go into the oven and brush low-fat teriyaki and barbecue sauces on meat and poultry before they're grilled or broiled."

The result is so tasty, she adds, that many people have actually come to prefer this style of eating to their old, high-fat diets.

Melons

The Benefits Are Big

Nothing beats hot weather better than an ice-chilled bowl of fresh melon chunks. Cantaloupe, watermelon, honeydew, casaba—all are low-fat, low-calorie sources of cool, natural sweetness.

But along with all that sweetness, melons also apparently contain a tough anti-tumor defense system that can help protect you from cancer of the colon and rectum.

In a study from Italy and Switzerland, researchers compared the diets of 575 men and women with colorectal cancer to those of 778 people who were free of the disease. The result? The more fresh fruits and vegetables people ate, the less likely they were to develop cancer. Melons had a particularly significant protective action, the researchers concluded, and regular consumption seemed to be associated with a 40 percent lower risk of colorectal cancer.

Scientists haven't yet figured out what it is in melons that soups up your cancer defenses. But they do know that most melons are good sources of vitamins A and C, with a hefty shot of potassium. Cantaloupes are probably the most nutritious, since a single eight-ounce serving has 100 percent of the Recommended Dietary Allowance (RDA) of vitamin C and at least 50 percent of the RDA of vitamin A.

A Bitter Treat

In the United States, the most popular melon is clearly the cantaloupe. But if you're passing by an Asian market, you might want to stop in and look for the melons that resemble bumpy cucumbers. Though technically a squash, they're called bitter melons (or sometimes balsam pears) and are generally available from April through September.

When fresh and unripe, they have a delicate, sour flavor. When ripe (you know they're ripe when they turn from yellow-green to yellow-orange), they're more likely to have a bitter flavor, which many people prefer. Both kinds are frequently used in Chinese cooking.

A preliminary study at Kansas

State University indicates that bitter melon contains a substance—mo-mordin—which can, at least in the lab, stimulate the immune system and activate naturally occurring killer cells to destroy both cancer cells and viruses.

Milk

A Calcium Cocktail

Milk's reputation has had its ups and down over the eons, to be sure. The cavemen who drew pictures on their dwelling walls of cows being milked may have thought the creamy white liquid was the best thing since water. And in the days before anybody knew anything about cholesterol and saturated fat, a tall glass of cold milk was considered as close to perfect as any food could come.

When milk was discovered to be high in cholesterol and fat, its producers did an admirable job of slimming their product down. Today, people drink about one-third more skim milk and low-fat milk than they do whole milk, and dietitians recommend you stick with the 1% low-fat or nonfat versions.

So now there's a choice of milk for just about everyone, and "moo-food" has settled into a comfortable niche on the menu. "Skim milk is a concentrated source of many essential nutrients, with practically no fat or cholesterol," says Colleen Pierre, R.D., a spokesperson for the American Dietetic Association. "Skim milk actually provides slightly more essential nutrients than whole milk. At only 90 calories a cup, it's hard to beat as an all-around healthy food."

Low-fat milk isn't a bad food choice either, says Pierre.

For babies, however, recommendations are a bit different. The American Academy of Pediatrics recommends only breast milk or infant formula for the first year of life, whole cow's milk between ages one and two, and low-fat or skim milk for children aged two and older.

Calcium Galore—And More

One of milk's chief benefits, of course, is its calcium. Three eight-ounce glasses of milk supply the 800 milligrams or so of calcium most people need each day.

We all know that calcium is used in the body to build and maintain bones and teeth. But calcium has many other functions, too. For example, it plays a role in maintaining a healthy heart and proper blood pressure. In several population studies (but not all), low calcium intake has been found to be the best predictor of high blood pressure.

Milk is also a great source of vitamin B_{12}, a nutrient essential for healthy blood and nerves. A one-cup serving offers more than 50 percent of the Recommended Dietary Allowance (RDA). A cup of skim or low-fat milk also contains about 20 percent of the RDA of riboflavin, along with about 15 percent of the RDA for vitamin A.

Cancer Fighter

Could milk cow cancer? No one knows for sure, but researchers at Roswell Park Cancer Institute in Buffalo, New York, interviewed al-

---

MILK ALTERNATIVES

For about one-fifth of American adults, drinking milk leads to gassiness and cramps. That's because milk contains a unique sugar called lactose, which some people, once they reach adulthood, simply can't digest. If you're one of those unfortunates, you may want to consider adding special enzymes to your milk, or you may want to consider one of these milk substitutes, available at some supermarkets and most health food stores.

Sweet acidophilus. This is real cow's milk, but it contains bacteria that break down lactose. The added acidophilus bacteria do not change the nutritional value or the taste.

Soy milk. This has no lactose or cholesterol. Brands vary widely in calcium content. Better Than Milk contains 50 percent of the recommended daily intake per serving, while others (such as Westsoy Lite) have as little as 2 percent. Westsoy Plus contains vitamin D, while others (such as Edensoy vanilla) do not. Regular formulas contain about as much fat as 2% milk; "lite" versions have about as much as 1% milk. The taste can be a bit chalky.

Rice milk. This has no lactose or cholesterol, very little calcium and riboflavin and no vitamin D. Fat and sodium content varies with the brand. It tends to be sweet but watery.

most 5,000 patients, with and without cancer, and came up with some interesting findings.

They found that people who drank 2% milk had a much lower risk of some types of cancer than those who drank whole milk. Risks were reduced for oral, stomach, rectal, lung, cervical and ovarian cancers. "That may be linked with a reduced rate of fat intake in the people who drink 2% milk," explains Curtis Mettlin, Ph.D., chief

of epidemiologic research at the institute.

But the researchers also found that the cancer risk for those who drank low-fat milk was lower than for those who drank no milk at all. How to explain that? "One possible explanation is that nutrients in milk may offer some cancer protection," Dr. Mettlin says. Calcium, riboflavin and vitamin A: All three nutrients have been linked to reduced risks for several cancers.

Nuts

Heart Protection by the Handful

POTENTIAL HEALING POWER
May help: • Protect against heart attack • Lower cholesterol

Squirrels hide them in trees. Elephants tuck them in trunks. Chickadees hold them between their toes. And to humans, they are dear to the heart. Yes, eating nuts—no more than a handful a day—may protect us from heart attacks.

In a study of more than 26,000 Seventh-Day Adventists in California, researchers from Loma Linda University found that those who ate a handful of nuts four or more times a week had *50 percent* fewer fatal heart attacks!

Why? "We really don't know,"

says chief researcher Gary Fraser, M.D., Ph.D., professor of medicine and epidemiology at the school. It may be because nuts contain fiber, vitamin E and monounsaturated fats. All are proven heart protectors.

"Or it may have something to do with the fact that a handful of nuts has two-thirds of the Recommended Dietary Allowance of magnesium—and there's evidence that magnesium protects the heart," says Dr. Fraser.

Nuts also contain a potent chemical that may relax arteries and prevent arterial spasms that could harm the heart, adds Dr. Fraser.

Nutritional Wonders

Before the Loma Linda study, doctors had been concerned that the high calorie content of nuts would make people gain so much weight that the weight itself would put them at risk for heart problems. But not only do Adventists who eat nuts not gain weight, they tend to weigh less than non-nut-eaters. The possible reason, says Dr. Fraser, may be that nibbling nuts discouraged snacking on fat-dripping foods like potato chips. Many Adventists also follow a vegetarian diet, which is naturally low in fat.

Which nut is most effective at protecting your heart? The Adventists in the study ate predominately peanuts, almonds and walnuts. And although the study didn't try to figure out which nut is best, another study by a group of California researchers may give us a clue.

In that study, researchers fed $3\frac{1}{2}$ ounces of almonds to a group of 19 people with high cholesterol every day for nine weeks. Three weeks into the study, the group's cholesterol levels had plummeted 20 points. Since high cholesterol levels put people at risk for heart disease, lowering cholesterol levels may be one way that nuts protect your heart.

Before you go nutty for nuts, Dr. Fraser suggests you consider how the Adventists eat them. "They tend not to just sit in front of the TV with a whole can of nuts. They eat them in a variety of ways—almost as a condiment. They sprinkle them over cereal, fruit, salad and desserts and even use them as an ingredient in vegetable entrées."

Oils

Good Guys, Bad Guys

You're standing in front of a supermarket shelf filled with row upon row of gleaming golden oils. Soybean oil. Corn oil. Safflower oil. Sunflower

POTENTIAL HEALING POWER

When used in place of saturated fats, monounsaturated fats such as those found in olive oil may help:

- Reduce cholesterol
- Lower blood pressure
- Regulate blood sugar in people with diabetes

oil. Canola oil. And at least three kinds of olive oil.

Each oil is a lovely color, a pure and shining testament to the healthy plant from which it has come. Each is priced not too far from the other, although some of the imported olive oils can get a little steep. So which one do you pick up off the shelf and take home to your family? Which is the healthiest choice?

"The thing to remember first is that all oils are 100 percent pure fat," says John C. LaRosa, M.D., director of the Lipid Research Center at George Washington University School of Medicine and Health Sciences in Washington, D.C. "The thing to remember second is that in countries where people live a long time, a key factor seems to be that they eat very little fat."

Making Wise Choices

So once you've realized that you're going to use these oils sparingly, the next step in your decision is to evaluate the pros and cons of each oil.

Generally, each oil—even those generically labeled with the ubiquitous "vegetable" oil—will contain vitamin E and a combination of two types of fat, says Dr. LaRosa.

Saturated fat is abundant in meat, cheese, butter and tropical oils. It's solid at room temperature, raises LDL or "bad" cholesterol levels in your bloodstream and lowers HDL or "good" cholesterol,

says Dr. LaRosa. LDL cholesterol is bad because it gloms onto your arteries, shuts them down and can cut off the blood supply to your heart and brain. HDL cholesterol is good because it actually puts a half nelson on the bad stuff and wrestles it to the liver for disposal.

Unsaturated fat is the predominant fat in vegetable oils. It's generally liquid at room temperature, lowers or at least does not raise LDL cholesterol and pretty much leaves HDL cholesterol alone.

But unsaturated fat is further divided into two different types, says Dr. LaRosa: *Poly*unsaturated and *mono*unsaturated fat.

What's the difference? Scientists once thought that polyunsaturates lowered cholesterol, while mononunsaturates didn't affect it one way or another. But today we know that monounsaturates are far from being a neutral party. In a study at Hadassah Hospital in Jerusalem, for example, researchers put 26 male rabbinical students on a diet that got 32 percent of its calories from fat—which is close to what the American Heart Association recommends.

The scientists studied rabbinical students because they eat all their meals at school and have little opportunity to buy outside food. For the first 12 weeks of the study, the fat in the students' diet was altered to contain mostly monounsaturates; for the second 12 weeks it was adjusted to contain mostly polyunsaturates. In both cases, saturated fats were kept low. When scientists compared baseline cholesterol levels to levels at the end of the study, they found that the students' cholesterol levels dropped 16 percent while on the polyunsaturates and 10 percent while on the monounsaturates. LDLs accounted for most of the drop, while the students' HDLs remained unaffected.

But what impressed researchers most was the discovery that the LDL roaming the students' bloodstreams while they were eating monounsaturates seemed to lose its ability to set in motion the chemical process that leads to clogged arteries and heart disease. In other words, the LDL cholesterol lost some of its punch.

How much did it lose? Subsequent animal studies at the Univer-

---

SMART SPREADS

Just about the only difference between the margarines lined up in your market's refrigerated dairy case and the oils lined up on a shelf in the baking aisle is a couple of hydrogen atoms. Yet those two microscopic entities could mean a big—and bad—difference to your heart and arteries.

The difference is that when you make margarine or any other solid fat from a liquid polyunsaturated oil, you change the molecular structure, explains John C. LaRosa, M.D., director of the Lipid Research Center at George Washington University School of Medicine and Health Sciences in Washington, D.C. You add two hydrogen atoms, which results in a certain chemical rigidity that allows the fat to assume a solid form.

But this process, called hydrogenation, changes the configuration—the shape of the molecules—of the fatty acids in oils. "And perhaps because of that changed configuration, a polyunsaturated fat *acts* like a saturated fat in your body," says Dr. LaRosa. It raises the levels of LDL cholesterol—the stuff that clogs your arteries—and reduces the levels of HDL cholesterol—the stuff that clears your arteries.

Unfortunately, says Dr. LaRosa, any solid margarine is going to have this problem to one degree or another. And that makes them more like butter, which is almost pure saturated fat.

His recommendation? Stick to the soft margarines that are sold in little tubs. They will have the least amount of hydrogenated oils. Or eat Italian. "Italians dip their bread in olive oil," he says. "Why shouldn't we?"

sity of California, San Diego, seem to indicate that monounsaturated fats may be able to reduce the heart-damaging potential of LDL cholesterol by as much as one-third.

Mono Magic

As if that's not enough to send your hand reaching toward one of the monounsaturated oils, further studies indicate that highly monounsaturated oils—olive oil, in particular—may also be able to reduce blood pressure and blood sugar as well. In a joint study of almost 5,000 men and women by the State University of New York at Buffalo and the Italian National Research Council, habitual use of olive oil was associated with lower levels of cholesterol, blood pressure and

blood sugar. Polyunsaturates were also associated with lower blood sugar, reported the researchers, but the polyunsaturates apparently had no effect on blood pressure.

There are even more reasons to favor monounsaturates: A concern among some scientists is that large amounts of polyunsaturates may somehow be implicated in the development of some cancers. And laboratory studies indicate that very large amounts of polyunsaturates may suppress the immune system, particularly in people who are already hurt or ill.

As a result of these concerns, Scott Grundy, M.D., Ph.D., director of the Center for Human Nutrition at the University of Texas Southwestern Medical Center in Dallas, suggests that the consumption of

---

KNOW THY ENEMY

Any oil you buy will contain a blend of saturated, polyunsaturated and monounsaturated fats. The percentages within the blends, however, vary greatly. Your heart-healthy mission: To steer clear of those oils with the highest amounts of saturated fat. Keep in mind, however, that *every* tablespoon of oil is 120 calories of pure fat. So use all of them sparingly.

Oils with the *least* saturated fat:	Oils with the *most* saturated fat:
Canola oil	Coconut oil
Safflower oil	Palm kernel oil
Sunflower oil	Palm oil
Olive oil	
Soybean oil	

linoleic acid—the specific ingredient in polyunsaturates that is causing concern—be kept to under 7 percent of calories. In an average diet of 2,000 calories a day, that works out to two tablespoons of corn oil a day.

Although some scientists suggest that you limit polyunsaturates, others point out that they *do* lower cholesterol and aid in vitamin absorption. Also, linoleic acid is an essential nutrient. And there may be other beneficial effects not yet discovered.

What's the bottom line? "Avoid adding any form of fat—including oil—to your diet as much as possible," says Dr. LaRosa. When you must use oil, he says, read labels and use those with the least amount of saturated fat. Keep polyunsaturates at least under 10 percent of calories a day—and let monounsaturates fill in when you need a little extra oil.

Okra

A Slick Southern Specialty

Okra blossoms year-round in gardens throughout the South. Its deep green pods add robust flavor and a thick texture to New Orleans–style gumbo and other Dixie favorites.

But okra is more than just an old Southern friend over which we wax nostalgic. It's also one of the richest sources of vegetable fiber you can find—which makes it one heck of a good fixin' to add to your menu.

POTENTIAL HEALING POWER

May help:
- Prevent irritable bowel syndrome
- Battle diverticulosis
- Fight off chronic constipation
- Prevent colon cancer
- Lower cholesterol
- Stabilize blood sugar in people with diabetes

Studies have shown that fiber is a major player in helping to prevent digestive diseases such as irritable bowel syndrome, diverticulosis and chronic constipation.

What's more, it's also likely to be an important factor in helping to protect against colon cancer, to lower cholesterol and to keep blood sugar levels under control in people with diabetes.

Battles Diabetes and Cholesterol

In studies at the University of Kentucky, researchers found that a high-carbohydrate, high-fiber diet can reduce the amount of insulin that people with Type I (insulin-dependent) diabetes need by 30 to 40 percent. And it can reduce the amount some people with Type II (non-insulin-dependent) diabetes need by 75 to 100 percent.

The reason? Researchers concluded that a high-carbohydrate, high-fiber diet apparently *doubles* the body's sensitivity to insulin. As a result, people with diabetes may need only about half as much auxiliary insulin as they normally would.

The insulin-preserving diet that was developed at the University of Kentucky calls for 40 to 50 grams of fiber a day. Of that amount, 10 to 15 grams a day should be soluble fiber—mostly oats, beans and fruit. The remaining 30 to 35 percent should be insoluble fiber—mostly found in vegetables and whole-wheat products, says Belinda Smith, R.D., a research dietitian with the university's metabolic research group.

"Okra is a good source of fiber compared to other vegetables not only because it's high in fiber but also because it has both kinds," says Smith. "It has four grams of total fiber per half-cup serving—three grams of insoluble fiber and one gram of soluble.

"That's a good amount," adds Smith, who is also quick to point out that adding just about that amount of fiber to anyone's daily diet may also help reduce cholesterol levels.

"A study we did here at the University of Kentucky indicated that even a small increase in the amount of fiber you eat can have an effect on your cholesterol," Smith explains. In this study, 146 healthy men and women increased their fiber intake by five grams per day—slightly more than what's supplied in a single half-cup of okra. The result was a drop in cholesterol levels of 13 percent.

Year-Round Nutrition

Besides its possible beneficial effect on blood sugar and cholesterol, a single, half-cup serving of okra also contains one-third of the Recommended Dietary Allowance of 400 micrograms of folate needed by pregnant women. Since folate plays an important part in cell division and tissue growth, doctors say, a deficiency during pregnancy may result in miscarriage or deformity. A single serving of okra also contains nearly 20 percent of an entire day's supply of vitamin C.

Ready to give okra a try? Look for pods that are firm, dark green and less than four inches long. Longer pods may be tough and fibrous; limp pods are past their prime.

Canned and frozen okra is available year-round throughout the country. Frozen okra is fine, but experienced cooks say canned okra is too gooey for anything but gumbo.

Onions

Layer upon Layer of Health

POTENTIAL HEALING POWER
May help: • Clear sinuses   • Prevent certain cancers   • Control high cholesterol   • Prevent heart attacks

You've just sliced up an onion bigger than a softball. Your eyes are tearing. Your nose is running. But take a deep breath and enjoy the flow. The very same compounds that seem to be dissolving your sinuses may also lower your chances of cancer, diabetes and a heart attack.

The sulfur compounds that give onions such distinctive tear-jerking abilities are the same ones that give them—and their odoriferous cousins like the leek and scallion—their therapeutic properties, says Barbara Klein, Ph.D., professor of food and nutrition at the University of Illinois in Urbana and an associate editor of the *Journal of Food Science*. These compounds are powerful disease fighters, says Dr. Klein. "Some scientists think that they could be a miracle drug for the future." A number of studies support the idea that onions help protect against stomach and colon cancer.

In a joint study performed by the National Cancer Institute and the Beijing Institute for Cancer Research, for example, scientists examined the eating habits of 564 people who had stomach cancer and 1,131 people who did not have the disease. Those who regularly ate onions, scallions and chives were about 60 percent less likely to have the disease than those who didn't eat them.

A similar study, this one involving 3,669 people from Belgium, found that those who ate onions were 84 percent less likely to develop colon cancer, while those who ate leeks were 66 percent less likely to develop the disease. Onions and leeks also appeared to provide protection against rectal cancer, the researchers reported, although the protective effect was not as dramatic.

How do onions protect against cancer? Scientists aren't really sure. However, with regard to stomach cancer at least, researchers suspect that allium vegetables—including onions, garlic, leeks, chives and scallions—may block the conversion of nitrates into cancer-causing agents.

Protect Your Heart from Blood Clots

Onions also have a dramatic effect on your body's ability to dissolve blood clots that can develop, lodge in an artery and cause a heart attack.

In one study in India, for example, researchers gave ten men between the ages of 35 and 50 a daily supplement of $3^{1}/_{2}$ ounces of butter. As you'd expect, the men's cholesterol levels rose, while the naturally occurring clot-busting activity in their blood dropped. Then, over the next week, the researchers periodically added the juice or oil extracted from roughly 2 ounces of raw onion to the men's daily allotment of butter.

The result? The onion extract completely prevented the expected fat-induced rise in cholesterol—and increased the men's clot-busting activity nearly 16 percent.

Think about that the next time you order a steak and the waitress asks, "With onions?"

Go South of the Border

Despite all the indications that onions are good for your health, most of us simply do not eat enough onions to get a therapeutic effect, says Martha Stone, Ph.D., professor of food science and human nutrition at Colorado State University in Fort Collins. "Onions are 91 percent water," she explains. "And although most of us eat a few slices now and then on a hamburger or a salad, how many of us are going to top them with half a cup?

"Eat enough onions to have a therapeutic effect and no one would want to be in the same room with you," says Dr. Stone.

But Marilyn Swanson, R.D., Ph.D., a nutritionist and extension food safety specialist at the University of Idaho in Moscow, suggests you stiffen your backbone, focus on your health and ignore the issue of social acceptability.

"Don't worry about what your breath smells like after lunch," she chuckles. "Eat as many onions as you can." The Mexican condiment, salsa, which often contains a lot of onions, is a great way to add onions to your diet. And it's popular, too.

Salsa now outsells ketchup as the most popular condiment in the United States. "Spoon it over baked potatoes, chicken or other foods and enjoy the flavor," suggests Dr. Swanson.

Parsley

Too Nutritious to Be Mere Decoration

POTENTIAL HEALING POWER

May help:
- Build healthy blood cells
- Stabilize blood sugar in people with diabetes
- Freshen breath
- Aid digestion

The succulent whitefish lies gleaming on your plate. All you have to do is remove that tiny bouquet of fresh parsley and the fish is ready to eat. But as you fork up the parsley and drop it to the side of your plate, you wonder: Is there any value to parsley other than just its looks?

There certainly is. Fresh parsley is a good source of disease-fighting vitamins A and C, plus the blood-building nutrients folate and iron. Most of us don't get a lot in that little bouquet on our fish, but if the chef had been smart enough to sprinkle the fish with *dried* parsley—ah, that's another story.

Dried parsley—even just a tablespoon's worth dusted over a salad—provides a very healthy dose of trace elements, says Curtiss Hunt, Ph.D., a research biologist at the U.S. Department of Agriculture's Grand Forks Human Nutrition Re-

search Center in North Dakota. That's because once the water content of parsley is removed, the nutrient content is concentrated. And gram for gram, it provides two to three times more copper, iron, magnesium and boron than almost any other food.

Copper and iron are involved with building healthy blood cells, while magnesium helps your body maintain muscle movement. And recent research at Grand Forks indicates that boron may be involved in stabilizing blood sugar.

A single tablespoon's worth of dried parsley provides 7 percent of your daily need for iron, 6 percent for vitamin A, about 3 percent for vitamin C, almost 2 percent for calcium and roughly 1 percent for magnesium.

And it wouldn't be fair not to mention that something about parsley also makes it a great natural breath freshener as well as a potent digestive aid. Not bad for a garnish, wouldn't you say?

Peas

Good Things in Small Packages

A rich, steaming bowl of pea soup on a cold winter's day may do more than defrost your nose and warm your insides.

"Pea soup is also a good source of protein," says Barry Swanson, Ph.D., professor of food science and human nutrition at Washington State University in Pullman. "I use it as a substitute for soups with meat, like beef soup. That moves me away from the high-fat diet most of us eat toward the low-fat diet I want."

What's more, there's some indication that the fiber in dried peas may be able to help those with diabetes stabilize their blood sugar. In a Danish study, for example, researchers asked eight healthy men and women between the ages of 23 and 30 to eat one of three meals on various days: five ounces of ground beef mixed with either wheat bran, sugar-beet fiber or pea fiber.

When the meat was mixed with pea fiber, blood glucose levels did not rise and fall as rapidly or as severely as they did in response to the other foods. What's more, meals eaten with pea fiber did not demand as much insulin from the pancreas to translate food into energy for the body. Since insulin is something that's either ineffective or in short supply among people with diabetes, pea fiber may be of help in handling the disease, concluded the researchers.

Unfortunately, fresh peas simply do not have the same nutritional value as their dried counterparts. In fact, to the doubtless joy of every kid who's ever been told to sit at the dinner table until he's finished his peas, Dr. Swanson admits: "Fresh peas are nutritionally hard to justify. They're 95 percent moisture with a little bit of fiber and a few minerals.

"The only reason to eat them," he adds, "is to add variety, flavor and color to the diet." Which, on occasion, isn't a bad idea.

Peppers

Piquant Power Pods

Although most of us will slice a green pepper on top of a pizza or a red pepper into a salad once in a while, peppers are too often left to wither on the shelf.

Yet scientists tell us that most peppers are bursting with cancer-fighting vitamin C and heart-healthy beta-carotene. A half-cup of sweet red peppers provides 150 percent of your daily need for vitamin C and one-fifth of your daily supply of beta-carotene.

Peter Piper Picked 'Em

How beneficial can the simple pepper be?

One study in northern Italy compared the eating habits of 339 people who had colon cancer with 778 people who did not have the disease. Although the researchers did note the possibility of a coincidence, their statistics indicate that those who regularly ate peppers had a 32 percent lower risk of colon cancer.

The researchers could not say what it was that may have protected people in the study, but a review of some 70 studies by Gladys Block, Ph.D., professor of public health nutrition and epidemiology at the School of Public Health at the University of California, Berkeley, indicates that vitamin C–rich foods such as peppers may significantly reduce the risk of many types of cancer—including cancers of the mouth, esophagus, stomach, pancreas, cervix, rectum, breast and even lung.

What's more, beta-carotene, which is found in both hot and sweet peppers, has been found to protect a diseased heart from further damage. In a study at Harvard Medical School, researchers followed a group of 333 men with serious heart disease for seven years. Some of the men received beta-carotene, others did not. The result? The men taking beta-carotene had 50 percent fewer strokes, heart attacks and deaths than those who did not get the beta-carotene.

A Rainbow of Health

Unfortunately, "very seldom do you eat enough peppers to reap their nutritional benefits," says Jodie Shield, R.D., a spokesperson for the American Dietetic Association. "Yet peppers are so versatile. You can add a good half-cup serving to your diet simply by adding them to such old standbys as vegetable pasta, tuna salad and chili."

But be aware that not all peppers are the same. One branch of the pepper family—which includes bell peppers—is characterized by its sweet personality. Its members start off green, but left on the vine a little longer, they turn yellow, then orange, then red. The color is determined solely by how long the pepper hangs on the vine. The longer it hangs, the sweeter it gets.

The other branch of the family—which includes more than 200 known varieties of chili pepper you're likely to find in Caribbean curries or Mexican salsa—is characterized by its hot, sometimes *very* hot, personality. Its members follow a ripening process similar to that of their sweet cousins.

But while the hot pepper is noted for its capsaicin—an ingredient that pharmaceutical companies are turning into a new drug to relieve various types of pain and itching—it is the sweet pepper that is noted for its cancer-fighting vitamin C. And both peppers are noted for being good sources of beta-carotene.

Pineapple

Rings of Healing Gold

Five hundred years ago Christopher Columbus discovered his first pineapple on the Caribbean island of Guadaloupe. He was intrigued not only by the fruit's succulent flesh and aromatic juice but also by the ways in which islanders claimed the plant could be used to heal.

"Pineapple has been thought of for centuries in the Caribbean as a cure for all kinds of diseases," explains Steven J. Taussig, Ph.D., a retired chemist from the University of Hawaii in Honolulu who spent 30 years researching chemicals in the fruit.

But pineapple ceased being a folk remedy and became a scientific discovery when a pineapple industry researcher absentmindedly rubbed his fingers together three decades ago and noticed that his fingerprints were disappearing.

"This is a true story," chuckles Dr.

POTENTIAL HEALING POWER

May help:
- Prevent blood clots
- Relieve stomachaches
- Reduce inflammation
- Aid burn healing
- Prevent certain cancers

Taussig. The researcher wasn't sure what was happening, but an enzyme called bromelain contained in the pineapple's fruit and stem can break down protein. Since fingerprints are essentially dead protein on the surface of the skin, the bromelain was dissolving them away day after day, as the researcher handled the plant.

Amazed scientists began looking into what else the pineapple's bromelain could do, says Dr. Taussig. And over the years he and others have discovered that various concentrations of the fruit's protein-dissolving enzyme can—either in the lab or in humans—prevent cancer cells from growing, aid in burn healing, relieve stomachaches, reduce inflammation, prevent the blood clots that lead to heart attack and stroke and even clean up arteries clogged up with plaque.

In one German study, for example, researchers gave 14 people with angina pectoris—chest pain that usually results from partially clogged arteries in the heart—between 1,000 and 1,400 milligrams of bromelain a day for several months. The result? The angina disappeared. It reappeared when the bromelain was discontinued.

"One whole, fresh pineapple would supply sufficient bromelain to have therapeutic value," says Dr. Taussig. Unfortunately, because pineapple is so acidic, most people's stomachs can't tolerate a whole pineapple.

But even a few chunks of fresh pineapple are a super source of valuable nutrients. A one-cup serving offers 40 percent of the Recommended Dietary Allowance of vitamin C and almost two grams of healthful fiber. You'll also find moderate amounts of thiamin, folate, vitamin B_6, iron and magnesium in every delicious bite.

Potatoes

Nutrition from the Soil

Mashed, diced, sliced or whole, potatoes may well be the most versatile vegetable in the world. You can whip them into a soup for lunch

POTENTIAL HEALING POWER

May help:
- Fight high blood pressure
- Control appetite
- Prevent kidney damage from high blood pressure
- Ward off certain cancers
- Prevent heart attack
- Protect against stroke

or add low-fat cheese and broccoli to make a dinner casserole. You can eat them cold in a salad, hot as a vegetable or baked whole as a healthy alternative to burgers at the local fast-food joint.

You can boil 'em, grill 'em, roast 'em, fry 'em or microwave 'em. But almost any way you prepare them (frying is the single exception), potatoes are hard to beat when it comes to their healing potential. They can help lower your blood pressure, reduce inflammatory disease and decrease your appetite. Not only that, they also can help to increase your anti-cancer defense systems and boost your resistance to heart attacks.

Potassium Galore

Potatoes are a nutritionally dense food that provides vitamin C, potassium and other assorted minerals," says Nell Mondy, Ph.D., professor of nutritional science, food science and toxicology at Cornell University in Ithaca, New York.

One baked potato offers almost one-quarter the recommended amount of potassium—that's more than *any* other food. And since all that potassium is locked into a food that's also low in sodium, potatoes are a terrific choice for people with high blood pressure, says Dr. Mondy.

Studies indicate that people with high blood pressure who do not get enough dietary potassium can worsen their troubles. In a joint study conducted by Temple University and the University of Pennsylvania in Philadelphia, researchers placed 12 men and women who had high blood pressure on a low-potassium diet for 10 days. Then on the 11th day the researchers intravenously glutted the bodies of everyone with salt—just as you would do with a burger and fries.

Had those in the group had an adequate intake of potassium, chances are nothing would have happened. That's because salt increases blood pressure by increasing the amount of fluid around your cells, while potassium seems to cancel out the effect. No one's quite sure how that happens, but when there's no potassium around to do the job, the result is clear: In this study, blood pressure readings jumped an average of six points.

That may not sound like much, the researchers noted, but if you have borderline or high blood pressure, six points could make the difference between whether or not you need to take medication. And it's enough of a leap to start scientists wondering whether a long-term potassium deficiency is actually a *cause* of high blood pressure to begin with.

Boosting Heart Health

Besides having a possible direct effect on blood pressure, a diet rich in potassium may also help ward off some of the complications of high blood pressure.

Animal studies at Cornell University Medical College in New York City indicate that a diet high in potassium may help delay the onset of kidney damage that often comes from high blood pressure. What's more, these same studies show that a potassium-rich diet may also be able to reduce the incidence of high blood pressure–related stroke.

And even among those who don't already have high blood pressure, potassium seems to exert a powerful effect on preventing the blood clots that can block arteries and trigger a heart attack or stroke. In a study of 260 people between the ages of 30 and 60, researchers at Umea University Hospital in Sweden found that eating potatoes

helps to keep blood from clotting up in the arteries. As a result, the more potatoes people ate, the less likely they were to have a heart attack or stroke.

How much less? Researchers don't know. But a study of 859 people at the University of California, San Diego, found that those who ate a *single* extra serving a day of a potassium-rich food like potatoes had a 40 percent lower risk of dying from stroke.

An All-Around Champ

As if that isn't enough to put potatoes in every pantry, scientists have also found that potatoes are rich sources of two substances that fight cancer at the source.

Potatoes contain protease inhibitors, which may prevent cancer

---

TO PEEL OR NOT TO PEEL

Peel a potato? Nonsense! The skin is the healthiest part—isn't it? Actually, no. "It's folklore that potato skins contain all the nutrients in a potato," says Nell Mondy, Ph.D., professor of nutritional science, food science and toxicology at Cornell University in Ithaca, New York. The lion's share of a potato's nutrition, especially the vitamin C, is found in the center of the potato.

So does it matter whether or not you peel? It may. Some experts, including those with the federal government, say there's nothing wrong with eating your potatoes whole. Other experts, like Dr. Mondy, express concern over the toxicity of both the agricultural chemicals used on potatoes and of the natural chemicals that potato skins produce themselves after being removed from the soil.

While scientists try to reach a consensus, Dr. Mondy is playing it safe and peeling her potatoes.

cells from blasting their way through the body to set up house-keeping in healthy tissue. And they contain quercetin, a substance that can not only inhibit the growth of cancer cells but also smother the inflammatory process, which damages eyes and nerves in people with diabetes. Quercetin may also be able to reduce the inflammation that makes allergies, bursitis, asthma and arthritis so uncomfortable. And it may decrease the infectiousness of such viruses as herpes and polio.

One of the potato's more unusual attributes, however, is that it may help you lose weight. In a study at the University of Leeds in England, researchers prepared lunch for 11 thin people. On different days, the researchers preceded their lunchtime service with either an appetizer, a plain soup or a soup to which a protease inhibitor extracted from potatoes had been added.

The result? Those who had plain soup ate 3 percent fewer calories than the appetizer group. But those who had the soup that included the potato extract ate *21 percent* fewer calories.

Preserve the Potato's Virtue

Clearly potatoes make good nutritional sense. But how we cook and serve them can neutralize many important benefits they have,

cautions Marilyn Swanson, R.D., Ph.D., a nutritionist and extension food safety specialist at the University of Idaho in Moscow.

"Plain potatoes are a real nutritional heavyweight," says Dr. Swanson. "Unfortunately, 50 percent of the potato crop in the United States goes to chips and fries." The rest are often mashed with butter or served with sour cream. We've turned a low-fat food into a high-fat food, says Dr. Swanson.

"We really should use more baked, boiled and mashed potatoes topped with healthy things to improve their nutrition even more," she says. If, for example, you top a baked potato with chili, particularly meatless chili, it's a great source of protein, iron, fiber and potassium—without excessive fat.

Or peel your potatoes, cut them into quarters and dot them with a small amount of oil—either olive or canola. Sprinkle them with rosemary, onions, oregano or basil and bake them in a hot oven—400° or so—until brown.

"You might even keep a windowsill garden so that you can snip fresh herbs for your potatoes every night," says Dr. Swanson. The result will be an endless variety of potato dishes that preserve the potato's nutritional virtue, with no added vice.

Prunes

A Plum of a Snack

The prunes your grandmother fed you as a child are not the prunes of today.

Today's prunes have no pits, a sweet, juicy flavor and a moist, chewy texture. And while they still have enough dietary fiber to effectively ward off constipation, prunes can also apparently give your cholesterol levels a good swift kick.

In one study, 41 men with total cholesterol levels ranging from a moderately high 201 mg/dl (that's milligrams of cholesterol per deciliter of blood) to a staggering 290 mg/dl were given 12 prunes a day for four weeks. Their cholesterol levels were then compared with those taken during a second four-week study period in which they drank grape juice instead of eating the prunes.

The result? Clearly, "prunes are a natural way to add fiber to the diet and lower cholesterol," says Bar-

PRUNING THE FAT IN DESSERTS

Food scientists have come up with a new idea for making prunes more appealing. They've put them in dessert.

The idea? Prune puree. And it has a big payoff. It can cut the fat in baked goods by as much as 90 percent—and eliminate much of their calorie count! You can make one cup of prune puree by blending eight ounces of pitted prunes with six tablespoons of water. It can be substituted for butter, margarine or oil in any recipe other than pastry crust or white cakes. If the recipe calls for two tablespoons of butter, try it with one tablespoon of puree instead.

If you're not up to making your own prune puree, check your supermarket shelves for Lekvar Prune Butter, in the jam and jelly section, or Lekvar Prune Filling, in the baking section. Both are essentially prune puree with a little added sugar. If you find your baked goods are sweeter than you'd like with either product, try cutting the amount of sugar in your recipe by about 25 percent.

bara O. Schneeman, Ph.D., who chairs the Department of Nutrition at the University of California, Davis. In her study the prunes were able to reduce total cholesterol levels by five points and LDL cholesterol—the cholesterol that clogs your arteries—by a good eight points.

Not bad, she says, for what amounts to two handfuls of fruit a day.

Fortunately, you need even less to prevent constipation. "Our advice is to include around six whole prunes a day in your diet," says Dr. Schneeman. "The whole fruit has more fiber than the juice and can work just as well as some of the stuff that is sold over the counter in drugstores."

And, of course, the benefits of eating foods high in fiber don't end with greater regularity and lower cholesterol. Studies also show that eating more high-fiber foods like prunes will decrease risk of overweight and certain cancers.

Pumpkin

A Harvest of Health

If Peter, Peter Pumpkin Eater really did keep all the pumpkin for himself, it's no wonder he "had a wife and couldn't keep her." Because aside from the kind of life she'd lead with such a selfish oaf, pumpkin hogging should be a punishable offense.

Not only does pumpkin bake up into one of the most popular pies ever made, it's also a blend of health-building nutrients that may reduce your chances of heart disease, cancer and constipation.

Just a half-cup of cooked pumpkin provides nearly three times the

POTENTIAL HEALING POWER
May help:
• Prevent constipation
• Ward off certain cancers
• Fight heart disease

daily requirement of heart-healthy beta-carotene, thus making pumpkin one of the best sources of this all-important nutrient. In addition, it contains as much fiber as most cereals and nearly 10 percent of the Recommended Dietary Allowance for vitamin C and folate.

"Pumpkin is one of the vegetables the National Cancer Institute is talking about when they say we should eat five a day to help prevent cancer," says Paul Lachance, Ph.D., chairman of the food science department at Rutgers University in New Brunswick, New Jersey.

"Pumpkin contains antioxidants that fight cancers and carotenoids that convert to vitamin A, which helps fight infection," he explains. "There's also some folate, which may be another cancer fighter."

As Easy as Pie

At this point, no one is sure how many forms of cancer can be warded off by eating yellow-orange vegetables such as pumpkin. But the list seems to be growing.

Take lung cancer, for example. In one government study, researchers compared the diets of 763 male smokers who had lung cancer with those of 900 who did not. They found that male smokers who ate the most dark yellow-orange vegetables such as pumpkin had half the risk of lung cancer compared to those who ate the least.

What was truly amazing, however, was the incredibly small difference in eating habits between those who got cancer and those who didn't: Men who ate only one serving of dark yellow-orange vegetables every ten days or less were more likely to get lung cancer. Men who ate one serving every other day were less likely to get lung cancer.

In other studies, the regular consumption of yellow-orange fruits and vegetables high in beta-carotene seemed to protect women from lung cancer as well.

Radishes

Fireballs of Protection

POTENTIAL HEALING POWER
May help: • Prevent certain cancers

Radishes are far more than elaborate rose-shaped decorations that lend color and elegance to a lunchtime buffet. These cruciferous root vegetables are loaded with naturally occurring substances that may fight cancer.

"All of the strong-flavored vegetables like radishes contain compounds that reduce the risk of cancer," explains Barbara Klein, Ph.D., professor of food and nutrition at the University of Illinois in Urbana and an associate editor of the *Journal of Food Science*.

In particular, radishes contain substances called isothiocyanates that can apparently help prevent cancer in two ways. First, when a cancer-causing substance invades your body, isothiocyanates can literally run interference and prevent a molecular marriage between your body and the invader. If that fails to prevent the malignant marauder from gaining a foothold, isothiocyanates can help suppress the growth of any resulting cancer.

Radishes also contain protease inhibitors, other substances that seem to fight cancer by suppressing its growth. Yet other cancer fighters in radishes include kaempferol, dithiolthiones and vitamin C—all of which are thought to have a protective effect against cancer-causing chemicals.

If you're interested in working a little more of this healthful vegetable into your diet, Dr. Klein suggests global thinking. "The French and the Japanese both make salads from little more than sliced-up radishes," she explains. "The French use a vinaigrette-type dressing and the Japanese use primarily soy sauce."

To prepare a Japanese radish salad takes only a few minutes. "You just slice up the radishes and mix them with a tablespoon or two of soy sauce and a dash of sugar—a little sherry if you like—and add some chopped-up garlic," says Dr. Klein. "It's very tasty!"

Rice

Pilaf Power

For half the world's population, life without rice would be hard to imagine. In Japan, the word for rice, *gohan*, means "a full meal." In India, the Sanskrit word for rice, *vrihih*, means "life-giving seed." In America, we might all be a bit healthier if we ate more of this "life-giving seed."

Whether you eat it brown or white, steamed or boiled, with a fork or with chopsticks, rice is good food.

POTENTIAL HEALING POWER

May help:

- Prevent colon cancer
- Ward off constipation
- Reduce high cholesterol

For starters, rice is a carbohydrate—the kind of starchy food the American Heart Association says should make up 55 percent of our calories. "It's also extremely low in fat, contains no cholesterol and has only about 90 calories in a half-cup serving," says Meghan Flynn, R.D., a spokesperson for the USA Rice Council.

Brown Power

Brown rice—simply white rice with its outer shell intact—has the reputation for being a health food, and there's no doubt it has a nutritional edge over white. "That brown outer layer is the most important part of the rice," says Christine Negm, spokesperson for Lundberg Family Farms, a California producer of brown rice and brown rice products. "Brown rice contains fibers and oils that are extremely important to human health."

A one-cup serving of cooked brown rice has about 3.5 grams of fiber, compared to less than 0.5 gram for white rice. "Fiber may help prevent colon cancer and constipation, and it seems to play a role in reducing blood cholesterol levels," Negm says.

In fact, several studies indicate that a component of the fiber found in brown rice—rice bran—is as effective as oat bran at lowering blood cholesterol levels.

In a study at Louisiana State University, for example, people who ate three servings a day of rice bran saw their cholesterol levels drop an average of 7 percent. Also, their harmful LDL cholesterol dropped 10 percent, but their good HDL was unaffected.

"The results indicate that people with borderline-high cholesterol levels may lower their cholesterol into the normal range with the addition of rice bran," says Maren Hegsted, Ph.D., associate professor of human nutri-

---

RICE EXOTICA

There are an estimated 7,000 varieties of rice in the world. Except for wild rice, which has substantially more fiber and potassium, most rices are nutritionally about the same. Where they differ is in texture and flavor. Here are a few rices you may find in your supermarket or in ethnic food markets.

Basmati. This aromatic rice contains oils that give it a nutty fragrance and flavor. It stands well on its own or as a pilaf.

Arborio. This Italian short-grain rice has an exceptionally creamy texture. Use it to make risotto, a buttery, saffron-scented dish.

Wild rice. Actually the seed of an aquatic grass, this black-hulled grain has a chewy texture and a strong nutty flavor. Wild rice is frequently mixed with other rices for cooking.

Sweet glutinous rice. Also called waxy rice, this Asian import cooks up very sticky. It is used in oriental confections, snack foods and noodles.

tion at the university, who headed the study.

In addition to its bounty of fiber, brown rice is loaded with vitamins and minerals. A cup of brown rice offers about 20 percent of the Recommended Dietary Allowance (RDA) for magnesium, 14 percent of the RDA of vitamin E and 21 percent of the RDA of selenium. Brown rice also has moderate amounts of several B vitamins. White rice has been stripped of most of its natural vitamins and minerals, but many companies fortify white rice with iron, thiamin and niacin.

Sea Vegetables

Neptune's Natural Fiber

When the sea crashes against the rocky shores of northern Maine, it first sweeps through the dark green beds of seaweed that cling to the North Atlantic's granite coast. Although few Americans think of seaweed as food, these wild sea vegetables are a flavorful source of fiber that may be able to reduce your cholesterol levels and help prevent cancer.

"The major sea vegetables harvested in this country are kelp, alaria, laver and dulse," says Alfred Bushway, Ph.D., professor of food science at the University of Maine at Orono. Historically, most sea vegetables consumed in this country have been dried and imported from

POTENTIAL HEALING POWER

May help:
- Prevent constipation
- Fight hemorrhoids
- Battle diverticular disease
- Lower cholesterol
- Ward off certain cancers
- Control blood sugar in people with diabetes
- Prevent obesity

Japan, although today they're increasingly dried and packaged in coastal areas such as Maine and California.

The four popular varieties of sea vegetables are as distinct in flavor and texture as turnips are distinct from asparagus.

Kelp, a green or brown leaf, is the all-around sea vegetable—great roasted, pan-fried, pickled, boiled or marinated, says Carl Karush, marketing team leader of Maine Coast Sea Vegetables, a company that harvests sea vegetables for sale in the United States. Related to a Japanese seaweed called *kombu,* kelp adds a fresh "of-the-sea" note to soups and stews.

Alaria, the made-in-America equivalent of another Japanese seaweed known as *wakame,* has a "wilder" taste. Its advocates say it works best as a flavor-enhancer for long-cooking grains and in miso soup.

Laver—which the Japanese frequently sell in dried sheets called *nori*—has a sweet, nutty taste. It works best crumbled into sautéed vegetables and salads or even over popcorn.

And dulse, a strong-flavored seaweed with a soft, chewy texture, is a native son. Harvested and sun-dried on an island off the Maine coast during the low tides of July and August, it is frequently tossed into chowders, chopped into green salads or eaten as a snack right out of the bag.

A Wave of Health

Although sea vegetables are frequently touted as a rich source of minerals, the fact is that they are rarely eaten in the large quantities that, on paper, make their roster of minerals look so impressive. What's more, the high potassium levels that occur naturally in sea vegeta-bles are generally lost when the vegetables are rinsed prior to cooking.

But when it comes to dietary fiber, ounce for ounce, sea vegetables offer more than many of their landlubber cousins.

"All of the sea vegetables are particularly rich sources of fiber," says Dr. Bushway. Dried alaria, for example, has over nine grams of fiber per ounce—that's $3^1/_2$ times the amount found in an ounce of dried figs.

Soluble and insoluble fiber—both of which are found in sea vegetables in roughly equal amounts—have been found to have important therapeutic effects. Soluble fiber may help lower cholesterol, help people with diabetes keep their blood sugar under control and help prevent obesity by turning off your appetite alarm for longer periods of time than other foods. Insoluble fiber may help prevent constipation, hemorrhoids, colorectal cancer and diverticular disease.

Want to work sea vegetables into your diet? They may be snipped into a broth to flavor miso soup, mixed with macaroni to color a pasta salad, wrapped around fish, rice and vegetables to create sushi or tossed into a stir-fry to zip up the flavor of tofu. If you can't find them in your local supermarket, check out health food stores and Asian markets.

Shellfish

Low-Fat Jewels of the Sea

> **POTENTIAL HEALING POWER**
>
> May help:
> - Prevent heart disease
> - Boost immunity
> - Ensure healthy nerves

Oysters, clams, lobster, crab—shellfish evoke the feel of warm sand, sharp breezes and saltwater.

Maybe that's why we love them. And maybe that's why we've increased our consumption of shellfish, as well as of finfish, nearly a quarter over the past two decades. Or maybe we've simply come to understand how they can contribute to a healthy lifestyle.

"Shellfish have negligible amounts of fat, even less than most finfish," says Lynne W. Scott, R.D., director of the Diet Modification Clinic at Baylor College of Medicine in Houston. These jewels of the sea can be used to replace fatty red meat and other foods that can set the stage for heart disease. In addition to being lean dreams, shellfish also have a trace of the same heart-healthy omega-3 fatty acids that are found in the oil of finfish.

Shellfish are a terrific source of vitamin B_{12}, which is essential for a healthy nervous system. A single serving of a dozen steamed clams, for example, has about *2,700 percent* of the Recommended Dietary Allowance of B_{12}, while six medium-size steamed oysters have "merely" 736 percent.

Most shellfish are good sources of iron and immunity-boosting zinc as well. A serving of 20 steamed clams supplies 140 percent of your daily need for iron and 17 percent of your daily need for zinc. A half-dozen oysters offers 510 percent of your daily need for zinc and 28 percent of your need for iron.

Don't Worry about the Cholesterol

Although most shellfish are generally recommended as part of a heart-healthy diet, concerns about their relatively high cholesterol content have kept many scientists in the past from giving them a full-fledged endorsement.

But a joint study between the University of Washington and Seattle Pacific University may have finally laid those concerns to rest—or at least sorted out the good, the bad and the ugly. In that study researchers alternately fed 18 men three different shellfish diets over three separate periods, each time comparing the men's blood cholesterol levels to their levels at the beginning of the study.

How'd these guys do? Replacing the high-fat meat, cheese and eggs in their diet with the low-fat oysters, clams, crab and mussels did what any low-fat substitution should: It lowered their collective cholesterol level, in this case by about a third. The cholesterol in these shellfish did not raise the men's blood cholesterol levels.

As a result of this and similar studies, the American Heart Association says you can eat as much shellfish as any other source of animal protein—up to six ounces a day, seven days a week—and still be on a heart-healthy diet.

The only exceptions are shrimp and squid. These shellfish have appreciably more cholesterol than other shellfish. Some doctors recommend that you eat them sparingly if cholesterol is a concern for you.

Soy

An Oriental Offspring

POTENTIAL HEALING POWER
May help: • Lower cholesterol • Fight certain cancers

Many of us think the only soy we buy is in a sauce, but the truth is that most of us eat at least a little every day.

Aside from its common use in traditional oriental foods such as tofu, miso and tempeh, soy is often used by the American meat industry to shore up its products.

Soy appears, for example, as "textured soy protein" in about 100 million pounds of meat products sold to the federal school lunch program every year. It's often found in hot dogs, hamburgers and sausages.

In recent years, most supermarkets have also begun to stock a wide variety of products that are made almost entirely from soy. These include soy cheeses, soy yogurts and soy milks (plain or chocolate).

Sales of soy-based foods are skyrocketing—and more than 200 new soyfood products enter the market every year. And that's good news, because soy may have some powerful preventive powers, particularly when it comes to fighting cancer and high cholesterol.

Powerful Nutrients

Five different compounds that may fight cancer are found in relatively high concentrations in soybeans, says nutritionist Mark Messina, Ph.D., former head of the National Cancer Institute's Designer Foods programs and a researcher and consultant on soy in Mt. Airy, Maryland. The most important of these are chemical compounds called *isoflavones,* and they have the ability, says Dr. Messina, to help discourage normal cells from turning into cancer cells. Isoflavones may also negate the effects of estrogen hormones that foster the development of breast, endometrial and ovarian cancer.

"I rarely get excited over one individual food," says Dr. Messina. "But soy is the single most important dietary source of isoflavones in the world. Numerous studies have found that eating as little as a single serving of soy a day on a consistent basis may reduce the incidence of cancer by 50 percent," says Dr. Messina.

"Almost as a side benefit," he adds, "soy also helps lower cholesterol." Studies have found that people with high blood cholesterol who give up meat and dairy foods for soy products experience drops in total cholesterol of 20 percent or more. One probable reason is that soy products, while relatively high in fat, are still lower in total fat than most cheeses and many meats. They are also much lower in

saturated fat and contain no cholesterol. What's more, soyfoods are good sources of blood-building folate and iron, bone-hardening calcium and magnesium. "Soybeans also are fairly high in fiber. This could explain the lowering effect on blood cholesterol and could be helpful to prevent colon cancer," says Kristi A. Steinmetz, Ph.D., consulting nutritional epidemiologist in the Division of Epidemiology at the University of Minnesota in Minneapolis.

Easy to Digest

Undoubtedly, many Americans are turning to soy as an alternative to milk products. Soy contains no lactose, the hard-to-digest milk sugar that leads to gut troubles for many. Soy-based dairy substitutes are found in many markets next to the milk and cheese. If you can't find them yet in your local market, try a health food store.

And while you're shopping, check out the frozen foods case. There are now many frozen soy products on the market—including tofu pizza and lasagna and even tofu "hot dogs."

Of course, you can skip the processed soyfoods entirely and go right to the bean itself. Soybeans are considerably higher in fat than most beans, but they are loaded with vitamins and minerals. A ½-cup serving of boiled soybeans offers up 44 percent of the Recommended Dietary Allowance of iron, about 23 percent of folate, 21 percent of magnesium and about six grams of dietary fiber. You can eat them as you would most other beans, or let them go to sprout and enjoy them atop your evening salad.

Squash

A Jolly Good Yellow

Squash does not squish. It can be whipped like potatoes, nested like spaghetti or grated like cabbage. It can even be fried like a potato or baked like bread.

Not all squash are created equal. Summer squash—zucchini or crookneck are generally what we find at the market—have little nutritional value except for a moderate dose of folate and fiber. But winter squash—the deep orange varieties including acorn, buttercup, butternut, hubbard and pumpkin—are full of cancer-fighting beta-carotene, vitamin C, folate and fiber.

A ½-cup serving of baked butternut squash, for example, serves up nearly three-fourths of your daily beta-carotene needs, over one-fourth of the Recommended Dietary Allowance for vitamin C, 10 percent of your daily folate need and nearly three grams of constipation- and cholesterol-fighting fiber.

"My household rule has always been that there's always a green vegetable, a yellow vegetable and a salad on the table," says Paul Lachance, Ph.D., chairman of the food science department at Rutgers University in New Brunswick, New Jersey. And chances are, he admits, the yellow is likely to be squash, which is one of the best sources of carotenoids—those substances in yellow-orange foods that help fight cancer.

"A lot of people just don't want to take the time to prepare it," he says. "But we peel it, slice it, steam it, add a little butter, salt and pepper," then enjoy.

"If time is of the essence," he adds, "we use it frozen. Frozen squash is cheaper, but fresh has the best taste."

Just how good for you is this tasty little vegetable? *Very* good, according to a government study comparing the diets of 763 male smokers who had lung cancer with those of 900 male smokers who did not. The difference between those who got cancer and those who didn't? Men who were more likely to get lung cancer ate only one serving of dark yellow and orange vegetables every ten days. Men who were less likely to get lung cancer ate one serving every other day.

And that's not all. A study conducted by the Cancer Research Institute in Beijing reveals that people in an area of China known for high rates of stomach cancer had only half the risk if they ate about five pounds of squash a year. What's more, in a study at the University of Washington, women who regularly ate dark yellow and orange vegetables such as squash had a 60 percent lower risk of cervical cancer than those who ate them less frequently.

Need any more reason to squish more squash into your diet?

Sweet Potatoes

Autumn's Natural Beauty

POTENTIAL HEALING POWER
May help: • Prevent constipation   • Ward off certain cancers   • Lower cholesterol

Whipped into sweet, moist mountains, chipped into colorful rounds, folded into luscious pies or baked into spice-flavored breads, sweet potatoes are as much a part of autumn as frosted spider webs under the porch or falling leaves in the backyard.

But aside from their glorious yellow-orange color and sweet taste, sweet potatoes are among the richest sources of beta-carotene, which can help ward off cancer, explains Jodie Shield, R.D., a spokesperson for the American Dietetic Association. One sweet potato, she adds, contains nearly 300 percent of the amount of beta-carotene experts say you need daily for good health.

A government study compared the diets of 763 male smokers who had lung cancer with those of 900 male smokers who did not have the disease. The study indicated that the men who ate the most beta-carotene-rich dark green and

99

yellow-orange vegetables such as sweet potatoes had half the risk of lung cancer compared to those who ate the least.

The difference between those men who had cancer and those who didn't? Those who ate only one serving of dark yellow-orange vegetables every ten days or less were most likely to develop lung cancer. Those who ate one serving every other day were least likely to develop lung cancer.

Fortunately, other studies indicate that women who consume a lot of foods rich in beta-carotene seem to receive the same protection from lung cancer as men and that both men and women may also be protected from other cancers as well.

In a study by the National Cancer Institute, the Beijing Institute for Cancer Research and the University of Southern California in Los Angeles, researchers compared the diets of 564 men and women who had stomach cancer with those of 1,131 people who did not. Once again, those with stomach cancer ate fewer sweet potatoes.

Researchers at the University of Washington have good reason to believe that sweet potatoes may also protect against cervical cancer among women. In their study, women who ate more dark green and yellow vegetables had a 60 percent lower risk of cervical cancer than those who ate less.

Although many scientists are convinced that beta-carotene is the specific nutrient in sweet potatoes

that combats cancer, sweet potatoes also contain vitamin C, fiber and folate—three nutrients that may very well have cancer-fighting properties of their own. In fact, one sweet potato has about 50 percent of the Recommended Dietary Allowance (RDA) for vitamin C, 13 percent of the RDA of folate and as much constipation- and cholesterol-fighting fiber as an average bowl of cereal.

"The nutrient density is quite good in most yellow-orange vegetables," says Paul Lachance, Ph.D., chairman of the food science department at Rutgers University in New Brunswick, New Jersey. "It's unfortunate that we're biased against these vegetables. Only 17 percent of us will have a yellow-orange vegetable once every four days. Yet these are the kinds of vegetables the National Cancer Institute is talking about when they say we should eat 'five a day' to prevent cancer."

The Southern Advantage

Unfortunately, sweet potatoes are eaten on a regular basis only throughout the South. No barbecue is quite complete without one version or another, no picnic quite up to snuff. But for the rest of us, well, the rest of us eat so few that we drag the national level of sweet potato consumption down to around five pounds a year per person.

If you'd like to take better advantage of these protective powerhouses, try mashing them with a

WHICH IS IT—SWEET POTATO OR YAM?

Many people think of yams and sweet potatoes as siblings. But they're not even distant cousins.

Sweet potatoes are what you typically find in your supermarket produce section. They come in two varieties: light yellow and dark orange. The darker variety, the sweeter and moister of the two, is often called a yam. But that's a misnomer. Any botanist will tell you that a dark sweet potato is very different from a yam.

A true yam is actually the tuberous root of a tropical vine. It is unrelated to the sweet potato. If you find a true yam in the United States—which is rare—it'll usually be chopped into chunks, because yams can grow anywhere from the size of a potato to a 7$\frac{1}{2}$-foot-long monster that weighs 120 pounds!

little skimmed evaporated milk as an alternative to the classic mashed potato. Or temper the sweetness by mashing them with some winter squash before baking in a casserole.

When you buy sweet potatoes, try to buy them fresh. Sweet potatoes that are mashed and canned have 25 percent less beta-carotene than their fresher cousins, and potatoes that are vacuum-packed lose nearly 60 percent.

Tomatoes

Saucy Sources
of Vitamin C

POTENTIAL HEALING POWER
May help: • Prevent certain cancers

Every gardener eagerly anticipates that sweet summer evening when he can step into the garden and harvest a beefy red tomato to add to his dinner.

Bursting with vitamin C–enriched juices and packed with pulpy fiber, tomatoes are also one of the richest sources of lycopene. A close relative of beta-carotene, the substance found in many fruits and vegetables that the body converts into vitamin A, lycopene is the plant pigment that makes tomatoes red. Just like beta-carotene, lycopene may enhance your ability to fight cancer—at least according to one study.

Researchers at the University of Hawaii compared the diets of 332 men and women who had lung cancer to those of 865 people who did not. The higher the consumption of tomatoes, the less likely the incidence of lung cancer, reported the researchers. Men who consumed the most tomatoes had half the risk of lung cancer compared to men who ate few tomatoes. Women who ate the most tomatoes were one-third as likely to have lung cancer.

Eating tomatoes can apparently help women in other ways as well. A second study found that women with a precancerous condition of the cervix had lower levels of lycopene

---

FRUIT OR VEGETABLE?

People have been arguing over whether the tomato is actually a fruit or a vegetable for at least a hundred years. In 1893 a tomato importer argued that the "love apple" (as it was known in those days) was a fruit, and because of that, not subject to duty. The case went all the way to the United States Supreme Court, where it was ruled that the tomato was actually a vegetable.

Unfortunately, the Supreme Court was wrong.

Although the tomato is used and thought of as a vegetable, botanically—which is how foods are actually classified—it is a fruit. More specifically, it is a berry, reports the United Fresh Fruit and Vegetable Association, since it contains both pulp and seeds.

in their blood—and a lower level of tomatoes in their diets—than women who did not have the condition. The women whose intake of lycopene-rich foods was highest had only one-fifth the risk of getting the pre-cancerous condition, reported the researchers.

The difference between low and high intakes? One tomato a day. Fortunately, even tomato sauce and tomato paste contain high amounts of lycopene.

Tropical Fruits

Sunny Selections

POTENTIAL HEALING POWER
May help:
• Prevent certain cancers
• Battle high cholesterol
• Lower blood pressure

Passionate purple, luminous green, vibrant yellow, Day-Glo orange—the colors of tropical fruits are as exotic as the places from which they come. And most of them are so packed with nutrients that a single serving is as healthful for you as a vacation to their place of origin.

Mangoes, for example, are those round or elongated greenish-yellow fruits that develop red mottling when ripe. Half a mango boasts nearly half your daily need of vitamin C and is packed with fiber and beta-carotene, which may help reduce your risk of cancer.

In a study at the University of Hawaii, for instance, researchers compared the diets of 404 men and women with lung cancer to those of 968 people who did not have the disease. "A significant difference between the two groups was that those who ate mangoes and other foods rich in beta-carotene were nearly *half* as likely to develop lung cancer as those who avoided such food," says Loïc Le Marchand, M.D., Ph.D., an epidemiologist at the university's Cancer Research Center who conducted the study.

And mangoes may have a protective effect that goes beyond their beta-carotene content. "We're wondering if perhaps there are other protective nutrients yet to be discovered," says Dr. Le Marchand. "Or perhaps the beta-carotene initiates some kind of health-promoting synergy when combined with other nutrients."

A Gold Mine of Vitamin C

Gladys Block, Ph.D., professor of public health nutrition and epidemiology at the School of Public Health at the University of California, Berkeley, has been thinking along similar lines. But while Dr. Le Marchand has been checking into beta-carotene, Dr. Block has been investigating vitamin C—a nutrient that pulses through every bite of almost any tropical fruit.

Dr. Block reviewed 29 different studies on eating fruits rich in vitamin C and found that there is a direct correlation between the amount of fruit people eat and whether or not they developed cancer. In particular, says Dr. Block, the consumption of vitamin C–rich fruits seems to protect against cancers of the esophagus, larynx, mouth, pancreas, stomach and cervix.

But Dr. Block doesn't claim that vitamin C alone is the protective agent. Instead, she points out that most foods that contain vitamin C are also a rich source of beta-carotene. And rather than either nutrient alone being responsible for the anti-cancer effects of fruit, it is far more likely that the two of them are working hand-in-hand to defeat a common enemy.

"Vitamin C seems to form the first line of defense with its ability to capture and inactivate maverick molecules of cancer-causing agents," explains Dr. Block. "And beta-carotene, which operates within the body at different oxygen pressures than vitamin C, seems to form another line of defense." Together the two may provide a bigger anti-cancer wallop than either one could on its own. Or it may even be that vitamin C works better at preventing one particular kind of cancer while beta-carotene works better at preventing another.

"The point is that you should eat fruits that are rich in both beta-carotene and vitamin C," says Dr. Block. Tropical fruits are right at the top of her list.

A Tropical Cast of Characters

Although mangoes are probably the best tropical source of both beta-carotene and vitamin C, other tropical fruits are also excellent sources of health-giving nutrients.

A single guava, for example, has nearly *300 percent* of the Recommended Dietary Allowance for vitamin C and almost five grams of fiber, both of which may protect against cancer. But it's in the effects it has on your cardiovascular system that guava really shines.

In a study at the Heart Research Laboratory in Moradabad, India, researchers asked 61 people with high blood pressure to add a pound of guava to their diets every day for 12 weeks. The result? The group lowered their cholesterol 27 points, dropped their triglyceride levels nearly 8 percent and knocked 11 to

13 points off their blood pressures—both top and bottom numbers.

Papaya, that golden yellow, pear-shaped fruit that can sometimes grow as big as a watermelon, is also a good source of fiber. In addition, half a papaya has more than an entire day's supply of vitamin C and 15 percent of the recommended daily amount of blood-building folate.

A single serving of either passion fruit, star fruit or breadfruit also contain almost half your daily need of vitamin C.

And most tropical fruit also contains between 250 and 500 milligrams of potassium per serving—in the same ballpark as bananas. Potassium may have a lowering effect on your blood pressure.

In a study of 54 people with high blood pressure at the University of Naples in Italy, for example, 81 percent were able to cut their medication in *half* when they added three to six servings a day of potassium-rich food to their diets.

Wheat

Amber Waves of Goodness

POTENTIAL HEALING POWER
May help:
• Reduce risk of certain cancers
• Protect the heart
• Lower cholesterol

Those amber waves of grain that cover our country's midsection are the source of our nation's most popular complex carbohydrate—wheat. Each year the average American gobbles up roughly 136 pounds of wheat, mostly in the form of breads, hot dog rolls and hamburger buns, cakes, cereals and pastas.

Wheat can be a good low-fat source of fiber, nutrients and energy. But even in today's health-conscious times, most people rarely take maximum advantage of this grain's nutritious benefits. The overwhelming preference is still for the stripped-down version—white wheat flour, rather than whole (brown) wheat flour. The healthiest of all forms of wheat—wheat germ, wheat bran and whole-wheat foods such as bulgur or wheat berries—are as alien to most Americans as are tropical fruits to Eskimos. But there's no reason to be left out in the cold when it comes to whole-wheat foods. They are readily available, and there are more good reasons than ever to put them on your menu.

Fiber Feast

Certainly among whole wheat's most important offerings is fiber.

Whole wheat contains a bit of cholesterol-lowering soluble fiber. Its main fiber component is the *in*soluble variety, known for its ability to relieve constipation and cut your chances of developing colon and rectal cancer.

Adding whole wheat may help cut your chances of cancer by shrinking precancerous polyps in the lower intestine, say researchers at the New York Hospital–Cornell Medical Center in New York City. In one study, people who ate regular servings of a cereal high in wheat bran saw a reduction in both the size and number of polyps compared to a low-fiber group. Wheat bran is what is left behind when wheat is turned into white flour.

It's possible that eating wheat bran may also reduce a woman's risk for breast cancer, a study by the American Health Foundation in Valhalla, New York, suggests.

In that study, 62 women were divided into three groups and fed either wheat-, oat- or corn-bran muffins that doubled their fiber intake from 15 to 30 grams a day. After two months of this fiber sup-plementation, only the women in the wheat-bran group had lower levels of circulating estrogen. In other studies, reduced circulating estrogen has been linked to lower rates of breast cancer.

It's possible that the fiber and other nutrients in whole wheat may also help to prevent heart attacks, says Gary Fraser, M.D., Ph.D., professor of medicine and epidemiology at Loma Linda University in California.

One study by Dr. Fraser and his colleagues at the university found that people who regularly ate whole-wheat bread had a 40 percent reduction in the incidence of heart attacks compared to those who normally ate white bread.

Making the Switch

Simply switching from white bread, which has about 0.5 gram of fiber per slice, to whole-wheat bread, with 2 grams per slice, could add substantially to your daily fiber intake, says Susan Finn, Ph.D., director of nutrition services for Ross Laboratories in Columbus, Ohio. Most people only get 10 to 12 grams of fiber a day, about half the recommended amount.

Look for bread labeled as 100 percent whole-wheat bread. Whole-wheat flour—*not* wheat flour—should be the first item on the list of ingredients. Don't rely on color as an indication of whole-wheat content, Dr. Finn warns. Some breads contain brown caramel coloring.

If you're choosing a wheat cereal, check the fiber content. A hot whole-wheat cereal, such as Wheatena, offers about five grams of fiber per one-cup serving. Cream of Wheat, on the other hand, has but one gram of fiber per cup.

A tablespoon of wheat bran contains about 1.5 grams of fiber. Bulgur, which is simply cracked wheat berries, contains about eight grams of fiber per one-cup serving. Bulgur can be served as a cereal or a side dish.

Sprinkle-On Health

Where vitamin E is concerned—a nutrient that may help protect us from cancer and heart disease—few foods dish up as much as wheat germ. The heart of the wheat berry, wheat germ, like wheat bran, falls by the wayside in the production of white flour. It has a pale gold color, a crumblike texture and a nutty taste. A quarter-cup serving provides 40 percent of the Recommended Dietary Allowance for vitamin E.

In a study at St. Luke's Medical Center in Chicago, researchers found that people with high cholesterol levels who ate about six to eight tablespoons a day of raw wheat germ had a drop in harmful LDL cholesterol of 15.4 percent and an 11.3 percent drop in triglycerides.

Wheat germ can be sprinkled atop breakfast cereals, yogurt or even vegetables. Be careful, however, as wheat germ spoils easily. It should be stored in an airtight jar in the refrigerator or freezer.

Yogurt

A Cultured Dairy Delight

For more than 4,000 years, people have been mixing certain bacteria and milk together to make yogurt. In fact, this sour, custardy concoction may be the world's first convenience food.

POTENTIAL HEALING POWER

May help:

- Prevent osteoporosis
- Battle high bood pressure
- Prevent certain cancers
- Fight vaginal yeast infections
- Avoid diarrhea that often comes as a side effect of antibiotics

---

Yogurt resists spoiling—and it's easier than milk to haul around on a donkey. That's why the nomads of eastern Europe who invented yogurt always kept a bit of yogurt culture on hand. With it, they could preserve any precious surplus milk by making it into yogurt.

These days, yogurt has a solid image as a health food, and for the most part, it's an image well deserved. Yogurt is easy to digest, for it contains only a quarter of the amount of lactose found in milk. (Lactose is a milk sugar that in some people leads to bloating and diarrhea.) Not only that, yogurt is crammed with powerful nutrients.

Calcium Countdown

Yogurt is a top source of calcium. Nonfat and low-fat yogurt are perhaps the best sources available. One cup of nonfat plain yogurt has about 450 milligrams of calcium, more than half the Recommended Dietary Allowance (RDA). In comparison, one cup of skim milk has about 300 milligrams, and a cup of low-fat cottage cheese, 150 milligrams.

Calcium is the proverbial white knight when it comes to strong bones. Studies suggest that eating lots of high-calcium foods may help prevent frail bones later in life—a condition called osteoporosis. Calcium may also play a role in preventing colon cancer and high blood pressure.

Aside from calcium, yogurt contains a healthy mixture of other nutrients—especially the all-important B-complex vitamins. One cup offers about 31 percent of the RDA of riboflavin, 23 percent of the RDA of B_{12} and 14 percent of the recommended amount of pantothenic acid. One cup also has about 575 milligrams of the mineral potassium. That's 125 milligrams more than a banana!

Yeast Eradicator

For years women have treated vaginal yeast infections with yogurt, inserting the yogurt into the vagina just as they would an anti-yeast cream, or making it a big part of their diets. "This would have been considered a folk remedy, but now there's some scientific proof that it works," says Eileen Hilton, M.D., infectious disease specialist at Long Island Jewish Medical Center in New Hyde Park, New York.

Dr. Hilton looked at the effects of yogurt in 13 women who'd had at least five vaginal yeast infections the previous year. The women ate one cup of yogurt containing live cultures (*Lactobacillus acidophilus*) every day for six months. At the end of that time, their incidence of infection had been cut to one-third. "In fact, the response was so good that some of the women who were supposed to go on a no-yogurt diet for another six months refused to do so," Dr. Hilton says.

If you're eating yogurt to battle

yeast infections, make sure the yogurt you select says "made with *Lactobacillus acidophilus* culture." Not all yogurts are.

Popular Culture

The virtues of live-culture yogurt may go well beyond the prevention of yeast infections.

Pure yogurt "cultures"—concentrated doses of certain live bacteria found in yogurt—have been found to protect against colon cancer and some other types of cancer in animals, says Georges Halpern, M.D., Ph.D., adjunct professor of medicine in the Department of Internal Medicine at the University of California, Davis. But does this mean that eating yogurt can protect humans against cancer?

"There are no studies of this sort in humans, at least not yet. But populations that consume large amounts of yogurt—Bulgaria, Turkey, Lebanon—do seem to have reduced rates of intestinal cancers," says Dr. Halpern.

Yogurts made with *Lactobacillus acidophilus* culture may also help ward off diarrhea that comes as a side effect of taking antibiotics, says Dr. Halpern. To gain the maximum therapeutic effect, he recommends two eight-ounce cups of low-fat yogurt a day. "The bacteria remain more viable in low-fat rather than nonfat," he says. Start your "yogurt therapy" while on the drug, and continue for a week to ten days after you stop taking it.

VITAMINS, MINERALS AND OTHER SUPPLEMENTS

Vitamins, Minerals and Other Supplements

Low-Cost Health Insurance

Gerald loves to eat. He loves sweet rolls and fried potatoes and thick steaks and gooey desserts. He also likes to spend several evenings a week downing brews at his favorite bar.

His wife, Gerda, eats a carefully balanced diet of whole grains, fresh fruits and vegetables, skim milk, fish and lean meats and takes 20 high-potency vitamin and mineral tablets a day.

Who's better off?

Actually, both members of this hypothetical couple are playing a dangerous nutritional game. Gerald's high-sugar, high-fat diet lacks several important nutrients, and his steady drinking puts him at even greater risk for nutritional deficiency.

Gerda, on the other hand, eats a healthy diet, but the handfuls of nutritional supplements she takes may in fact be injuring her health. Some nutrients are dangerous in large doses, and too much of one nutrient can actually cause a deficiency of another.

Truth or Consequences

There is a lot of hype out there about vitamins and minerals— if you believed everything you read in a health food store you'd wonder how anyone existed before bottled supplements. What's the truth?

Supplements *won't* make up for poor eating or other unhealthy habits. "Some people expect to get good health out of a bottle," says Donald B. McCormick, Ph.D., chairman of the Department of Biochemistry at Emory University in Atlanta. That's not a realistic expectation, he says.

On the other hand, some of us— whether because of inadequate diet, physical stress or other special needs—may not get an optimal amount of nutrients in our food. "Taking supplements is a practical way for a person to make sure he's

UNDERSTANDING RDAs, U.S. RDAs AND DVs

How do you know how much of a nutrient you need? Today we use something called the Recommended Dietary Allowance (RDA) to help determine how much of each essential nutrient we need daily. These amounts, considered ample to prevent deficiency in healthy people, vary according to your age and gender and whether or not you're pregnant or nursing. They were first established in 1941 and are revised periodically by the Food and Nutrition Board of the National Research Council.

These figures are by no means cast in stone, however. The 1989 RDAs, for example, included vitamin K and selenium for the first time. They also included lowered requirements for vitamin B_{12} and folic acid.

Because there are so many different RDAs that depend on age and gender—far too much information to fit on the side of a supplement bottle—most manufacturers use another set of figures called the U.S. RDA. When the U.S. RDA was set by the Food and Drug Administration in 1973, it was based on the highest recommended nutrient level for any age and sex group (excluding children under four and pregnant and lactating women).

The U.S. RDA is meant to be used as a guideline for your daily nutritional needs. The U.S. RDA for vitamins and minerals does not take into consideration your age or sex or any special needs you may have.

The most modern term for vitamin and mineral requirements is the Daily Value, or DV. The DV is exactly the same as the U.S. RDA. Government officials introduced the term because "U.S. RDA" looks so much like "RDA" that people were continually confused.

getting all the vitamins and minerals he needs," says Jeffrey Blumberg, Ph.D., associate director of the U.S. Department of Agriculture's Human Nutrition Research Center on Aging at Tufts University in Boston. "You still need to concentrate on eating right, but you can look at supplements as a low-cost form of health insurance."

But even beyond basic health insurance, some nutrients, when taken in large doses, can apparently prevent certain diseases. "Many of the scientists I know who are working in the field of aging take supplements of vitamins C and E and beta-carotene," says Bruce Ames, Ph.D., director of the National Institute of Environmental

NATURAL VERSUS SYNTHETIC

It seems an easy choice: "Natural" conjures up an image of a nutrient gently coaxed from fresh vegetables. Synthetic, on the other hand, brings to mind an image of a bubbling stew of chemicals.

But the reality of the situation may surprise you. "Your body doesn't know the difference between a 'natural' and a 'synthetic' vitamin," says Howerde E. Sauberlich, Ph.D., professor of nutrition in the Department of Nutrition Sciences at the University of Alabama at Birmingham.

And while your mind may still yearn for natural over synthetic, it's tough to say exactly what *is* natural. Even when a vitamin comes from a plant, extracting that vitamin from the plant often requires the use of chemical solvents—not really a "natural" process. Sometimes manufacturing a supplement combines natural and synthetic methods: The nutrient is made by yeast or bacteria in a lab.

The word *natural* may also mean that only a small percentage of the ingredients are natural. You could find a bottle of vitamin C, for example, labeled "natural" because part of the ingredients come from rose hips, yet most of the contents could be synthetic.

One exception: The natural form of vitamin E (called d-alpha-tocopherol or d-alpha-tocopheryl acetate) is about one-third more potent than the synthetic form (d*l*-alpha-tocopheryl acetate). Both forms are effective, but you have to take more of the synthetic form.

Minerals, of course, most often come from their natural sources, so it's no surprise that they're labeled "natural." For two minerals, however, you may fare better by seeking out labels that say "organic." The organic forms of the minerals selenium and chromium (made from yeast) may be better absorbed by the body.

Health Sciences Center at the University of California, Berkeley.

But nutrition experts know where to draw the line. They know how to use supplements to enhance the health benefits of a good diet. And they know how much is too much. In the following pages, you will learn enough to make wise decisions for yourself.

What Are Vitamins and Minerals?

Before you make your way to the health food store and wander up and down the aisles, let's take a closer look at vitamins and minerals. You probably have a pretty good idea they're essential for good health, but chances are you're not quite sure exactly what they *do*.

Vitamins and minerals don't supply energy or calories—you get those from carbohydrate, protein and fat. What vitamins and minerals do is help release energy from foods so your body can use it. And they have other vital functions as well. They play a role in the health of every organ in the body—including the heart, brain and skin—as well as your bones, immune system and nervous system.

There are 13 vitamins that are considered essential to good health. Four of those vitamins—vitamins A, D, E and K—are fat-soluble, and any excess you take can be stored in your body. The other vitamins are water-soluble, and you won't store any excess amounts (you lose the excess through your urine). These are vitamin C and the B vitamins: thiamin (B_1), riboflavin (B_2), niacin, pantothenic acid, vitamin B_6 (pyridoxine), B_{12} (cobalamin), folic acid and biotin.

Essential minerals include calcium, copper, chromium, iodine, iron, magnesium, manganese, molybdenum, phosphorus, potassium, selenium, sodium and zinc.

Without adequate amounts of these vitamins and minerals, deficiency diseases can develop. A deficiency of vitamin C causes scurvy, a lack of vitamin D causes rickets, too little niacin causes pellagra, and a lack of thiamin causes beriberi—all serious diseases. People with a diet excessively low in iodine commonly experience swelling in the neck, called a goiter. And the pallid maidens of days past who swooned frequently probably had iron-deficiency anemia.

Who Needs More?

Are you getting all you need of every nutrient? "The average American doesn't have any outright deficiencies, but a lot of people are just barely getting by," says John Erdman Jr., Ph.D., director of the Division of Nutritional Sciences at the University of Illinois in Urbana. Deficiency diseases such as rickets and beriberi are almost unheard of in this country. On the other hand, many Americans may not have enough nutrients stored to meet the extra nutritional demands placed on the body by things like a viral invasion. "As a result, they may get more colds or take longer to recover from setbacks to their health," says Dr. Erdman.

The elderly quite often are at risk for marginal deficiency, points out Howerde E. Sauberlich, Ph.D., professor of nutrition in the Department of Nutritional Sciences at the University of Alabama at Birmingham. "Their bodies' ability to use nutrients may be impaired by age," he says. The elderly also often don't eat as much as they did when younger—but their nutrient needs diminish only slightly.

Other groups who may be at risk for specific deficiencies:

- Pregnant or nursing women, who need extra nutrients

- Frequent aspirin takers, because aspirin interferes with metabolism of vitamin C and folic acid

- Heavy drinkers, because alcohol depletes the B vitamins and vitamin C

- Smokers, who apparently use more vitamin C than non-smokers

- Strict vegetarians, who eat *no* foods from animals, may be low on vitamin D, riboflavin, B_{12}, calcium, zinc and iron

Disease Prevention

There's a whole array of health benefits that may be possible from taking certain nutrients in amounts above the Recommended Dietary Allowance (RDA).

"We used to think of vitamins strictly in terms of what you needed to prevent short-term deficiencies," says Simin Nikbin Meydani, D.V.M., Ph.D., chief of the Nutritional Immunology Laboratory at the Research Center on Aging at Tufts University. "Now we're starting to think about what the optimal level of vitamins is for lifelong health and the prevention of age-associated diseases."

Much of the exciting news is about nutrients that act as antioxidants. In your body you have compounds known as free radicals. These are unstable molecules that can damage your body in much the same way rust attacks metal. Scien-

tists believe that free radicals contribute to cancers, heart disease and respiratory problems. They're formed by everyday reactions in your body or from environmental influences such as smog, sunlight and cigarette smoke. Antioxidants, however, can latch onto the free radicals and render them harmless.

Nutrients that act as antioxidants include beta-carotene (which converts to vitamin A in the body), vitamin C and vitamin E.

What exactly can these nutrients do? In a Harvard University study, 165 male doctors with signs of heart disease took beta-carotene supplements every other day for six years. They had *half* the number of strokes, heart attacks and heart-related deaths compared to a similar group of doctors who didn't take supplements. And nurses who took daily supplements of vitamin E had less risk of heart attack.

The anti-cancer evidence is also strong. "There is no doubt in my mind that vitamins C and E and beta-carotene are effective in protecting against a whole array of cancers," says researcher Gladys Block, Ph.D., professor of public health nutrition and epidemiology at the School of Public Health at the University of California, Berkeley.

Beyond the Antioxidants

But anitoxidants aren't the only headline-grabbers in the nutrient world. Other nutrients have vital health roles as well. Calcium

YOUR EASY GUIDE TO NUTRIENT TERMS

Antioxidant: A compound that may protect against cancer and other diseases by neutralizing free radicals (unstable molecules) within the body. Beta-carotene, vitamin C and vitamin E are antioxidants.

Fat-soluble: Dissolves in fat (rather than water); excess intake is stored in the body. Fat-soluble vitamins include A, D, E and K.

International Unit (IU): A measurement term for fat-soluble vitamins A, D and E.

Microgram (mcg): One-millionth of a gram or one-thousandth of a milligram. (There are approximately 28 grams to the ounce.)

Milligram (mg): One-thousandth of a gram.

Trace element: An essential mineral that you require in very small quantities, less than 100 milligrams a day.

Water-soluble: Dissolves in water (rather than fat); excess intake is generally excreted in the urine.

---

and vitamin D are crucial in preventing osteoporosis. Zinc may improve wound healing. Folic acid apparently can help prevent serious birth defects. And the list goes on.

You may think of all fats as bad for you, so you may be surprised to learn that some fats, in moderation, may help fight diseases such as cancer and heart disease. On supplement shelves you'll find many types of fats. In this section, we discuss two of the most promising, fish oil and primrose oil.

A few other common supplements don't fit into any of the categories above but nonetheless may offer substantial health benefits. Brewer's yeast, for example, is packed with many valuable nutrients. Fiber supplements may help fight constipation and high cholesterol. Garlic tablets may help battle cancer and improve cardiovascular health. And some enzyme supplements can help your digestion.

Supplement with Care

If you decide to take any supplement, you should choose it carefully and in consultation with your doctor. As you'll find explained in the following pages, some nutrients can interact with each other, making one less or more available. And you can overdose on certain supplements, with potentially serious consequences. For example, vitamin A, vitamin D, niacin and iron should all be taken with extreme caution.

And because supplements are regulated by the Food and Drug Administration as foods, not as drugs, their quality is not as rigorously controlled as that of drugs. Consumers have become ill from taking mislabeled or misformulated supplements. You should select products marketed by manufacturers and retailers you trust. If you have specific questions, write or call the company.

In the chapters that follow, you'll find information on many nutrients, including what foods they're found in, the RDA for men and women aged 25 to 50 and advice for supplement use. As you read, keep in mind that supplements cannot make up for poor nutrition or an unhealthy lifestyle. They may, however, fill in any nutrient gaps in your diet and help ensure your optimal health.

Vitamin A

Best in Small Doses

Vitamin A ranks on the Dean's List of nutrition: It plays a key role in vision and the development and growth of cells. It also keeps skin healthy, assists the immune system and may even help protect you from cancer.

But when it comes to this necessary nutrient, too much of a good thing can be bad. In fact, excess vitamin A can be downright dangerous, and vitamin A supplements are rarely recommended.

A Host of Benefits

Vitamin A has many virtues. It stimulates wound healing, especially in people taking steroid drugs. (Steroids are often prescribed to control inflammation, but this makes skin slower to heal.) So if you've been wounded or severely burned, or are either planning for or recovering from surgery, it's important to get plenty of vitamin A.

Vitamin A also has been found to help decrease the severity of measles in children, adding to the reasons that it's been a literal "lifesaver" in African and Asian countries, where many suffer from poor nutrition, says Harinder Garewal, M.D., Ph.D., assistant director of cancer prevention and control at the Department of Veterans Affairs Hospital and the Arizona Cancer Center in Tucson.

Vitamin A has also long been linked to a lower risk of certain eye diseases that can result from the natural aging process. Researchers at the University of Illinois found that people who fail to get enough vitamin A in their diets are twice as likely to develop macular degeneration, a condition that causes vision problems in many people over 60. Vitamin A is also important for younger people, as a deficiency can impair night vision.

Researchers in Belgium found that stroke victims fared better when their diets included plenty of vitamin A. Closer to home, vitamin

AT A GLANCE

VITAMIN A

RDA: Men: 5,000 IU. Women: 4,000 IU.

Good food sources: Orange, yellow, and green leafy vegetables and orange and yellow fruits.

Who's at risk for deficiency: Virtually no one in the United States or other Western countries except poverty-stricken people with extremely poor diets and people with certain diseases of the liver, pancreas or intestines.

Possible signs of deficiency include: Night blindness, trouble focusing in changing light and glare sensitivity.

Advice for use: Supplements should be avoided. It's possible to get enough vitamin A in a balanced diet or by taking a multivitamin.

A is being intensely researched as a possible cancer fighter. Additionally, it may protect the lining of the lungs—one reason that it's especially useful to smokers.

Two Forms, Two Effects

Despite the many benefits of vitamin A, the typical American has "no compelling reason to take specific vitamin A supplements," says Keith West Jr., Dr.P.H., associate professor at the Dana Center for Preventive Ophthalmology and director of the Vitamin A Program at Johns Hopkins Hospital in Baltimore. The reason for not taking vitamin A supplements, in addition to their potential dangers, is that you are undoubtedly already getting enough. Most experts agree that it's difficult for Americans to experi-

ence vitamin A deficiency.

You can get vitamin A from many different foods—but some sources are better than others.

One form of vitamin A abounds in organ meats such as beef liver. This form is called retinol and is "preformed," meaning it's ready for your body to use.

"If you get too much vitamin A, it may overwhelm the liver's capacity to store it," says Robert M. Russell, M.D., professor of medicine and nutrition at Tufts University in Boston and director of human studies at the U.S. Department of Agriculture's Human Nutrition Research Center on Aging there. "The problem is, the liver has a huge capacity to store retinol vitamin A and a limited capacity to get rid of it, so it tends to accumulate. This can result in a whole list of symptoms: severe headaches, nausea, dry skin, hair loss or an enlarged liver." In severe cases, cirrhosis, nerve damage, achy joints or bone pain can also result.

Fortunately, you can also get "precursor" vitamin A from your diet by eating fruits and vegetables that are rich in beta-carotene. The advantage of this form is that it's turned into vitamin A inside your body as needed. In fact, many experts recommend that you concentrate on getting your vitamin A from produce such as sweet potatoes, carrots, apricots and cantaloupe because there's little chance of toxicity. Plant food sources of beta-carotene also don't pose the same health risks as retinol-rich, high-cholesterol animal sources such as liver.

Caution Advised

So with all the risks of pure vitamin A supplements, why are they sold over the counter?

"Good question," says Dr. Russell. "If I had my druthers, high-dose vitamin A would be available only by prescription." Most multivitamins have 5,000 international units of vitamin A, a safe amount, he adds.

"Vitamin A is definitely necessary and is very useful," says Dr. West. But a little goes a long way: "Most people don't need anything more than what you'll find in a decent diet or multivitamin supplement."

Acidophilus

Bacterial Hero

Just like people, there are all kinds of bacteria in this world. Some are bad. Some are good. Some are *so* good that we just can't seem to get enough of them. One form of bacteria that nearly always deserves a warm welcome is *Lactobacillus acidophilus*.

Commonly known simply as acidophilus, these bacteria occur naturally in our bodies. We can also eat

POTENTIAL HEALING POWER

May help:
- Aid digestion of milk products
- Prevent some yeast infections
- Restore bacterial balance in the intestines
- Fight gastrointestinal cancer
- Control cholesterol levels

acidophilus in certain dairy products or get them in supplement form. Studies show that you're in good company when there's lots of acidophilus around. They may help protect you from indigestion, yeast

AT A GLANCE

ACIDOPHILUS

RDA: None established.

Good food sources: Acidophilus milk and some yogurts.

Who's at risk for deficiency: Acidophilus is not considered essential, although people who take antibiotics may benefit from adding it to their diet.

Possible signs of deficiency include: Women who have frequent yeast infections may have low levels of acidophilus.

Advice for use: Because it can alter the intestinal "ecosystem," people who have serious (medically treated) intestinal problems should check with their doctor before trying acidophilus.

infections, diarrhea and possibly more.

Taking the Burp out of Dairy

If you're one of the unfortunate folks who can't digest milk products, you *know* what lactose intolerance is. It means you lack sufficient quantities of the enzyme lactase, which is necessary to break down the lactose, or sugar, in dairy products. The result can be indigestion, bloating or worse.

For minor cases of lactose intolerance, acidophilus milk may digest more easily, says Georges Halpern, M.D., Ph.D., adjunct professor of medicine in the Department of Internal Medicine at the University of California, Davis. The busy little bacteria work to help break down lactose before it causes havoc in your gut.

You could buy acidophilus in health food stores in powder form, sprinkle it in milk and drink up. Or, in some markets, you can buy milk with acidophilus already in it. (For severe lactose intolerance, you may prefer to use a lactase enzyme, available at drugstores and many health food stores.)

The Antibiotic Antidote

For women plagued with recurrent yeast infections, acidophilus can be a real boon. These vaginal infections occur most often when helpful bacteria in your system are killed off, often by antibiotics. At these times, eating extra acidophilus bacteria can help restore the balance.

When 13 women in a study at the Long Island Jewish Medical Center ate yogurt with acidophilus bacteria every day, they had only 4 yeast infections among them over a period of six months. In a six-month period when they didn't eat yogurt, the same women had *32* yeast infections among them.

Our bacterial good-guy can also help restore balance in the intestines. "Acidophilus milk or yogurt is a good way to repopulate the bacteria in the intestines when you're on antibiotics," says Dr. Halpern. Acidophilus can sometimes help control the diarrhea that comes as a side effect of taking antibiotics.

Acidophilus may someday be an approved remedy for other ailments as well. For instance, there's some suggestion that acidophilus can help fight cancer in the gastrointestinal tract. A study at Tufts University in Boston found that oral acidophilus helped kill off certain enzymes that help convert chemicals in our bodies into cancer-causing substances. Some preliminary studies also suggest that acidophilus may help reduce cholesterol levels.

Scouting Out Acidophilus

If you want to up your acidophilus intake, you've got several choices. Dr. Halpern leans toward yogurt and acidophilus milk as your most reliable sources. Before you begin scarfing down that tub of yogurt, however, get out your reading glasses and check the fine print: All yogurts are not created equal. Even if the label says "Contains Active Yogurt Cultures," this could mean critters other than acidophilus. You're looking for the words *Lactobacillus acidophilus* or *L. acidophilus*.

What about frozen yogurt? That depends. Many bacteria are killed off during the pasteurization and freezing process, but many companies add them *back* to the yogurt afterward. If you want to know for sure, you'll need to call the manufacturer.

Amino Acids

Protein at Its Purest

POTENTIAL HEALING POWER

May help:
- Fight depression
- Battle liver damage
- Treat Raynaud's disease

W hat's for lunch, Mom? "Well, dear, we're having isoleucine, leucine, lysine, methionine, phenylalanine, threonine, tryptophan, valine and histidine."

"Yuck!"

Actually, what Mom rattled off shouldn't taste so bad. It could describe a chicken breast, a tuna salad or even a bean burrito. The scientific-sounding names identify amino acids, the chief components of protein. Animal and plant products are full of these amino acids. And that's a good thing. Without them, and without protein, your body would run down like a machine without oil.

But don't worry. Protein and amino acids are so easy to come by that very few people in the United States are deficient. About the only people who might be low in an amino acid are people with genetic defects that prevent them from making or utilizing certain amino acids, people with liver damage or people with very low protein intake, notably vegetarian children who consume no milk, eggs or fish.

So if we all get plenty of protein, and therefore all the essential amino acids, why would anyone ever want to take more?

Good question. Some studies have found that specific amino acids—including ones that aren't considered essential—may help manage ailments ranging from depression to liver disease. And if you pick up a bodybuilding magazine, you'll find that advertisers are trying hard to convince would-be Arnold Schwarzeneggers that supplemental amino acids will build bulging muscles.

A Bodybuilder's Boondoggle

F lip through that bodybuilding magazine, and you'll find claims that amino acid formulas will pump you up and out. "Build muscles of steel!" and "Grow bigger, faster, and harder!" are typical claims.

These claims are at least *based* on fact. Protein does build muscle. And the nonessential amino acids arginine and ornithine can stimulate the output of growth hormone (a substance that stimulates body growth). But if you're already getting adequate amino acids from your normal diet, will supplemental amino acids do anything to help build muscle?

Absolutely not, says G. Harvey Anderson, Ph.D., professor and former chairman of the Department of Nutritional Sciences at the University of Toronto in Ontario and former chairman of an expert advisory committee on amino acids established by Health and Welfare Canada. "The body has an enormous capacity to get rid of any excess amino acids," says Dr. Anderson. "Your liver and enzyme systems chew them up."

In other words, amino acid supplements are no more likely to turn you into Arnold Schwarzenegger than into a polka-dotted unicorn!

Therapy—Or Hazard?

Bodybuilding hoopla aside, many studies have found positive effects from specific amino acids. For instance, one doctor in India reports great success treating Raynaud's

AN AMINO ACID GONE ASTRAY

It's the classic nighttime soother and sleep inducer: a glass of warm milk. If the milk helps you become drowsy, it's likely an essential amino acid called tryptophan that pushes you over the edge into Slumberland.

Studies have consistently found that tryptophan helps you go to sleep. It has also been used to treat depression and premenstrual problems, reduce drug and alcohol craving and suppress appetite. It seemed a safe, drug-free treatment—until 1989, when some users began to develop a painful muscle problem called eosinophilia-myalgia syndrome. By August 1990, 1,536 cases and 27 deaths had resulted.

In 1989, the Food and Drug Administration removed tryptophan supplements from the market and started a study of other amino acid supplements.

While you can't buy tryptophan supplements in this country, you're still safe with natural tryptophan, which you can get from meat, fish and, of course, a nighttime glass of warm milk.

AT A GLANCE

AMINO ACIDS

Estimated daily requirement (for a 150-pound person):

Histidine: 545–817 mg

Isoleucine: 680 mg

Leucine: 955 mg

Lysine: 820 mg

Methionine (plus cystine)*: 885 mg

Phyenylalanine (plus tyrosine)*: 955 mg

Threonine: 480 mg

Tryptophan: 240 mg

Valine: 680 mg

*One can substitute in part for the other.

Good food sources: Animal products provide all the essential amino acids, as does a meal that combines any legume and any grain.

Who's at risk for deficiency: People with liver damage, people with specific genetic defects and people with unusually low protein intake.

Possible signs of deficiency include: There are no known signs of amino acid deficiency.

Advice for use: Supplements should not be taken without a doctor's okay.

disease (a blood vessel problem that results in cold fingers and toes) with supplemental arginine.

Supplemental amino acids also have been used successfully in some cases to treat various behavioral problems. Priscilla Slagle, M.D., associate clinical professor in the Department of Psychology at the University of California, Los Angeles, and author of *The Way Up from Down*, prescribes specific amino acids for depression. Other nutritionists tout specific amino acids for anxiety, addiction and more. And there may be some merit to this: Phenylalanine has helped cheer up depressed patients and control addictive cravings, while tyrosine has been used to help cocaine users withdraw. Amino acids also may help control food cravings and allergies.

Other preliminary findings suggest that supplemental arginine can improve immunity, fight cancer growth in animals and accelerate wound healing. Certain amino acids (leucine, isoleucine and valine) have also helped treat a form of liver damage known as hepatic encephalopathy.

Why Not Self-Dose?

All pretty exciting stuff, right? But before you even *think* about buying supplements, consider this: Some studies indicate that many of the amino acids that have promising therapeutic effects *also* have negative effects, including nausea and diarrhea.

There's also a question of quality control. In England, amino acid supplements are prescribed and regulated just like drugs, but in the United States they're sold as food supplements, which means they're poorly regulated.

Such poor regulation became a serious concern after many people became seriously ill and 27 people died from bad tryptophan supplements in 1989 and 1990. The U.S. government ordered tryptophan off the market and shortly thereafter issued a warning about the safety of *all* amino acid supplements.

Experts agree that we just don't know enough about these things. "We've got information on rats and mice and frogs, and people who have taken a couple of grams of supplemental amino acids daily for a month, but we don't have information on people who have taken these things long term," says John Brosnan, Ph.D., professor of biochemistry at Memorial University in St. John's, Newfoundland.

Because of the quality-control factor alone, Dr. Brosnan recommends leaving supplements on the shelf. "You've got to wonder what in the name of heaven you're taking in," he says. "It might be 99.7 percent amino acid that won't harm you, but you have to wonder about the other 0.3 percent."

Experts generally agree: Don't try self-dosing. If you have a condition that could be treated by a supplemental amino acid, your doctor should be the one prescribing the supplement *and* monitoring your progress.

Vitamin B$_6$

A Jack of All Trades

If they gave out awards for the nutrient with the largest number of reported benefits, vitamin B$_6$ would win hands down. This vitamin has been suggested or used as treatment for conditions ranging from A (autism) to Z (zinc deficiency), with carpal tunnel syndrome, herpes, kidney stones, worms (yes, worms) and more in between.

"This vitamin has been linked with an amazing list of conditions, diseases and disorders, some of them really bizarre, but very few of these claims have scientific support," says James E. Leklem, Ph.D., professor of human nutrition at Oregon State University in Corvallis.

There's some disagreement among experts as to exactly what B$_6$ can and can't accomplish. Experts *do* agree, however, that too much B$_6$ can be dangerous, so indiscriminate pill popping is definitely out.

> ### POTENTIAL HEALING POWER
>
> May help:
> - Keep the nervous system healthy
> - Strengthen the immune system
> - Treat premenstrual syndrome
> - Lessen harmful effects of diabetes
> - Prevent one type of kidney stones
> - Treat carpal tunnel syndrome

Catering to Basic Needs

You need vitamin B$_6$, also called pyridoxine, for many important functions, including making red blood cells, helping your body use protein, fats and carbohydrates and keeping your nervous system working right. B$_6$ also helps convert the amino acid tryptophan into another essential B vitamin, niacin.

And B$_6$ helps you fight off disease. When eight healthy people over age 60 were fed a liquid diet with essentially no B$_6$, the activity of disease-battling cells decreased, lowering their immune power. "When their B$_6$ intake was then increased one step at a time, immunity gradually returned to normal," says Jeffrey Blumberg, Ph.D., associate director of the U.S. Department of Agriculture's Human Nutrition Research Center on Aging at Tufts University in Boston.

How much B$_6$ is enough? The Recommended Dietary Allowance (RDA) is 1.6 milligrams for women and 2 milligrams for men. While B$_6$ appears in many foods, including meats, nuts, poultry, fish, whole grains and a few vegetables and fruits like potatoes, avocados, and bananas (a large banana boasts about a milligram of this vitamin), many older people apparently aren't getting enough of this nutrient. One study of nearly 200 people aged 60 to 96 found that at least three-fourths of them fell short of getting the RDA for B$_6$ from their diets.

It's possible that people use B$_6$ less efficiently as they age. A small study at the Research Center on Aging at Tufts suggested that older people may need *more* than the RDA levels of B$_6$ to meet their daily needs. This doesn't mean a huge dose, however. "I think there probably is a small increase in need," says Dr. Leklem, "but certainly less than double the RDA."

The Front Line

What about *treatment* with this vitamin in larger doses?

There have been some reports of doctors successfully treating carpal tunnel syndrome and premenstrual syndrome (PMS) with B$_6$. Carpal tunnel occurs when you've got too much pressure on a nerve that passes through a narrow opening in your wrist bones. The result is pain, numbness and tingling, which can become sharp bolts of

---

AT A GLANCE

VITAMIN B$_6$

RDA: Men: 2 mg. Women: 1.6 mg.

Good food sources: Walnuts, unpolished rice, peanuts, bananas, tuna, beef, chicken, pork, herring, whole-wheat products and cauliflower.

Who's at risk for deficiency: Alcoholics, people with a genetic defect that prevents them from using B$_6$ properly and possibly the elderly.

Possible signs of deficiency include: Anemia, weakness, nervousness, irritability, insomnia, difficulty walking and later, convulsions.

Advice for use: High doses should be taken only under the supervision of a doctor.

pain that shoot up into the elbow, upper arm and shoulder. PMS symptoms can include headache, dizziness, bloating, nausea and vomiting, breast heaviness and backache.

But for both of these syndromes, B$_6$ seems to work only sometimes. "I've seen four to five studies where B$_6$ has seemed to help PMS, and eight to ten where it did not," says Dr. Leklem. In the cases where B$_6$ did help some of the symptoms, the doses were so high that they should be taken only under a doctor's supervision.

Some promising research suggests that B$_6$ may be a ticket to better health for those with diabetes, says Dr. Leklem. About 20 to 30 percent of people with diabetes have low blood levels of vitamin B$_6$, he says. For these people, a large daily dose of B$_6$ may help protect the heart and blood vessels from premature wear and tear by minimizing the harmful effects of high levels of blood sugar on blood vessels.

"If I had diabetes, I'd make darn sure that my B$_6$ intake was at the RDA level or slightly above it," says Dr. Leklem. Experts agree, however, that people with diabetes should *not* take single supplements of B$_6$ without consulting with their doctor.

Second String

What about the rest of the alphabetic list of possible benefits? Researchers have found promising

results in using very high doses of B$_6$, combined with magnesium, to treat autism, a disorder marked by withdrawal, daydreaming, hallucinations and failure to relate to others. "There are some promising results," says Dr. Leklem, "but it's still iffy."

Some people use B$_6$ to help prevent kidney stones, chunks of accumulated mineral salts. One five-year study of 100 people showed that a daily dose of 40 milligrams of B$_6$ eliminated calcium oxalate crystals in the urine. Stones can be formed from a variety of minerals, however, and B$_6$ only prevents calcium stones caused by too much oxalate in the urine.

Some researchers have used B$_6$ to treat schizophrenia. In the laboratory, B$_6$ inhibits the growth of skin cancer cells, and there's some suggestion that B$_6$ may help prevent heart disease.

Playing with Fire

As mentioned previously, this vitamin can be dangerous in high doses. While you can find supplements of B$_6$ in 200-milligram tablets, you're playing a dangerous game if you're taking these. "Don't fool yourself," says Dr. Leklem. "This is serious stuff."

What can happen? Doses as low as 300 to 500 milligrams have caused nerve damage. Less serious effects have occurred in people even at 100 milligrams daily. Studies have noted unstable gait, numb feet and eventually numbness and clumsiness of the hands in people taking high-dose B$_6$ supplements for two months.

And surprisingly, you can get "hooked" on this vitamin. A study conducted at Fitzsimons Hospital in Denver found that when people stop using vitamin B$_6$ supplements, they may have abnormal electroencephalograms (recordings of the electrical impulses in the brain). If you're currently using vitamin B$_6$ supplements, reduce your dose gradually rather than going off cold turkey.

While most of us can get adequate B$_6$ from our diets without any trouble, older people and those with diabetes should make an effort to eat foods rich in B$_6$, such as lean meat, poultry or bananas. Taking a balanced vitamin and mineral supplement containing the RDA of B$_6$ or slightly above offers added insurance. But pure B$_6$ supplements should be taken only under the supervision of a doctor.

Vitamin B$_{12}$

The Vitality Vitamin

Back in the 1920s, two doctors made a lifesaving discovery. They found that people with pernicious anemia, a rare and sometimes fatal blood disorder, could survive, as long as they ate at least ⅔ pound of *raw liver* daily. No doubt it took more than a little coaxing to keep patients on this unappetizing diet.

The doctors who discovered this treatment won the Nobel Prize in medicine. But it wasn't until 1948 that researchers isolated (from raw liver, of course) the small red crystals of the nutrient we now call vitamin B$_{12}$.

POTENTIAL HEALING POWER

May help:
- Prevent anemia
- Counteract fatigue
- Reverse neurological symptoms such as tingling hands and feet, memory loss, unsteady gait and muscle weakness

---

Since that time, this vitamin, sometimes called cobalamin, has been the subject of some controversy. The argument isn't so much over what vitamin B$_{12}$ does as over who's deficient in it and who might need supplements.

Until recently, much of the medical establishment looked upon B$_{12}$ supplementation as a needless frivolity for anything except pernicious

SHOULD YOU GET A B$_{12}$ TEST?

The only *sure* way to find out if you're running low on B$_{12}$ is to have a blood test, experts agree. Most say that it's wise to have your blood B$_{12}$ levels checked:

- If you exhibit unexplained nerve or blood problems of the kind associated with a B$_{12}$ deficiency. These include "pins and needles" sensations in the hands or feet, muscle weakness in the legs or arms, incoordination or abnormal gait, memory loss, fatigue, changes in personality or mood, or disorientation.

- At age 60, and every few years thereafter, whether or not you show signs of deficiency.

Most also agree that, for starters, you should have a serum B$_{12}$ test. This test has been used for years to measure B$_{12}$ status. It measures all the B$_{12}$ circulating in your blood. "This test is effective at detecting a B$_{12}$ deficiency in about 90 percent of people," says Robert H. Allen, M.D., professor of medicine and biochemistry and director of hematology at the University of Colorado Health Sciences Center in Denver.

If you fall into the "low but normal" range or you're showing signs of blood abnormalities associated with B$_{12}$ deficiency, your doctor may suggest a second test. He may suggest that, along with the B$_{12}$ test, your blood be tested for a folic acid deficiency. That's because a folic acid deficiency can cause what looks like a B$_{12}$ deficiency.

anemia, the classic symptom of deficiency. Now, though, studies are showing that more people than previously realized—particularly the elderly—are low in vitamin B$_{12}$ and may require supplements.

Diet's Not the Problem

Most nutritional deficiencies occur because people aren't eating enough of the foods that contain a particular nutrient to meet their needs.

But that's *not* the case with B$_{12}$, explains Howerde Sauberlich, Ph.D., professor of nutrition in the Department of Nutrition Sciences at the University of Alabama at Birmingham. "In the U.S., most people do get the Recommended Dietary Allowance (RDA) of B$_{12}$ by eating just a few ounces of meat or dairy products a day," he says.

Then why are so many deficient?

"A small number are strict vegetarians—they eat no meat or dairy products, and they haven't for years," Dr. Sauberlich explains. "But the big reason is that many older people simply can't absorb B$_{12}$ from their intestines. And the older you get, the more of a risk that becomes."

It has been known since the 1960s that by age 60, about 5 percent of people have stopped absorbing B$_{12}$ from their food. "And that figure goes up by another 5 to 10 percent every five years after that," says Victor Herbert, M.D., J.D., professor of medicine at Mount Sinai School of Medicine in New York City. That means a substantial number of older people are running low on this nutrient and showing signs of deficiency that may sometimes be shrugged off as old age.

Warning Signs

A classic sign of deficiency is, of course, fatigue, the kind caused by pernicious anemia.

Your body makes about 200 million red blood cells a *minute*. If you go too long without B$_{12}$, your red blood cells become large, immature and unable to carry oxygen. Production of red blood cells also decreases, and their numbers plummet. Your tail is dragging. You have pernicious anemia.

Your body also requires B$_{12}$ to manufacture the fatty sheaths that cover and protect nerves. A B$_{12}$ deficiency eventually leads to nerve damage as this sheath, called the myelin, breaks down and is not

properly repaired. "Tingling of the feet or hands is a very common symptom," says Robert H. Allen, M.D., professor of medicine and biochemistry and director of hematology at the University of Colorado Health Sciences Center in Denver. Other signs of nerve damage may include muscle weakness, unsteady gait, memory loss and changes in mood and personality.

It's now apparent that these neurological disorders can be the first and sometimes the *only* signs of a B$_{12}$ deficiency, experts agree.

If You're Deficient

Of course, not all fatigue and not all nerve damage is due to a lack of vitamin B$_{12}$. If you're experiencing constant tiredness or any other signs of possible B$_{12}$ deficiency, see your doctor. "The only sure way to detect a B$_{12}$ deficiency is with a blood test," says Dr. Allen.

And what if your doctor finds that you are deficient? Time to eat more foods high in B$_{12}$? No, probably not.

As mentioned earlier, most Americans eat some meat, eggs, fish or dairy products, so getting enough B$_{12}$ in their diets isn't a problem for most. The problem more likely is in your gut, where you should absorb B$_{12}$ from food. Most people who are deficient in B$_{12}$ can't absorb the nutrient properly because their stomachs don't produce a substance called intrinsic factor, which is required for B$_{12}$ absorption, or

AT A GLANCE

VITAMIN B$_{12}$

RDA: 2 mcg.

Good food sources: Liver (although doctors recommend you limit your liver intake because of its high cholesterol content), beef, oysters and tuna.

Who's at risk for deficiency: People who have digestion problems or have had intestinal surgery or radiation, anyone aged 60 or older, strict vegetarians, breast-fed infants of vegetarian mothers, drinkers and people taking drugs to lower cholesterol.

Possible signs of deficiency include: Fatigue, "pins and needles" sensation in the hands and feet, apathy, light-headedness, loss of appetite, labored or difficult breathing and personality changes.

Advice for use: Although dangers of overdose are very low, it's best to use supplements only under a doctor's supervision.

they may have low stomach acid, a condition called achlorhydria, due to old age, surgery or other health problems. Or they have problems in their small intestine that hinder absorption.

How about people who don't eat meat? For years, nutritionists warned that strict vegetarians (those who avoid all meat, dairy products and eggs) were at risk for B$_{12}$ deficiency, because plants don't contain B$_{12}$. But very few vegetarians actually become deficient, perhaps because, unless there's an absorption problem, the body is very good at hoarding B$_{12}$. "Some people may remain strict vegetarians for 20 to 30 years before they begin to have symptoms of B$_{12}$ deficiency," Dr. Sauberlich

says. Still, to be on the safe side, many doctors do recommend a B$_{12}$ supplement for their vegetarian patients.

Smokers, heavy drinkers, pregnant women and people taking drugs can also have B$_{12}$ problems, and they may need supplements, Dr. Sauberlich adds. People who are low in B$_{12}$ who don't have absorption problems can take oral B$_{12}$ supplements that provide the RDA.

"People with clear-cut B$_{12}$ deficiencies begin to feel far more energetic once their problem is diagnosed and they are treated with B$_{12}$," Dr. Allen says.

People with absorption problems need to bypass their gut to get adequate vitamin B$_{12}$, Dr. Allen says.

The surest way is with monthly B$_{12}$ injections.

Vitamin B$_{12}$ gel, which is squeezed into the nose and absorbed through the nasal membranes, is sold in some health food stores. But the gel is not medically proven. Experts agree that people with B$_{12}$ absorption problems are much better off getting the injections.

Beta-Carotene

A Pigment on Patrol

POTENTIAL HEALING POWER
May help: • Prevent certain cancers   • Boost immunity   • Protect against heart disease

It used to be that beta-carotene was best known for the orange or dark green color it gave all those "healthy" vegetables that Mom nagged you to eat: carrots, broccoli, brussels sprouts and others whose bright hues made them difficult to hide in the mashed potatoes.

But it's no longer just Mom urging you to consume more beta-carotene. Now she has the National Academy of Sciences, the American Cancer Society and an army of health researchers to back her up.

Why such universal support for this nutrient? Because studies have shown that beta-carotene may fight cancer, boost immunity, help protect against heart disease and even slow the effects of aging!

"There is great excitement over news that consuming more beta-carotene may prove to be *extremely* beneficial in preventing chronic, life-shortening diseases, because it seems to do so many things," says Harinder Garewal, M.D., Ph.D., assistant director of cancer prevention and control at the Department of Veterans Affairs Hospital and the Arizona Cancer Center in Tucson. Dr. Garewal's own research found that boosting beta-carotene intake can reverse precancerous changes in the mouth and may improve immunity in those with HIV, the virus that causes AIDS.

New Findings, New Promise

Amazing stuff, this beta-carotene. Yet it wasn't too long ago that except for the fact that it's a source of vitamin A, beta-carotene was virtually ignored by nutritionists and little known by the general public. "A decade or so ago, the idea that beta-carotene might prevent diseases such as cancer or heart attacks was not generally considered scientifically respectable," recalls Richard B. Shekelle, Ph.D., professor of epidemiology at the University of Texas Health Science Center in Houston and one of the first researchers to study the nutrient's cancer-prevention abilities. "Even as recently as a few years ago, most people incorrectly referred to vitamin A as meaning both beta-carotene and vitamin A."

The confusion existed because beta-carotene converts into vitamin A in our bodies as needed. That's important because preformed vitamin A from animal food sources, although necessary, can be dangerous in large doses. Vitamin A is a fat-soluble vitamin that is stored primarily in the liver, and high intakes can be toxic. But beta-carotene is much safer. Excess amounts generally pass through the body with no side effects. This is one of the reasons that beta-carotene may be the best way to get your vitamin A.

Cancer Killer

Perhaps beta-carotene's greatest power is in preventing certain cancers, particularly those caused

---

AT A GLANCE

BETA-CAROTENE

RDA: None established. Some experts recommend daily supplements of 15 mg.

Good food sources: Orange, yellow and dark green leafy vegetables such as carrots, pumpkin, sweet potatoes and spinach, and orange and yellow fruits such as oranges, peaches, cantaloupe and apricots.

Who's at risk for deficiency: Heavy drinkers and smokers may need extra beta-carotene to maintain good health.

Possible signs of deficiency include: There are no known signs of beta-carotene deficiency.

Advice for use: Most preliminary results suggest no harm and possible benefits from supplementation, particularly for people who don't eat the recommended five servings of fruits and vegetables each day.

by cigarette smoking. "The evidence shows, very consistently, that smokers who eat the most foods rich in beta-carotene have the lowest incidence of lung cancer, and those who rarely eat foods rich in beta-carotene have the highest," says Dr. Shekelle. "In fact, the risk difference is about eightfold between those eating the most and the least beta-carotene."

The protective effects of beta-carotene are not limited to lung cancer. In the United States and abroad, researchers have reported that low beta-carotene intake is associated with a higher risk of cancers of the stomach, cervix, bladder, breast, colon, mouth and throat.

With the increasing evidence supporting preventive activity, researchers have gone hog-wild studying beta-carotene—and in the process have learned that it may ward off, or even *cure,* a host of ills from cataracts to hardening of the arteries.

"That's because beta-carotene acts as an antioxidant and blocks out oxidation," says Ishwarlal Jialal, M.D., associate professor of clinical nutrition and internal medicine at the University of Texas Southwestern Medical Center in Dallas.

Your Body's "Rustproofing"

Oxidation is the chemical reaction that coats an unseasoned skillet with an orange film of rust or turns a freshly cut apple brown. Inside your body, this oxidation or "rusting" occurs when oxygen merges with hydrogen and other substances to form molecular menaces called free radicals. These are molecules wounded by exposure to life's nasties—pollution, ultraviolet light, cigarette smoke, alcohol, radiation and other environmental hazards—that feed off other molecules and initiate a chain reaction that can eventually damage cells and organs.

But antioxidants—which include beta-carotene, along with vitamins C and E—help prevent oxidation, stopping free radicals before they can ravage your body, says Dr. Jialal. These free radicals are thought to trigger certain types of cancer and cause LDL cholesterol—the "bad" kind—to oxidize where it's more likely to line arterial walls, clog the arteries and lead to heart disease.

In addition, beta-carotene and other antioxidants may also boost the immune system by producing changes such as an increase in the number of beneficial "natural killer cells" that gobble up harmful bacteria and viruses and help keep the immune system strong.

Where to Find It

As Mom knew, beta-carotene is most abundant in orange and yellow vegetables like carrots, green leafy vegetables like spinach and in many fruits. Unfortunately, it may take more carrots than you'd find on Liz Taylor's engagement ring to get the prime protection from beta-carotene. There is no Recommended Dietary Allowance (RDA) for beta-carotene, but the RDA for vitamin A is 4,000 international units for women and 5,000 international units for men. This is the equivalent of 2.4 milligrams of beta-carotene for women and 3 milligrams for men. While you can get this amount of beta-carotene by eating just two carrots or ¼ pound of sweet potatoes, some experts recommend taking higher doses, usually around 15 milligrams, to prevent oxidation.

That's where supplements can be beneficial.

The Role of Supplements

Although researchers are well aware of the wide-ranging wonders of beta-carotene, most studies have only examined it in *dietary* form—getting it from fruits and vegetables. Only lately have researchers begun studying the nutrient in supplement form. Beta-carotene is now sold over the counter (usually in doses of 15 milligrams). So far, the supplements appear promising, but additional studies need to be completed.

"My point of view is that if you can get enough beta-carotene from your diet, do it," says Dr. Garewal. "But since the requirements for beta-carotene's protective powers haven't been adequately studied, it's hard to make an across-the-board recommendation of what constitutes 'enough.'"

Adds Dr. Garewal, "Once you get beyond a certain point, high doses (usually over 15 milligrams) probably won't help you anymore. But they don't seem to hurt, either. This is why the doses selected for clinical studies have often tended to be on the high side, since the primary concern is to be sure enough is being taken. The only known side effect, which occurs only after taking high doses over some time, is a yellow look (actually more like a suntan) which results from excess pigment collecting under the skin.

"Many physicians now don't think twice about advising people to take an aspirin a day to prevent heart attack. And beta-carotene supplements are actually less toxic than aspirin—and may do more," says Dr. Garewal.

One Finnish study found that large doses of beta-carotene seemed to increase lung cancer risk among heavy smokers. But most studies show no potential harm from supplements.

The authors of the Physicians Health Study, which found that aspirin helps prevent heart attacks, are now looking into the matter.

While awaiting final results, most experts agree that you should do what Mother said: Eat plenty of vegetables to make sure you're getting enough beta-carotene. But if you decide to take supplements, doses of 15 milligrams are reasonable and may prevent cancer and reduce risk of heart disease.

Bioflavonoids

The Rookie Healers

POTENTIAL HEALING POWER

May help:
- Strengthen capillaries
- Improve immunity
- Fight cancer
- Reduce inflammation

Hey, it's tough out there: Fame doesn't just happen overnight. You wait and wait to be discovered, and at last comes your lucky break. Suddenly you're hot stuff, the darling of the media—and then . . . Poof! You're back to the bottom of the heap—a nobody.

That's what things have been like for the bioflavonoids, plant substances closely linked to vitamin C. The bioflavonoids were first considered vitamins, then medicine. Today they're neither—and you have to search through the shelves of health food stores to find them (although most of us swallow about a gram a day, primarily in fruit juices).

Bioflavonoids are tiny colored crystals that give many fruits and vegetables their hues of red, blue and yellow. There are more than 800 known bioflavonoids; some of the most common are quercetin, hesperidin and rutin.

"The bioflavonoids certainly seem to have some beneficial actions on lower forms of life, such as crickets," says Donald B. Mc-Cormick, Ph.D., chairman of the Department of Biochemistry at Emory University in Atlanta. "But early hopes that those benefits would extend to humans just haven't worked out."

Don't be too quick, however, to cross these nutrients off your list as has-beens. Studies are still going on, and it's quite possible that the bioflavonoids may someday be dubbed as comeback kids.

Fighting for Respect

Bioflavonoids were discovered in 1936 by Albert Szent-Gyorgyi, the same fellow who discovered vitamin C. He found that extract from lemon juice or red pepper was more effective than pure vitamin C at curing scurvy, a vitamin C deficiency that causes bleeding, among other symptoms. The active ingredients in the extract were bioflavonoids—but at the time they were called vitamin P.

Studies found that this newly

THE VITAMIN C CONNECTION

Most of the supplemental bioflavonoids you'll find today are sold in combination with vitamin C, and some people think bioflavonoids help increase C's effectiveness. It's not true.

"There's absolutely no valid scientific evidence that bioflavonoids enhance the absorption of vitamin C," says Donald B. McCormick, Ph.D., chairman of the Department of Biochemistry at Emory University in Atlanta. There's a *possibility*, however, that bioflavonoids do work with vitamin C to help keep small blood vessels healthy.

discovered nutrient strengthened the small blood vessels called capillaries. Doctors eventually began to prescribe drugs containing bioflavonoids for various bleeding problems, such as heavy menstrual bleeding and easy bruising.

In 1950 a committee of nutritionists and biologists changed the name of this apparently nonessential food item from vitamin P to bioflavonoids. (No studies have ever shown that the bioflavonoids are essential for our health or that we develop any deficiency symptoms when we don't have them.) The real blow to bioflavonoids' character came in 1968, when the Food and Drug Administration yanked all drugs containing bioflavonoids off the market, saying their beneficial effects had not been proved. Today bioflavonoids are sold in the United States only as nutritional supplements.

Although bioflavonoids are no longer prescribed as medicine in the United States, some researchers

still believe they may help control bleeding problems. In other countries, the bioflavonoid rutin is used to treat varicose veins and hemorrhoids, for example.

The Comeback Attempt

Several studies in past years have focused on things other than bleeding. They suggest that the bioflavonoids quercetin, hesperidin and catechin may help fight the viruses that cause herpes, respiratory ailments and flu and may help battle allergic reactions. And that's not all: In a study at the State University of New York School of Medicine and Biomedical Sciences at Buffalo, the bioflavonoids nobiletin and tangeretin inhibited the growth of cancer cells in the lab. Other researchers have found that bioflavonoids improve immunity and help reduce inflammation.

All of this sounds pretty promising, but none of these studies were done with *people*. And, as Dr. Mc-

BIOFLAVONOIDS

RDA: None established.

Good food sources: Fruit juices, citrus fruits, green peppers, cherries, grapes, apricots, papaya, tomatoes and broccoli.

Who's at risk for deficiency: Bioflavonoids aren't considered essential, so deficiency is unlikely.

Possible signs of deficiency include: There are no known signs of bioflavonoid deficiency.

Advice for use: Supplements are not recommended.

Cormick points out, what happens in the lab and in animals doesn't necessarily happen in humans.

You should also realize that some of the existing studies have turned up negative effects. Certain bioflavonoids, for example, may damage cells' genetic material. And tanin, a bioflavonoid found in red wine, may be linked to cancer of the esophagus.

In short, bioflavonoids *may* help us, but doctors just aren't sure yet—nor are they entirely sure how safe they are. "Right now there's no scientific proof of benefit to humans," says Dr. McCormick. "That's not to say that there might not be some effect or some benefit proved in the future."

In the meantime, most experts agree: If you want to consume more bioflavonoids, your best bet is to eat more fruits and vegetables and drink more fruit juice—and wait until conclusive research comes out before reaching for supplements.

Biotin

The Bountiful B Vitamin

Her doctor suggested that she needed more protein, so, like the movie hero Rocky, the 62-year-old woman started gulping down raw eggs: Six a day, seven days a week.

Bad move. Within weeks the woman had lost her appetite and her tongue was sore. Then came swelling, fatigue and scaly skin—all signs of a raging deficiency of the B vitamin biotin. Unwittingly, the woman was eating the very food that would send her biotin levels plummeting.

Raw egg white contains avidin, a protein that latches onto biotin and keeps it from being absorbed and digested.

Fortunately, however, biotin deficiency is not only rare but reversible. When this woman stopped dining on raw eggs à la Rocky and revamped her diet to include more biotin-rich foods such as nuts, milk, whole grains and vegetables, her symptoms disappeared.

Benefits Inside and Outside

Even when a biotin deficiency is relatively severe, symptoms can be reversed. An 11-year-old who was biotin deficient because of eating raw eggs was completely bald, with reddened skin and scaly eruptions on his face. After his diet was improved, his skin quickly began to clear up and he began to grow hair.

From these people's misadventures, you can see that we need biotin to help keep our hair and skin healthy. Biotin is also required for many enzymes that kick off many important reactions in our bodies. For example, biotin-containing enzymes help our bodies make glucose, a sugar we use for fuel, and also help us use fat and other nutrients.

We make some of the biotin we need, courtesy of certain friendly bacteria that reside in our intestines. We also need to eat some biotin—from 30 to 100 micrograms daily, estimates the Food and Nutrition Board of the National Research Council. Biotin is found in many foods. A cup of oatmeal, for instance, gives you 58 micrograms, and a cup of cooked cauliflower provides 21 micrograms.

Biotin is so prevalent, in fact, that most of us get plenty without even trying, says Donald B. McCormick, Ph.D., chairman of the Department of Biochemistry at Emory University in Atlanta. "I wouldn't give a thought to my biotin intake unless I was locked in a jail cell eating bread and water for weeks on end," he says, tongue-in-cheek.

When Deficiency Looms

But a few folks *do* have to be aware of their biotin intake—obviously those who gulp down raw egg whites (which isn't a recommended practice in the first place). Even then most people would have to get almost a third of their daily calories from those egg whites before showing any signs of deficiency.

Who else may be at risk? There's some evidence that people on limited or very-low-calorie diets *may* not be getting enough biotin, especially if they're on antibiotics (which may kill off the intestinal bacteria that help produce it). And, although there's no definite proof, some researchers suggest that low biotin in some babies' diets may

---

AT A GLANCE

BIOTIN

Estimated Safe and Adequate Daily Intake: 30 to 100 mcg.

Good food sources: Molasses, brewer's yeast, soybeans, wheat bran, oats, peanuts, walnuts, eggs, cauliflower and lentils.

Who's at risk for deficiency: People who eat lots of raw egg white (a third of their daily calories), people who take antibiotics frequently and do not eat a balanced diet and people with a genetic defect that prevents them from using biotin properly.

Possible signs of deficiency include: Lack of appetite, inflamed skin and tongue, nausea and depression.

Advice for use: Danger of overdose is low.

contribute to sudden infant death syndrome.

And one very small group of people, who have a genetic defect that won't let them use biotin properly, must take biotin supplements.

Enter Dr. Biotin

In a few cases, doctors have used biotin to treat specific problems, even where no deficiencies were evident. For example, supplemental doses of biotin have been claimed to clear up "uncombable hair syndrome" in children. This is exactly what it sounds like: stiff hair that sticks up and can't be combed.

And biotin has been reported to help strengthen fingernails: Swiss researchers found that brittle nails became 25 percent stronger after six to nine months of biotin supplements. Richard K. Scher, M.D., head of the Nail Section at Co-

lumbia Presbyterian Medical Center in New York City, treats brittle fingernails with biotin. Because the weak nails could be a sign of another health problem, however, he cautions that you should see a doctor rather than self-dosing with biotin.

Biotin has also been used by doctors to treat acne, eczema and hair loss, with some limited success, although professionals agree that more studies need to be done before treatment with biotin becomes routine.

In summary, if you're in doubt about your biotin intake, a supplement of up to 100 micrograms daily won't hurt you. But, says Dr. McCormick, don't try to treat a health problem with biotin unless advised to do so by your doctor. In general, however, as Dr. McCormick says, most of us don't have to give this vitamin a second thought.

Boron

A Fruitful Nutrient

Mavis was past 55. She'd heard about older women having bones crumble due to osteoporosis, and she wanted to keep her bones healthy. So Mavis reached for a big, juicy apple.

POTENTIAL HEALING POWER

May help:
- Prevent osteoporosis
- Improve reflexes and mental alertness
- Treat arthritis

Yes, you read that right. Research by the U. S. Department of Agriculture (USDA) found that eating three milligrams of boron a day reduced the urinary loss of calcium and magnesium, two nutrients essential to bone health. And—you guessed it—boron abounds in apples, as well as other fruits. The researchers concluded that a diet high in boron-rich fruits and vegetables may help avert bone breakdown in women who are past menopause.

"We suspect boron is important in the prevention of osteoporosis," says Curtiss Hunt, Ph.D., research biologist with the USDA's Human Nutrition Research Center in Grand Forks, North Dakota. He adds that boron may be particularly helpful if you happen to be low in vitamin D, a nutrient you can get from fortified milk and fish, which also plays an important role in protecting aging bones.

Sifting Fact and Fantasy

Boron is something of a latecomer to the field of human nutrition. It wasn't considered essential even for animals until scientists discovered in 1982 that it affected bone growth in chicks. No one has yet proved that humans require boron, but if nutritionists laid bets, boron would be a strong candidate for eventual "essential" status, says Dr. Hunt.

One of the things that kept scientists from discovering the role of boron sooner is that if an animal gets plenty of other nutrients, boron isn't as crucial. The most common sign of boron deficiency in animals is decreased growth, but symptoms vary as the diet varies in calcium, copper, magnesium, phosphorus, potassium and other minerals. Apparently boron helps the body utilize minerals.

Boron may also serve as a kind of marriage counselor between your body and your mind. A study at the Grand Forks Human Nutrition Research Center found a marked improvement in reflex action and mental alertness when people low in boron were given three milligrams a day. "Women with a low boron intake could not tap their finger as fast, follow a target as accurately using a joystick or respond as quickly when asked to search a field of letters for specific letters," says James Penland, Ph.D., research psychologist at the center.

Finally, a lone researcher in Great Britain says that a dietary deficiency of boron may contribute to arthritis. The theory doesn't have huge support, but nutritionist Rex E. Newnham—who recommends five to six milligrams of boron a day—found in a study at the Royal Melbourne Hospital that half the people with osteoarthritis who took boron reported some improvement.

One claim often made about boron *without* scientific merit is that boron will help men develop bulging muscles. This idea sprang from a USDA study that found that when elderly postmenopausal women took boron, their levels of the male hormone testosterone doubled, says Dr. Hunt. (Levels of the female hormone estrogen also doubled, a fact some chose to ignore.) But women have such tiny amounts of testosterone to start with, says Dr. Hunt, that the amount was still insignificant when doubled—and had no connection to what might happen in male bodybuilders.

Counting It Up

Wondering if you're getting enough boron? If you're eating at least five servings of fruits and vegetables a day, you're probably getting 1.5 to 3 milligrams, says Dr. Hunt. In fact, the average American man takes in about 1.5 milligrams daily. But those of us who only encounter vegetables in

the form of french fries may not be getting even that much. "A steak-and-potatoes diet is quite low in boron," points out Dr. Hunt.

No one yet knows how much boron we *need*, and as mentioned earlier, deficiency in humans has never been seen. But if you want to boost your intake to the three-milligram dose that shows promising results in many studies, don't reach for supplements, says Dr. Hunt. Not only are they unnecessary, but concentrated boron can be dangerous. Boric acid, for example, is a potent pesticide that can be deadly if eaten.

To boost your boron intake, just eat more fruits and vegetables, says Dr. Hunt. Boron is simple to get in food. Eating one big juicy apple will give you an extra 0.5 milligram.

Brewer's Yeast

A Bounty of Nutrition

Picture two Madison Avenue men bent over their desktops, dreaming up a hot ad campaign for their new brewer's yeast account. They're scribbling slogans as fast as they can: *Lowers cholesterol! Helps fight diabetes! Keeps skin healthy! Repels biting insects!*

"Whoa!" says one of them at last, raising his hand. "We've gone too far. *Nobody's* going to believe all this."

It does sound farfetched, but in fact some pretty good studies on brewer's yeast can back up some of these seemingly outrageous claims. And in cases where there's no scientific evidence—such as the bit about repelling insects—there are plenty of people who will swear that it works.

A Powerhouse of Vitamins

Yes, this is the same stuff used to brew beer. You can buy it in drugstores or health food stores as powder or tablets. (The powder tends to have a bitter taste.) It happens to be chock-full of vitamins and minerals, including thiamin, riboflavin, niacin, vitamin B_6, pantothenic acid, folic acid, biotin, chromium and selenium. It's this wealth of nutrients that makes brewer's yeast such a popular supplement.

"The most convincing research with brewer's yeast has to do with chromium and blood sugar levels," says Karen Miller-Kovach, R.D., manager of nutrition services for Weight Watchers International in New York City.

In one study in Denmark, people with low blood sugar (hypoglycemia) improved after taking two tablespoons of brewer's yeast a day for three months. The key factor: chromium. Two tablespoons of pure dried brewer's yeast serves up about 120 micrograms of this healthful mineral.

AT A GLANCE

BREWER'S YEAST

RDA: None established.

Good food sources: None.

Who's at risk for deficiency: Brewer's yeast is not considered essential, so deficiency is unlikely.

Possible signs of deficiency include: There are no known signs of brewer's yeast deficiency.

Advice for use: Doses should not exceed the amount recommended on the label, which varies according to the source of the brewer's yeast and how the product is formulated. Because brewer's yeast may alter insulin requirements, people with diabetes should check with a doctor before taking it.

And chromium does more than help regulate sugar levels in people who are hypoglycemic, says Richard Anderson, Ph.D., lead scientist in vitamin and mineral research at the U.S. Department of Agriculture's Human Nutrition Research Center in Beltsville, Maryland. It may also help keep diabetes from developing in people who have problems processing blood sugar or have a family history of diabetes. And in some studies, brewer's yeast has helped reduce symptoms in people who already have diabetes. If you have diabetes, however, check with your doctor before using brewer's yeast, as it may alter your insulin requirements.

Brewer's yeast also may help lower cholesterol. In a study at Syracuse University in New York, people taking two tablespoons of brewer's yeast daily for two months saw a 10 percent drop in their cholesterol. Several other studies show that brewer's yeast may cause both a decrease in overall cholesterol and an increase in HDL, the "good" cholesterol that helps transport the "bad" cholesterol out of your system. No one's quite sure what is in the yeast that causes the changes in cholesterol levels, however.

Some people also claim that brewer's yeast makes their skin healthier. "If you happen to be deficient in B vitamins, then, yes, brewer's yeast might be good for your skin," says Jerold Z. Kaplan, M.D., medical director of the Alta Bates-Herrick Burn Center in Berkeley, California. One tablespoon of brewer's yeast contains approximately 1.25 milligrams of thiamin, 0.34 milligram of riboflavin and 3 milligrams of niacin.

The Power of Repulsion

Another possible benefit from brewer's yeast is its ability to repulse. Although there's no scientific backup, many people report that giving brewer's yeast to dogs and cats helps repel fleas. Whether or not it gets rid of unwanted guests, yeast certainly won't harm your pet, says Amy Marder, V.M.D., clinical assistant professor at Tufts University School of Veterinary Medicine in Medford, Massachusetts. For cats, you can try one teaspoon of yeast a day mixed into food; for dogs, use about one teaspoon per 15 pounds of body weight. Many animals actually relish the taste.

What works for your pet might even work for you. Some people taking large amounts of thiamin—an important component of brewer's yeast—report that critters such as mosquitoes find them less appealing, says John Yunginger, M.D., professor and pediatrics consultant at the Mayo Clinic in Rochester, Minnesota.

So what's the lowdown on brewer's yeast?

"You should never rely on a supplement to replace a good diet," says Miller-Kovach, "but brewer's yeast isn't likely to do any harm." The nutrients it's rich in are relatively nontoxic, she says, and because it provides a mixture of nutrients, you're unlikely to overdose on any one. She recommends, however, not exceeding the dosage listed on the label, which will vary according to the brand or formulation.

Vitamin C

Certifiable Cancer Conqueror

POTENTIAL HEALING POWER
May help:
• Prevent certain cancers
• Fight heart disease
• Reduce severity of colds
• Protect against cataracts
• Reduce blood pressure

This high-profile nutrient has quite a reputation to live up to. Probably featured in more front-page newspaper stories than any other nutrient, vitamin C has been touted at one time or another for just about every illness known.

Admittedly, some of the claims

AT A GLANCE

VITAMIN C

RDA: 60 mg.

Good food sources: Citrus fruit and juices, red or green bell peppers, strawberries, broccoli, cantaloupe and tomatoes.

Who's at risk for deficiency: Smokers and elderly people on limited diets.

Possible signs of deficiency include: Bleeding gums, easy bruising, bumps around hair follicles, painful or swollen joints, fatigue, frequent infections and slow healing of wounds.

Advice for use: Some experts recommend limiting the use of chewable tablets. They can cause enamel loss from the surface of the teeth and other dental problems.

   People who have an iron absorption disorder or take large amounts of iron (above the U.S. RDA of 18 mg), should be careful when taking vitamin C. It can enhance the absorption of iron and lead to an unhealthy iron overload.

made for vitamin C over the years may have been exaggerated, and others remain to be proven. Nevertheless, evidence is accumulating that vitamin C does indeed have remarkable talents.

Without doubt, this nutrient, as an antioxidant, plays an important role in preventing disease. "An antioxidant helps protect the body's cells from oxidation, a chemical reaction that creates highly reactive substances, called free radicals, that can attack and damage cells," explains Jeffrey Blumberg, Ph.D., associate director of the U.S. Department of Agriculture's Human Nutrition Research Center on Aging at Tufts University in Boston.

The cell damage caused by free radicals can in turn trigger a number of health problems, including cancer, heart disease and cataracts. It's also part of the aging process.

Cancer Roadblock

Studies done in the last decade or so confirm that vitamin C's ability to clobber free radicals offers strong protection from cancer.

To date, of several dozen population studies that have looked at vitamin C intake, almost all of them have found a reduced risk for cancer in people with the highest intake.

"In many of these studies, people getting the most vitamin C had about half the risk for cancer as people with the lowest intake," says

Gladys Block, Ph.D., professor of public health nutrition and epidemiology at the School of Public Health at the University of California, Berkeley. How much is enough? While the cutoff point for cancer protection can't be determined from these studies, it was clear that people who ate more fruits and vegetables had less cancer. People eating a diet rich in these foods can easily get 200 to 400 milligrams of vitamin C per day. That's a lot more than the U.S. average of 70 milligrams per day. But it is not too hard to do—½ cup of orange juice or a single serving of broccoli provides about 60 milligrams of vitamin C each.

Most studies that assess fruit consumption—considered a good indicator of vitamin C intake—also find a cancer-fighting effect, Dr. Block says.

The protective effect of vitamin C seems to be clearest for cancers of the esophagus, mouth and stomach. The nutrient also seems to provide some protection against cancers of the rectum, pancreas, breast, cervix and perhaps even the lungs, Dr. Block says.

Vitamin C's ability to neutralize free radicals may not totally explain the nutrient's cancer-fighting abilities, Dr. Blumberg says. Vitamin C can also neutralize chemical compounds such as nitrosamines, which can increase your odds for gastrointestinal cancer. These compounds are formed in the body during diges-

tion of nitrites, preservatives used in meats such as cold cuts and bacon. And vitamin C may help your body's immune system track down and destroy precancerous cells, Dr. Blumberg adds. "These are your best possible defenses against cancer," he says.

In addition, vitamin C's role in the production of tough, fibrous connective tissue means it may offer help in walling off tumors and in limiting the spread of individual cancer cells to other parts of the body.

Halting Heart Disease

When it comes to preventing the fat-clogged arteries that can lead to heart disease, a hefty intake of vitamin C is like money in the bank, says Dr. Blumberg. Vitamin C helps prevent what can be a first step in the clogging of arteries—the oxidation of blood cholesterol. "If cholesterol is not oxidized, the process of fatty buildup is reduced," Dr. Blumberg says. Oxidized cholesterol triggers a chain of events that gums up arteries.

Studies also indicate that increased intake of vitamin C may lower blood pressure, which could also help protect your arteries and heart.

Given the possible effect of vitamin C on blood pressure and cholesterol, it's not surprising that one study found high intake of vitamin C may translate into fewer deaths from heart disease. Researchers at the School of Public Health at the University of California, Los Angeles, found that men who consumed an average of 300 milligrams a day of vitamin C lowered their risk of fatal heart disease by 45 percent compared to men who consumed less than 49 milligrams a day.

"In this study, high vitamin C intake was a stronger predictor of reduced risk than either low blood cholesterol levels or low dietary fat intake," says James Enstrom, Ph.D., the study's main researcher. "This finding could have profound effects, because it's easier to increase people's vitamin C intake than to reduce their blood cholesterol or dietary fat."

"C" Eye to Eye

We've all learned the hard way that a long day in the sun can fry our hides. Actually, a sunburn occurs not from the heat of the sun's rays but from oxidative damage caused by ultraviolet sunlight. That same oxidative reaction over a period of many years can damage the lens of the eye, Dr. Blumberg says. The result is cataracts, a common cause of vision problems in older people. Cataracts occur when proteins in the eye's lens oxidize and turn an opaque, milky white.

In animal studies, vitamin C has been found to protect the eye's lens against ultraviolet damage, reducing the incidence of cataracts.

And in a study of 77 people with cataracts and 35 without, an important difference between the two groups seemed to be the amount of foods rich in vitamin C that were consumed by each group. Eating fewer than 3½ servings of fruits and vegetables a day increased cataract risk 5.7 times.

"We've detected vitamin C levels in the eye as much as 60 times what there is in the blood. It must be there for a good physiological reason," says Allen Taylor, Ph.D., professor of biochemistry, nutrition and ophthalmology at Tufts University. It's possible, he says, that the high levels of vitamin C in the eye may protect enzymes that remove oxidation-damaged proteins, helping the eye heal itself.

Bring a Sneeze to Its Knees

Some people swear that orange juice does to colds and sniffles what garlic does to vampires— keeps them at bay.

In fact, an analysis of over a dozen studies showed a reduction in the duration of colds treated with at least one gram of vitamin C. The decrease in duration ranged from 5 percent to 75 percent, but all of the studies showed some decrease. The studies also reported a reduction in the nastiness of the beast—big sneezes became little sneezes and sniffles turned to snifflettes.

Two of the studies indicated that benefits are greatest with larger amounts of vitamin C (1,000 to

3,000 milligrams a day). In one study, vitamin C started within 24 hours of the onset of cold symptoms had the greatest impact.

Vitamin C may reduce cold symptoms a number of ways, Dr. Blumberg says. It is known to lower blood levels of histamine, a chemical released by immune cells that can trigger runny noses. It may also shield both immune cells and surrounding tissue from the oxidative reactions that occur when immune cells fight infection.

Unfortunately, while the evidence is good that vitamin C may reduce cold symptoms, preventing colds is another matter. A few studies have found a small decrease in the number of episodes of colds in people taking vitamin C; the majority, however, have found no significant effect.

High C Sounds Good

When it comes to optimal protection, many doctors say you'll have to get more than the Recommended Dietary Allowance of 60 milligrams of vitamin C. Just how much more may depend on your individual needs, but for most people, 250 to 1,000 milligrams is safe and adequate.

Unfortunately, half of all American adults get less than 70 milligrams of vitamin C a day in their diets. And if you overcook your vegetables, you may get even less.

To make up the difference, Dr. Block recommends that we all try to eat more fruits and vegetables— at least five servings every day. Supplements providing 100 milligrams or more of vitamin C would provide added insurance.

Vitamin C is considered quite safe, even in large amounts. For healthy people, the only risk of taking very large amounts is the possibility of diarrhea. Vitamin C can also affect the results of some medical tests. If you need a test for blood sugar levels or blood in stool, you should stop taking your supplements two to three days beforehand.

Calcium

A Bona Fide Bone Builder

The frivolous Grasshopper lived for the moment. She paid no heed to her friend the Ant, who warned her that a balanced diet and regular exercise were necessary to build strong bones. Instead, the Grasshopper turned up her nose at dairy products and spent her spare time loafing.

The industrious Ant, however, ate a balanced diet that included milk, yogurt and cheese, and she exercised regularly. When the Ant and the Grasshopper became elderly, the Ant's regimen had paid off handsomely. She had strong, healthy bones—while the poor Grasshopper's bones were fragile and broke easily.

The calcium in your bones is like savings in a bank. You deposit calcium through the foods you eat, and when your blood needs calcium—which it uses for many important functions, such as regulating muscle contraction, heartbeat and blood clotting—it's "withdrawn" from the bones. Should withdrawals exceed deposits—as the Grasshopper's did—eventually bones weaken and become fragile.

Assessing Your Deposits

The most important time for calcium consumption is in childhood and adolescence, when your bones are being formed and you can build up stores for future use, says Jack M. Cooperman, Ph.D., former clinical professor of community and preventive medicine at New York Medical College in Valhalla.

Even after you're an adult, however, you still need calcium. Although your bones are already formed, there is a continuous turnover of calcium in your bones.

How much calcium do you need? The Recommended Dietary Allowance (RDA) is 800 milligrams a day for adults and 1,200 milligrams for those aged 11 to 24 and pregnant and nursing women. Some nutritionists, however, believe that most women need at least 1,000 milligrams and postmenopausal women need 1,500 milligrams.

Unfortunately, many young people—especially girls—don't get enough calcium, and neither do many adult women. The average calcium intake for women aged 45 to 54 is 474 milligrams daily, and a University of California study found that 137 postmenopausal women who *believed* they were getting plenty of calcium were actually averaging only 560 milligrams daily.

The Osteoporosis Issue

Weak and fragile bones that result from many causes, including long-term lack of calcium, are all too common among America's elderly, particularly women. This condition is known as osteoporosis, and it's a serious problem, causing an estimated 1.5 million fractures a year in the hips, spine, wrist and other bones. Spine fractures can actually make those with osteoporosis grow shorter.

Most of us begin to lose bone around age 35—but additional calcium may help slow that loss. For example, a study of women aged 30 to 40 at the University of Massachusetts Medical Center found that those who took in 1,500 milligrams of calcium a day lost no bone mass in a three-year period, while women getting 800 milligrams a day lost 3 percent.

CALCIUM AND PMS

Menstrual problems cramping your lifestyle? Boosting your calcium intake may be the ticket to relief.

In a 5½-month study at the U.S. Department of Agriculture's Nutrition Research Center in Grand Forks, North Dakota, women who got 1,300 milligrams of calcium daily reported far fewer menstrual woes than those who got 600 milligrams daily.

Nine of the ten women had fewer mood changes such as irritability and depression, while seven had fewer cramps and backaches, says James G. Penland, Ph.D., research psychologist at the center. Calcium supplements also led to less water retention and less difficulty concentrating.

CALCIUM

RDA: 800 mg.

Good food sources: Milk, cheese, yogurt, leafy green vegetables and salmon and sardines with bones.

Who's at risk for deficiency: People who don't drink milk or eat dairy products, pregnant or nursing women and the elderly.

Possible signs of deficiency include: Muscle cramps or contractions and low backache.

Advice for use: Doses in excess of 2,500 mg daily should not be taken. High intakes may cause constipation, kidney stone formation and problems absorbing iron, zinc and other minerals.

For many women, a dramatic loss of bone comes after menopause, when they're no longer making the estrogen that helps bones absorb calcium. Hormone replacement therapy—low doses of estrogen—will help slow this loss, but not all women can take or choose to take hormones.

Although calcium intake is most important before menopause, calcium is also necessary to help reduce bone loss after menopause—whether or not a woman chooses hormone replacement therapy. In one study of people over 60, those who consumed more than 765 milligrams of calcium a day had fewer hip fractures than those getting less than 470 milligrams. And women whose lifetime dietary consumption was about 1,000 milligrams a day had between 60 and 75 percent

fewer hip fractures than women getting around 500 milligrams a day.

Beyond Bone Benefits

Calcium is more than just a bone builder. "There are tentative findings that link higher levels of calcium intake with lower colorectal cancer risk," says Martin Lipkin, M.D., head of the Irving Weinstein Laboratory for Gastrointestinal Cancer Prevention at Memorial Sloan-Kettering Cancer Center in New York City.

And calcium may help keep blood pressure low. Evidence suggests that getting at least 800 milligrams of calcium a day reduces the risk of high blood pressure. And in the Nurses Health Study—a four-year study of 60,000 women—those who consumed more than 800 milligrams a day were at less risk of developing high blood pressure compared to those who consumed less than 400 milligrams a day.

Calcium supplements may prevent premature births in teens. In one study, only 7 percent of pregnant teenagers who received 2,000 daily milligrams of extra calcium from late in their fifth month of pregnancy on had premature babies, while 21 percent of a similar group who didn't take the additional calcium supplements gave birth prematurely.

Making the Calcium Connection

Calcium needs vary from person to person—and so does each person's ability to absorb calcium. "The body is wonderful in that it will, to an extent, increase the absorption of calcium from foods as you need more," says Karen M. Chapman, R.D., Ph.D., assistant professor of nutrition at the University of Illinois at Urbana. Absorption also decreases as we get older, she explains. Breast-fed infants may absorb almost 70 percent of the calcium in breast milk, while normal absorption for adults is about 30 percent of what is eaten.

Regardless of age, the calcium in milk is the most available to the body, says Richard J. Wood, Ph.D., chief of the Mineral Bioavailability Laboratory at the U.S. Department of Agriculture's Human Nutrition

Research Center on Aging at Tufts University in Boston. An additional advantage of milk—whether regular or with extra calcium added—is that it provides vitamin D, which we need to help us use calcium.

Other dairy products, such as cheese and yogurt, are also good sources. If you don't eat dairy products, you could get your calcium from canned sardines and salmon (if you eat the bones), broccoli, kale, collard greens, turnip greens and tofu. Another source is calcium-fortified orange or grapefruit juice.

Various foods and beverages can make calcium less available to your body. "Caffeine can increase calcium losses through urinary excretion," points out Dr. Chapman. One study found that middle-aged women who drank more than 6 cups of caffeine-containing coffee daily had almost three times higher risk of hip fracture than those who downed less than 1½ cups daily.

Another calcium inhibitor is alcohol, which seems to reduce calcium deposition in bone. It also increases the amount lost in the urine. High protein intake from supplements or special diets can do the same. Fiber binds calcium, so you may want to avoid eating your calcium with high-fiber meals.

Who needs supplements? Pregnant or nursing women, the elderly and people who consume few dairy products—especially adolescents and young women, says Dr. Cooperman.

But you should check with a doctor before taking a supplement. Calcium can cause kidney stones in some people. And too much calcium can cause a serious condition called hypercalcemia (too much calcium in the blood), particularly in people with chronic kidney disease or hyperparathyroidism. Calcium can also interfere with the absorption of iron, zinc and other minerals.

The Lowdown on Supplements

Once you've decided you're in need of supplemental calcium, and your doctor has approved, you need to pick a supplement. You trek to the drugstore and gaze at the row of calcium supplements in every form imaginable. Which one of these many forms do you choose?

Calcium carbonate, available in capsules, is the cheapest and most concentrated form, says Dr. Cooperman.

You may have heard of people taking Tums for calcium. That's fine, says Dr. Cooperman. They contain 500 milligrams of calcium carbonate. But don't take just *any* antacid to up your calcium intake: Those with aluminum and magnesium hydroxide can cause loss of phosphate, which you need to use calcium.

Calcium gluconate and calcium lactate are other popular forms. They're less concentrated *and* more expensive. Steer clear of calcium chloride, though, suggests Dr. Cooperman. It irritates the gastrointestinal tract.

People with low stomach acid, such as the elderly and those taking acid-lowering medication for ulcers, should consider taking calcium citrate. It is more easily digested than many of the other forms.

Doctors agree that if you take a supplement, it's better to take it in small doses throughout the day rather than all at once. You should also take care to drink six to eight eight-ounce glasses of water daily. Calcium supplements *can* have a constipating effect, and drinking lots of water can help avoid that.

Because you need other nutrients such as vitamin D, magnesium and boron to use calcium, it's good to take a multivitamin/mineral supplement at the same time that you take your calcium supplement.

Chromium

More Than Just Glitter

Suzy's health problems came on slowly and then became so bad she couldn't get through the day at work. She felt tense and nervous. Her vision was blurred and she had frequent sweating spells.

After several years of going from doctor to doctor, none of whom could figure out what was wrong with her, she made one last lucky visit. The doctor thought her symptoms of hypoglycemia—low blood sugar—might be caused by a chromium deficiency.

Within weeks of receiving a chromium supplement, Suzy was feeling better and was able to return to work.

Chromium—also known as chrome—is the stuff that makes the trim on your car glitter. It's also an essential mineral.

"We've seen really dramatic changes in people in our work with hypoglycemia," says Richard A. Anderson, Ph.D., lead scientist in vitamin and mineral nutrition at the U.S. Department of Agriculture's Human Nutrition Research Center in Beltsville, Maryland. "Chromium supplementation can help immensely."

As you'll see, chromium supplementation may be helpful in other important ways as well.

Help for Diabetes, Cholesterol and More

Scientists know that chromium is part of something called the glucose tolerance factor, which helps us to turn carbohydrates into glucose, an important energy source. Studies have shown that chromium can not only help people with hypoglycemia but can also help prevent some people with mild glucose intolerance from getting diabetes.

In one study conducted by Dr. Anderson, eight people with glucose intolerance received 200 micrograms of chromium daily for five weeks. Seven showed dramatic

AT A GLANCE

CHROMIUM

Estimated Safe and Adequate Daily Intake: 50 to 200 mcg.

Good food sources: Meats, whole grains, grape juice, orange juice, broccoli, black pepper, thyme, brewer's yeast, barbecue sauce.

Who's at risk for deficiency: Drug or alcohol abusers, people on low-calorie diets, the elderly, pregnant women and athletes.

Possible signs of deficiency include: Blood tests may show elevated insulin, low HDL cholesterol and elevated triglycerides. Later symptoms can include overweight, fatigue, excessive thirst and frequent urination.

Advice for use: Experts recommend a multivitamin/mineral supplement containing 50 to 200 mcg of chromium. Overdosing is unlikely, but doses in excess of 600 mcg daily are not recommended.

improvement in their blood sugar levels. Another study in London indicated that bread made with barley—which is high in chromium—may help control symptoms of diabetes.

Chromium can also apparently help protect your heart and arteries. Animal studies indicate that chromium helps reduce arterial plaque, and research in North Carolina showed that two months of supplementation with 600 micrograms of chromium daily significantly increased HDL cholesterol (the "good" cholesterol) in a group of 63 men.

And, based on very preliminary studies, it's possible that chromium can help increase muscle mass. "There might be something to it," says Dr. Anderson.

A Tough Mineral to Find

Unfortunately, virtually none of us gets enough chromium in our daily diet, says Dr. Anderson. "We've had nutritionists make up diets designed to be nutritious, and when we analyzed these diets they still didn't have enough chromium." Most of us take in about 25 micrograms of chromium a day, far below the 50 to 200 micrograms estimated by the Food and Nutrition Board of the National Research Council to be an adequate daily intake.

Have we always been low in chromium, or has our diet changed? "Both our diet and our preparation of foods has changed," says Dr. Anderson. Today we eat many processed foods high in sugar, which increases the amount of chromium we excrete. And few of us cook in the iron kettles our grandmothers did, a process that also contributed chromium.

And the scourge of this decade—stress—may also be taking its toll. "We have many different forms of stress: strenuous exercise, physical trauma, work stress," says Dr. Anderson. "All these have large effects on chromium metabolism and chromium losses." Researchers say that inadequate chromium intake may affect us more as we get older and stresses on our bodies accumulate, and that older people absorb and use chromium more poorly.

The bottom line, says Dr. Anderson, is that unless you're a Sumo wrestler eating 5,000 calories, you're not getting adequate chromium in your diet. He recommends a multivitamin/mineral supplement containing 50 to 200 micrograms of chromium along with other nutrients. He *doesn't* recommend a supplement of pure chromium, because nutrients often work best in teams, he says.

Is it possible to overdose? Over-exposure to chromium in industrial processes—such as electroplating, steel-making and glass-making—can cause problems and has been linked to bronchial cancer. Nutritional chromium, however, is one of the safest minerals around, with no apparent adverse effects even in high doses.

Copper

The Cents-ible Mineral

Copper, copper, everywhere. In your kitchen you may have a copper pot or copper-plated tea kettle. The plumbing and wiring in your house may be made of copper. And if you can locate a penny made before 1982, you've found a coin that's almost all copper (today's pennies are

POTENTIAL HEALING POWER

May help:
- Prevent heart rhythm problems
- Regulate blood pressure
- Balance cholesterol levels
- Protect against cancer
- Boost immunity
- Prevent anemia
- Protect bones

made of copper-plated zinc).

But where you may *not* find copper—or at least an adequate amount—is in your diet. Two-thirds of Americans may get less than 1.5 milligrams daily, while the recommended range set by the Food and Nutrition Board of the National Research Council is 1.5 to 3 milligrams. "We have a hard time finding U.S. diets that reach the recommended range," says David K. Y. Lei, Ph.D., professor of nutrition and food science at the University of Arizona in Tucson.

You may not even know you're supposed to be eating copper— what's the big deal?

The big deal is that consuming too little copper may contribute to numerous health problems, such as heart rhythm problems, increased blood pressure and glucose intolerance, points out Leslie M. Klevay, M.D., of the U.S. Department of Agriculture's Human Nutrition Research Center in Grand Forks, North Dakota.

Dr. Lei's work supports the theory that a lack of copper can also contribute to cholesterol problems. His studies, as well as others, have found high total cholesterol levels in copper-deficient animals. And one study showed that feeding young men a copper-deficient diet caused a lowering of HDL ("good") cholesterol levels. High total cholesterol levels or low HDL cholesterol levels can eventually gum up your arteries and lead to heart problems.

The other big deal about copper is that it helps us absorb and use iron. A severe copper deficiency can result in anemia similar to that observed in iron deficiency. Most of us don't have to worry about this, although copper deficiency has been observed in infants who are fed only cow's milk. And although serious deficiencies have occurred in people being fed intravenously, today's intravenous preparations contain copper.

ALL IN THE WRIST

The more skeptical among us chortled at people who wore copper bracelets to help their arthritis. Now it looks as if those arthritis sufferers may have the last laugh: There may be something to copper bracelets after all.

Researchers in Australia found that people who were suffering from arthritis became worse after removing the bracelets, and they suggested that copper from the bracelets *could* be absorbed through the skin when dissolved in sweat.

Scientists think that copper absorption might be useful for fighting some forms of arthritis. Copper apparently helps neutralize harmful free radicals that may worsen arthritis symptoms.

AT A GLANCE

COPPER

Estimated Safe and Adequate Daily Intake: 1.5 to 3 mg.

Good food sources: Nuts, cocoa, cherries, shellfish (especially oysters), crustaceans, mushrooms, whole-grain cereals and gelatin.

Who's at risk for deficiency: Malnourished premature babies, infants fed only cow's milk and people taking high levels of zinc or vitamin C for prolonged periods.

Possible signs of deficiency include: Anemia, osteoporosis, low white blood cell count, loss of pigment from hair and skin and nervous system impairments.

Advice for use: People with Wilson's disease, a liver disorder, should not take supplements.

Cop These Added Benefits

Some animal studies suggest that copper helps protect against cancer. How does it help? Two copper-containing substances in our bodies work as antioxidants, disease fighters that neutralize potentially harmful forms of oxygen that can lead to the disease.

Copper's also important to your immune system, says Adria R. Sherman, Ph.D., chairman of the Department of Nutritional Sciences at Rutgers University in New Brunswick, New Jersey. This theory, Dr. Sherman says, is supported both by animal studies and the observation that people suffering from Menkes' disease—a rare genetic disease that doesn't allow efficient metabolism of copper—have frequent heart and urinary tract infections and often die in childhood of bronchopneumonia.

Copper may also be linked—along with calcium, vitamin D, manganese and zinc—with the formation of healthy bones, point out researchers at the University of California, La Jolla. Bone abnormalities that may be caused by copper deficiency have been seen in animals. And people with Menkes' disease have had skeletal problems.

A Proper Intake

Because some of us may not get enough copper in our diets, some professionals advise reaching for a daily multiple supplement that contains 1.5 to 3 milligrams of copper. Even if you're taking in enough, copper deficiency can be caused by overzealous supplementation with zinc, which interferes with copper utilization, says Dr.

Sherman. (Some experts suggest that if you use supplements, you should take in ten times as much zinc as copper—and no more—to maintain a proper balance.)

Needless to say, people who should *not* take copper supplements are those with Wilson's disease, a rare, inherited condition that inhibits proper copper metabolism. Symptoms include a golden brown or greenish ring around the cornea of the eye, cirrhosis of the liver and mental deterioration. If you suspect you may have this condition, see your doctor.

Vitamin D

The Solar-Powered Nutrient

After her painful fall last winter, your elderly neighbor Mildred has been reluctant to go outside. Some of her friends have ended up with a broken bone after a fall, and she doesn't want to risk another slip.

But Mildred may be *increasing* her odds of breaking a bone by staying inside. In fact, just going out on her porch occasionally and sitting in the sunlight for less time than it takes for a rerun of *The Cosby Show* might help strengthen and protect her bones.

What's the connection? You probably know that we need calcium to make strong bones, but we also need vitamin D in order to *use* that calcium. And our bodies can actually make vitamin D from the ultraviolet rays of the sun. You can also get vitamin D from some foods, but sunlight is perhaps the easiest way to get this nutrient.

Straighter, Stronger Bones

Vitamin D's pivotal role in bone health is no secret to doctors. A severe shortage of the nutrient in children causes the classic deficiency disease known as rickets, which results in stunted, bowed limbs and unhealthy teeth. Today rickets is rare in this country, thanks in part to milk fortified with vitamin D. But a lack of vitamin D in adults can cause osteomalacia, another condition marked by defective bone formation. It can also worsen osteoporosis, a thinning and weakening of the bones that's common in postmenopausal women.

Women who spend more time in the sun have more vitamin D and thus have stronger bones than women who don't spend time in the sun. But if there's not much sun or you don't go outside, you're not as likely to get enough vitamin D—and your bones can suffer.

Supplemental vitamin D, however, can apparently forestall the damage. In a group of healthy postmenopausal women in Boston, for example, those who took a special form of vitamin D daily for a year lost less bone mass during the winter months than those who didn't get the vitamin.

Getting ample vitamin D appears to help even women who already have osteoporosis. In a New Zealand study, women with diagnosed osteoporosis who took daily supplements of a special form of vitamin D for three years had just one-third as many fractures of the vertebrae as women who didn't take extra vitamin D.

Who's at Risk?

How do you know if you're getting enough vitamin D? "It only takes 10 minutes of midday

---

AT A GLANCE

VITAMIN D

RDA: 200 IU (5 mcg).

Good sources: Food sources include milk and fatty fish such as tuna and salmon; vitamin D is also added to baby formulas, breakfast cereals, rice and many baked goods. The other significant source is sunlight.

Who's at risk for deficiency: People who don't drink milk or eat fish, elderly people who avoid the sun, alcoholics and people with gastrointestinal, liver or kidney disease.

Possible signs of deficiency include: In children, vitamin D deficiency causes rickets (bowed legs, malformed joints or bones, retarded growth, late development of teeth). In adults, deficiency can cause osteomalacia (pain in the ribs, lower spine, pelvis and legs; muscle weakness; brittle bones) or worsen osteoporosis (bone thinning and weakening). Slow hearing loss could also occur.

Advice for use: Doses in excess of 400 IU daily should not be taken without a doctor's supervision. Larger doses could raise calcium levels in the blood and cause kidney disease, kidney stones, stomach problems and possibly muscle spasms and heart problems.

summer sun to give you your full daily requirement," says Hector DeLuca, Ph.D., chairman of the Department of Biochemistry at the University of Wisconsin in Madison and a pioneer in vitamin D research. While that 10 minutes is enough during the summer (assuming your skin is sunscreen-free), during the winter you need 30 minutes of midday sun. You can also get vitamin D in fatty fish such as tuna and salmon and in fortified milk. Other foods—including breakfast cereals, bread, pasta, rice and oils—often have vitamin D added as well.

Elderly people like Mildred tend to be at risk because they often have limited exposure to sunlight and eat few foods rich in vitamin D. They also may be taking drugs to lower cholesterol or other drugs that can interfere with vitamin D metabolism. In one study at a nursing home, researchers checked

MEDICINE OF THE FUTURE?

In the not-too-distant future, vitamin D—traditionally known as the vitamin that helps us build and maintain strong bones and teeth—may become a standard treatment for some types of cancer as well as for psoriasis, a skin condition.

Scientists have known since 1985 that vitamin D might help battle cancer, but its possible uses were limited because of side effects from high doses. Vitamin D causes the body to store calcium, so too much D meant too much calcium and potentially serious side effects. A new synthetic form of vitamin D, however, doesn't cause people to store calcium, and preliminary studies indicate that it may treat or help prevent various cancers.

In animal studies at the University of California, Los Angeles, for example, scientists found that this new form of vitamin D helped treat myeloid leukemia, a cancer of the white blood cells. Vitamin D apparently slows the rate of reproduction of the cancer cells.

And another new form of the vitamin has helped relieve some types of psoriasis, a stubborn skin condition that can be difficult to treat. When 40 people with psoriasis at Osaka University Medical School in Japan took vitamin D orally or rubbed it on their skin, their condition improved. In the future, new forms of vitamin D may provide safe and effective therapy for psoriasis, says Michael F. Holick, M.D., Ph.D., director of the Vitamin D Laboratory at Boston University School of Medicine.

22 people over age 65, none of whom had been outside for six months. Although they all were getting ample vitamin D in their diets, 7 had low blood levels of vitamin D and the rest were at the low end of normal. The conclusion? These researchers believe that elderly people not exposed to sunlight need *more* than the current Recommended Dietary Allowance of 200 international units daily.

Other people who need to take special care that they get enough vitamin D are residents of areas without much sun, vegetarians who don't eat dairy products, and alcoholics.

Considering Supplements

Perhaps you don't like being outdoors, or you have very sensitive skin and can't go without sunscreen for even brief periods. Or maybe you don't drink milk or eat the foods that have vitamin D in them. Or perhaps you're over 65 and concerned that you need *more* vitamin D than you can get from your diet and sunlight.

In these circumstances you could consider taking supplements, says Jeffrey Blumberg, Ph.D., associate director of the U.S. Department of Agriculture's Human Nutrition Research Center on Aging at Tufts University in Boston. Doctors caution, however, that you should never take more than 400 international units of supplemental vitamin D daily except under a doctor's supervision.

The problem is that too much vitamin D could result in excess levels of calcium in your blood. This could cause deposits of calcium in soft tissues, setting you up for a host of problems, including heart damage and kidney failure. (If your physician has told you that you already have elevated blood calcium, don't take supplemental D.) A synthetic form of vitamin D has been developed that doesn't cause calcium storage problems, but it isn't yet commercially available.

Vitamin E

Your Body's Rustproofer

<table>
<tr><td colspan="1">POTENTIAL HEALING POWER</td></tr>
<tr><td>May help:
• Reduce risk of heart disease
• Protect against cancer
• Stop cataracts
• Boost immunity</td></tr>
</table>

It comes in squishy little amber-colored capsules. Pinch one open and out comes a brownish goop that looks like something you might feed into the engine of your lawn mower. But don't be fooled by appearances. Vitamin E is powerful medicine.

The health benefits ascribed to this nutrient are numerous, ranging from improved circulation to cancer control to freedom from heart disease and cataracts.

Vitamin E's disease-fighting powers are due to its status as a star antioxidant. An antioxidant is to your body what a coat of wax is to your car. It's a kind of dietary "rustproofer," explains Jeffrey Blumberg, Ph.D., associate director of the U.S. Department of Agriculture's Human Nutrition Research Center on Aging at Tufts University in Boston.

"An antioxidant helps to protect the body's cells from oxidation, a chemical reaction that creates highly reactive substances called free radicals," Dr. Blumberg explains. Over time, free radicals can tarnish your once-shiny car. That is, they have the ability to attack and harm cells and introduce disease into your body.

Stopping Heart Disease

Two large studies suggest that vitamin E supplements substantially reduce the risk of heart disease. Conducted by researchers at Boston's Brigham and Women's Hospital and the Harvard School of Public Health, the studies found that women who took at least 100 international units of supplemental vitamin E a day for at least two years had a 41 percent drop in heart attack risk. Men who took over 100 international units for two or more years reduced their risk by 40 percent.

Vitamin E may help prevent heart disease several ways, Dr. Blumberg says. Its most important role may be helping to prevent the oxidation of cholesterol. The slowing of this oxidation process may limit cholesterol's propensity to clog up arteries.

Vitamin E may also help prevent what's called platelet aggregation, Dr. Blumberg explains. Platelets are disk-shaped blood components that promote blood clotting. They can also clot in blood vessels when they shouldn't. Getting adequate amounts of vitamin E may prevent platelets from clumping together and from sticking to blood vessel walls.

Cancer Shield

Many population studies show a link between vitamin E and cancer. People with lower blood levels of vitamin E tend to have higher risks for a variety of types of cancer. In one large study by researchers in Finland, the risk for several types of cancer was 1½ times higher in those with low blood levels of vitamin E than in those with high levels.

And a study by researchers at the National Cancer Institute found that people who took vitamin E as a separate supplement (containing about 100 international units) cut their risk of oral cancer in half.

Vitamin E may help to prevent cancer at least three ways, Dr. Blumberg says. First, by shielding a cell from free radicals, vitamin E may prevent the kind of damage in cells that can lead to cancer.

Second, by combining with cer-

AT A GLANCE

VITAMIN E

RDA: Men: 15 IU (10 mg). Women: 12 IU (8 mg).

Good food sources: Soybean oil, corn oil, wheat germ, sunflower seeds, hazelnuts, whole-grain cereals and eggs.

Who's at risk for deficiency: People with fat malabsorption problems, premature infants with very low birthweight, the elderly, people on very low-fat diets and people with chronic liver disease or cystic fibrosis.

Possible signs of deficiency include: In adults, vitamin E deficiency can cause lethargy, depressed immunity, ataxia (staggering gait, loss of balance) and anemia. In infants, deficiency can cause irritability, fluid retention and anemia.

Advice for use: People taking anti-clotting drugs should not take vitamin E supplements without a doctor's okay.

tain substances in the intestines, vitamin E, like vitamin C, can inhibit the formation of carcinogens—substances that can cause cell changes that lead to cancer. For instance, vitamin E helps stop the formation of cancer-promoting nitrosamines in the stomach. Nitrosamines are produced during the digestion of nitrites, which are found in especially high concentrations in preserved meats such as hot dogs and bacon.

And third, by enhancing the body's immune response, vitamin E helps keep the body's cancer "early surveillance system" in peak operating order. "Having adequate vitamin E in your blood helps keep your immune cells in a vigorous state, ready to attack the first cancer cells they see, which in fact is your primary defense against cancer," Dr. Blumberg explains.

Cataract Protection

If you're smart, you're already socking away money for your golden years. Similarly, you might want to invest in some vitamin E security for the golden years of your vision.

In both animal and human studies, supplemental vitamin E, like vitamin C, helps prevent cataracts, a condition where the normally clear lens of the eye becomes milky-white and opaque. World-wide, cataracts are one of the most common causes of vision problems among older people.

Vitamin E works by protecting proteins in the lens from oxidative damage from sunlight. In one study, says Dr. Blumberg, people who took supplements of vitamin E were found to be three times less likely to have cataracts than those who didn't take supplements.

The Protective Edge

It's becoming increasingly clear that more than the Recommended Dietary Allowance of 15 international units of vitamin E is necessary to provide maximum health benefits, Dr. Blumberg says. "My general recommendation is to get somewhere in the range of 100 to 400 international units of vitamin E daily."

There is absolutely no way you can get that amount of vitamin E through your diet, Dr. Blumberg says. "Most people get between 6 and 12 international units a day through their diet. People who try really hard might get up to 40 to 50, but that's about as high as anyone can go by diet alone," he says. "The rest should come from supplements."

Enzymes

Digestion Defenders

Janet loves beans, but beans make her gassy. Paul adores cottage cheese, but milk products make him bloated.

If only they had the necessary enzymes.

Our bodies abound with enzymes, feisty little molecules that make reactions happen. They help break down food, among other things. We make some of our own enzymes, and others come prepackaged in the food we eat. But—as Janet and Paul know all too well—sometimes some of us don't get enough.

Enzyme supplements to the rescue!

Bean Defuser

Beans and other legumes and cruciferous vegetables such as cauliflower and cabbage are oh-so-good for you, but they can make things oh-so-unpleasant afterward.

The problem is that these foods contain hard-to-digest sugars. When these sugars reach your intestines, they can produce gas, diarrhea and other unpleasant symptoms.

Luckily, you can buy an enzyme, called alpha-galactosidase, that should end your troubles. You'll find it on store shelves under the brand name Beano. "This enzyme works by breaking down indigestible sugars in the beans while they're still in your stomach," says Joseph Maga, Ph.D., director of the Food Research and Development Center at Colorado State University in Fort Collins. "These sugars then end up being absorbed into the bloodstream, where they can't cause any more trouble."

Beano, which is made from a mold, helps de-gas a variety of foods, including legumes, grains and vegetables such as brussels sprouts and parsnips. Results can

AT A GLANCE

ENZYMES

RDA: None established.

Good food sources: Fresh pineapple provides bromelain; fresh papaya supplies papain.

Who's at risk for deficiency: Many adults may need lactase enzyme supplements to help properly digest dairy products. A few people, such as those with chronic pancreatitis, may lack pancreatic enzymes helpful to digestion.

Possible signs of deficiency include: Lactase deficiency can cause indigestion, gas, cramps and diarrhea after drinking milk or eating milk products.

Advice for use: Because Beano alters the way the body processes sugar, people who have diabetes or galactosemia (inability to use galactose, a form of sugar) should not use it without a doctor's okay. People who are sensitive to mold or penicillin should also check with a doctor before using Beano, as it is made from mold.

---

vary from person to person, but just about everyone will experience *some* relief.

In one study in Guatemala, 38 volunteers gobbled up bowls of refried black beans and then waited for the inevitable results. The gassiest of the gassy then ate more beans, this time topped with Beano. As more and more Beano was added, gas production, to the certain relief of the volunteers, dropped. In another study, people who ate ½ pound of black beans averaged two episodes of diarrhea, gas or belching after the meal. With the enzyme, only 45 percent had symptoms, and the symptoms were not as bad.

To use Beano, add three to eight drops for every ½ cup of food, adding it to your first bite. You can't use it during cooking, because heat zaps the enzyme, but you can add it as soon as the food is cool enough to put in your mouth. It won't affect the food's taste or add any calories.

Because Beano alters the way you process sugar, you shouldn't use it without checking with your doctor if you have diabetes or have been diagnosed as galactosemic (meaning you're unable to use galactose, a form of sugar). And because Beano is made from a mold, you shouldn't use it if you are sensitive to mold or penicillin.

And if the gas in your house is coming from a four-legged member of the family, be aware that the alpha-galactosidase enzyme is available for pets, too! It's sold by veterinarians under the brand name CurTail. Just add CurTail to your pet's food. "You won't be able to blame the dog anymore!" jokes Betty Corson, a spokesperson for A. K. Pharma, the company that makes both Beano and CurTail.

Dairy Delight

You're sitting down to a meal of cheese-topped pasta, and you can spy a chocolate ice-cream cake in the kitchen. "Do you have any lactase enzyme?" you ask your hostess, just as you might ask her to pass the pepper.

You can't expect every kitchen to stock this enzyme, but it *does* make life easier for a large group of people. Lactase, an enzyme that normally occurs in the intestines, breaks down lactose, the sugar that occurs in dairy products. If you don't have enough lactase, you can't digest lactose properly, and the result can be bloating, cramping, diarrhea and worse.

If you have these unpleasant symptoms and don't know the cause, it's wise to check with your doctor. But if you do know that you're one of the 70 percent of the world's population who are lactose intolerant, lactase supplements can be very effective. You can take capsules right before a meal that contains dairy products, or you can buy drops to add to your milk. Use the amount recommended on the box. Or you can buy your milk with the lactase already added. The most common brand is Lactaid, available at most supermarkets.

The Tropical Enzymes

The healing effects of enzymes may go beyond helping digestion.

Folklore has long attributed healing qualities to the pineapple, and studies show that bromelain, an enzyme in pineapple, may help fight cancer, improve circulation and treat inflammation. It also can apparently improve the effect of some antibiotics.

If you're shopping for bromelain, be aware that commercial supplements can vary enormously, says bromelain researcher Steven J. Taussig, Ph.D., former research scientist at the University of Hawaii in Honolulu. "If the manufacturer doesn't know how to put it together, he has probably inactivated some of the therapeutic ingredients." If you want to take bromelain supplements, make sure you purchase them from a reputable company. Follow the directions on the label.

Sometimes you'll find bromelain mixed with papain, an enzyme from papaya, or you may find papaya enzyme tablets alone, promoted as a digestive aid. Papain also appears in meat tenderizers. In meat tenderizer, papain is fine, says William B. Ruderman, M.D., chairman of the Department of Gastroenterology at the Cleveland Clinic–Florida in Fort Lauderdale. But he doesn't recommend papain as a supplement. Because of the lack of standardization in the supplement market, you won't know how much papain you're getting in a capsule. And even if you did, says Dr. Ruderman, papain's ability to promote digestion is unproven.

You may also find pancreatic enzymes, which are also reputed to aid digestion. Normally you make these nutrient-digesting enzymes in your pancreas. A few people, however—such as those with chronic pancreatitis—don't make enough enzymes or have problems absorbing certain nutrients. For these people, doctors sometimes recommend supplements of pancreatic enzymes. For the rest of us, they're a waste of money, says Dr. Ruderman.

Fiber

A Natural Medicine

Your neighbor Denny, the astronaut, is going on a year-long space flight. In addition to the tubes of nutritional goop he'll eat in flight, he can choose one medication, food or supplement to take.

"What did you pick, Denny?" you ask at his going-away party. "Aspirin? Peanut clusters? Ginseng?"

"Nope," Denny says. "Fiber."

Denny just happens to be well aware of the many health benefits of fiber. He knows it can help reduce cholesterol levels, control diabetes, prevent constipation and

---

POTENTIAL HEALING POWER

May help:
- Prevent constipation
- Reduce cholesterol
- Lower risk of colorectal cancer
- Aid weight loss by reducing appetite
- Prevent and treat diverticulosis
- Battle hemorrhoids
- Prevent gallstones
- Control blood sugar levels in people with diabetes

---

colon cancer and possibly help with gastrointestinal problems, gallstones and ulcers as well. And just in case Denny is tempted to gulp down too many tubes of

TAKING IT SLOWLY

Okay, you're convinced of the benefits of fiber. So in the morning you munch high-fiber cereal, at lunch you sprinkle bran on your vegetable soup, and for your afternoon snack you gobble high-fiber cookies.

Whoa! Loading up on fiber too quickly can cause an array of uncomfortable symptoms—for both you and the folks around you. Doctors agree it's important to increase your intake gradually to avoid gassiness and a bloated feeling.

Start with five grams of added fiber a day, suggests George Blackburn, M.D., Ph.D., chief of the Nutrition/Metabolism Laboratory at New England Deaconess Hospital in Boston. After five or six weeks, try adding another five grams (the amount of fiber you'd find in, say, three tablespoons of wheat bran). If at any point you encounter problems, back off a bit.

If one type of fiber causes problems, switch to another, says Buck Levin, R.D., Ph.D., assistant professor of nutrition at Bastyr College in Seattle. "For example, people who have trouble with wheat bran may not have trouble with oat bran," he says.

---

space-goop food, fiber can help curb his appetite.

Health in Bulk

No one really connected fiber with health until 1969, when a researcher noted that Africans who eat lots of fiber in cereals, legumes and root vegetables had less colon and rectal cancer than Westerners, who typically eat little fiber. Since then, other researchers have found that eating fiber can also help ward off hemorrhoids, gallstones, intestinal diseases such as irritable bowel syndrome, and even heart disease.

The funny thing is that fiber—which abounds in whole grains, fruits, vegetables and legumes such as beans—isn't a nutrient at all. In fact, it passes through you without even breaking down.

Nonetheless, it has many benefits. Insoluble fiber, found in wheat bran, whole grains, legumes, fruits and seeds, helps prevent colon cancer and digestive disorders. It also makes your stool bulkier and helps speed it through the intestine. Soluble fiber, found in vegetables, fruits, brown rice, barley, oats and oat and rice bran, zaps cholesterol and may help control the symptoms of diabetes.

AT A GLANCE

FIBER

RDA: None established.

Good food sources: Apples, whole-grain products, brown rice, strawberries, pears and vegetables.

Who's at risk for deficiency: People who eat few fruits, vegetables and whole grains.

Possible signs of deficiency include: People on fiber-poor diets tend to be constipated and have hard, dark stools.

Advice for use: A few people have an allergic reaction to psyllium, a fiber-rich seed used in supplements. Discontinue use if rapid heartbeat or rapid breathing, swelling of the face, itching or tightness of the throat occurs. Additional fiber should be introduced slowly into the diet, and at least 8 8-ounce glasses of fluids, primarily water, should be consumed daily.

Arresting Two Potential Killers

There is strong evidence that soluble fibers such as oat bran and psyllium help lower harmful LDL cholesterol levels in the blood. In a study at the University of Kentucky College of Medicine in Lexington, when 105 people with high cholesterol took high-fiber psyllium supplements for eight weeks, their LDL cholesterol fell almost 9 percent more than when they ate a special cholesterol-lowering diet with no supplements. Another study found that a low-fat diet plus high-fiber oat cereal lowered cholesterol 10 percent, and the same diet plus 13 grams (about ½ ounce) of psyllium cut cholesterol 16 percent.

Experts say that for those with elevated blood cholesterol levels, every 1 percent drop can mean a 2 percent reduction in the risk of heart attack.

Fiber also helps prevent certain cancers. A Swedish study looked at 41 people with cancer of the colon or rectum and compared their diets over 15 years with the diets of people with no cancer. The healthier group tended to eat more fiber. And the colon cancer rate for people in Japan, who eat a low-fat, high-fiber diet, is about one-fifth that of Westerners—but when Japanese immigrate to the United States and change their eating habits, cancer rates leap.

Fat is probably not the deciding factor: People in Finland, who match American fat intake but eat more whole grains and fiber, have one-third as much colon cancer.

Vanquishing Diabetes and Intestinal Ills

In some cases diabetes can be managed by eating a high-carbohydrate, high-fiber diet rather than taking medication. Soluble fiber forms a gel in the gastrointestinal tract, explains Marion Franz, R.D., vice president of nutrition at the International Diabetes Center in Minneapolis. This makes food absorb more slowly and helps keep blood sugar levels stable.

Fiber can also help prevent diabetes in some susceptible people by aiding in weight loss. Not only does fiber help fill you up, it also helps slow the body's response to insulin, the hormone that stimulates appetite and promotes fat storage.

Fiber can help eliminate constipation and sometimes prevent hemorrhoids. It also may help prevent and treat diverticulosis, small pouches in the wall of the colon that can become inflamed.

Small amounts of fiber may help people with Crohn's disease—a gastrointestinal problem that can cause fever, pain and diarrhea—after symptoms have subsided. Fiber has also been used to treat stomach ulcers, and it may help prevent gallstones.

Fitting In Fiber

With all these great potential benefits, you'd think every man, woman and child would fill up on fiber. But the modern American's highly processed diet provides only 11 to 12 grams a day. The American Dietetic Association recommends 20 to 35 grams.

Note that sprinkling a fiber supplement onto your morning jelly doughnut *isn't* the best way to go, says Buck Levin, R.D., Ph.D., assistant professor of nutrition at Bastyr College in Seattle. "I haven't found it helpful to decorate a crummy diet with fiber," he says. Nutritionists agree it's best to get fiber in foods rather than in supplements, partly because fiber binds with some nutrients, such as calcium, making them less absorbable. High-fiber foods, however, come packaged with enough of their own nutrients to compensate for the loss.

But supplements are better than no fiber. "If you're definitely not going to get your fiber through foods," says Dr. Levin, "then supplements make a lot of sense."

Surveying the Supplement Selection

At your grocery store you'll find several varieties of high-fiber cereal: Fiber One boasts 13 grams of fiber per one-ounce serving, for example, and All Bran has 15 grams. Or you can choose high-fiber hot cereals made with wheat or oat bran. At health food stores you'll find choices ranging from high-fiber cookies to fiber tablets, which often contain crushed psyllium seeds as a primary ingredient.

What's your best choice?

It depends on your goal. "If you're targeting cholesterol reduction, stick to soluble fibers," says Dr. Levin. For regulating your bowels, choose insoluble fibers, which may also lower colon cancer risk. You'll have to read labels to figure out if you're getting soluble or insoluble fiber. Many supplements, like psyllium and oat bran, contain both. Pectin and gums are soluble; cellulose and lignin are not. If you're not trying to treat a specific condition, use a mixture of fiber types.

High-fiber cookies may not be a good choice nutritionally, warns Dr. Levin, as they may be high in fat and sugar. Fiber pills also aren't your best bet: Pressing the fiber to get it into a pill can reduce its effectiveness. And the amount of fiber in one daily dose of about nine tablets equals about the amount of fiber you'd get in an apple, which is cheaper and tastes better.

Fiber can also form a plug inside you if you don't drink enough water: Some doctors have reported rare cases of people whose esophagus became blocked from fiber pills that expanded after being swallowed. Whatever form of fiber you choose, be sure to drink eight eight-ounce glasses of fluids, primarily water, a day.

Fish Oil

Whale-Size Heart Protection

POTENTIAL HEALING POWER

May help:
- Reduce risk of heart disease
- Lower triglyceride levels
- Treat Raynaud's disease
- Slow rheumatoid arthritis
- Relieve psoriasis and eczema
- Lower blood pressure

For a period back in the 1970s, fish oil was in the headlines as often as Watergate. It was then that a series of landmark studies showed that Eskimos—who typically chow down on a diet high in fat and cholesterol—nonetheless had low rates of heart disease. How so? Eskimos eat lots of fish, and hence lots of fish oil.

As later studies have corroborated, fish oil can help keep your heart healthy. Researchers have also found that oil from fatty, cold-water fish such as mackerel and tuna may help fight diseases such as psoriasis, arthritis and Raynaud's disease.

The Magic Explained

You're probably used to thinking of fats and oils as enemies rather than friends. But all fats are not created equal.

You may have read that *polyunsaturated* fats are better for you than *saturated* fats, which come mostly from animals. But even in the world of polyunsaturated fats, there are differences.

The polyunsaturated fat in vegetable oils and grains consists of substances that scientists call omega-6 fatty acids. By contrast, the polyunsaturated fat in cold-water fish consists of omega-3 fatty acids. Two of the most significant of these omega-3 fatty acids are eicosapentaenoic acid (EPA) and docosahexaenoic acid (DHA).

When you eat any of these fatty acids, they change in your body to important substances such as prostaglandins, which influence important cellular functions. But the *types* of substances EPA and DHA make are different from the ones made by the omega-6 fatty acids in vegetable oil. As far as your health is concerned, these substances born of fish oil are in many ways superior.

Protecting the Heart and Arteries

It's a sure bet: Eating more omega-3's in fish or fish oil can help prevent heart disease, says Artemis P. Simopoulos, M.D., president of the Center for Genetics, Nutrition and Health in Washington, D.C. A study of 12,866 men aged 35 to 57 at high risk for heart disease backs this up. The men who ate more omega-3 fatty acids turned out to be 40 percent less likely to die from heart disease.

Fish oil battles heart disease on many fronts: It makes the blood less likely to clot and the blood vessels less likely to constrict. It also helps the body eliminate harmful blood fats called triglycerides. Also, fish oil may prevent lesions in the artery walls that provide a home for cholesterol deposits, according to Alexander Leaf, M.D., professor of clinical medicine at Harvard Medical School.

Fish oil may also help lower blood pressure. One study of 32 men with mild high blood pressure found that blood pressure fell in the 8 men who received a high dose of fish oil for four weeks.

Fish oil also apparently helps keep coronary arteries open after they've been cleared by a procedure known as balloon angioplasty. In a study of 205 people at Laval University and the Quebec Heart Institute in Canada, those who got a large dose of fish oil daily before and after surgery had fewer arteries clog up again later.

"We are able to decrease the rate of reblockage after angioplasty by one-third with fish-oil supplements," says Louis Roy, M.D., director of the institute and one of the authors of the study. "So far,

FISH OIL

RDA: None established.

Good food sources: Cold-water fish such as mackerel, tuna, salmon, sardines, herring, cod and bluefish.

Who's at risk for deficiency: Fish oil is not considered essential, so deficiency is unlikely.

Possible signs of deficiency include: There are no known signs of fish-oil deficiency.

Advice for use: Experts recommend eating fish rather than taking capsules. For those who do take capsules, intake should be limited to 3 grams of fish oil a day (equal to 1 gram of omega-3 fatty acids). Fish oil may raise blood sugar, so people with diabetes should check with a doctor before taking supplements. People taking anti-clotting drugs should also check with a doctor before considering supplements.

nothing else has been shown to be as effective."

A Plethora of Benefits

Not all of fish oil's benefits concern the heart and arteries. There's some evidence, for example, that fish oil can slow the advance of rheumatoid arthritis. In an Australian study, 23 people with arthritis who took fish oil daily for three months had less joint soreness and could grip more strongly than people not taking fish oil.

Many studies have shown that fish-oil supplementation may also help treat skin problems such as psoriasis and eczema. In a 12-week study at the Skin Research Foundation of California in Santa Monica, some of a group of 24 psoriasis patients took six one-gram capsules of fish oil daily, in addition to their standard treatment with a medication derived from vitamin A. The people who took fish oil improved more than those who didn't.

Fish oil also enhances the effects of light therapy for skin problems, says Nicholas J. Lowe, M.D., clinical professor of dermatology at the University of California at Los Angeles School of Medicine and director of the Skin Research Foundation.

And several studies show that daily high-dose fish-oil supplements may help control the diarrhea, cramping and pains of ulcerative colitis. People with colitis should *not* undertake this treatment on their own, however.

Fish oil may also help prevent preterm deliveries, suggest Danish researchers. Their study of 533 pregnant women found that fish oil in the last three months of pregnancy increased the number of days the women carried the babies, without making labor more difficult. Pregnant women, however, should consult with their doctor before taking *any* supplements.

Finally, many studies on animals have shown that very large doses of fish oil may slow or halt some cancers. For now, this has to stay on the "wish list" of therapeutic benefits, because scientists still don't know for sure what effect fish oil has on human cancers.

A Word to the Wise

The heart disease research alone may be enough to make you want to start gulping fish-oil supplements. But supplements aren't

---

A WARMING STORY

Imagine being five years old, living in Boston and being unable to stay outdoors more than a minute when it's chilly out. *Not* a fun life.

"This boy's fingers and toes initially would turn blue and painful within one minute of exposure to cold," says psychiatrist Margarita M. Woodbury, M.D., of her young patient. He had Raynaud's disease, a blood vessel disorder that causes extreme cold and loss of feeling in the hands and feet. Dr. Woodbury, who is now in private practice in Walnut Creek, California, was treating the child for psychiatric problems at the Children's Hospital in Boston, but she thought some of his behavorial problems might be linked to the disease and its effects on his social life.

She began treating the Raynaud's with a daily dose of fish-oil supplement. Within six weeks, the boy could stay outside for 30 minutes at a time, and once he could go outside and play, notes Dr. Woodbury, both his mood and his social life improved. Researchers theorize that fish oil helps reduce blood vessel spasms that cause blood flow to fingers and toes to shut down.

After three years of supplementation the boy could tolerate the cold for three hours, and now he can even go skiing with his family. "This child's quality of life increased tremendously," says Dr. Woodbury. "It was really incredible." The boy experienced no side effects from the fish oil, but the doctor cautions that treatment of Raynaud's with fish oil is still experimental and should only be done under a doctor's supervision.

for everyone. Studies have shown that fish oil can raise blood sugar, and therefore people with diabetes should take supplements only under a doctor's supervision. People on anti-clotting medications should also check with their doctors, warns Dr. Simopoulos. Because of its blood-thinning qualities, fish oil may dangerously augment the effects of these drugs.

Both because fish is a healthy alternative to meat and because of potential problems with supplements, most experts say that it's best to get fish oil directly from the source—preferably by eating three fish meals a week. And while all fish have at least some oil, cold-water fish such as mackerel, tuna, salmon, sardines and bluefish abound in the type of oils that you want.

The more you substitute these fish for dishes like hamburger and pork chops, the better. In fact, some researchers believe you won't benefit much from fish oil unless you also cut back on other kinds of fat, such as animal fat.

Selecting Your Dose

For treating diseases, large doses of omega-3 fatty acids may be needed. To get this amount of fish oil, you would have to eat fish all day.

In these cases, fish-oil supplements are an acceptable substitute, says Dr. Simopoulos. "For disease prevention, eating fish two to three times a week is advisable, or fish-oil supplements are an acceptable substitute," he says. A good dosage of omega-3 fatty acids is one gram per day, or three grams of fish oil, she says. Three one-gram fish-oil capsules that contain 180 milligrams of EPA and 120 milligrams of DHA each would give you this healthy measure. It's true that in studies EPA seems more beneficial than DHA, but it's likely that DHA can convert to EPA in the body. So don't waste time searching out supplements with higher levels of EPA.

What you do want to search out is a supplement that contains both fish oil *and* vitamin E, because the fish oil will spoil quickly without it, says Sheldon Saul Hendler, M.D., Ph.D., assistant clinical professor of medicine at the University of California, San Diego, and author of *The Doctor's Vitamin and Mineral Encyclopedia*. Another reason to seek out a combination capsule is that some studies have found that large doses of fish oil without E may cause you to become deficient in that essential vitamin.

Folic Acid

A Cellular Hero

This B-complex vitamin gets its name from the word "foliage"—and with good reason. The researchers who initially isolated this nutrient in 1941 waded through *four tons* of spinach to come up with enough folic acid to test its properties.

Fortunately, it only takes a single cup of cooked spinach to supply you with the Recommended Dietary Allowance (RDA) of 200 micrograms. And spinach is only one of many good sources.

Yet some nutrition experts think that too little folic acid (sometimes known as folate) could be the number-one nutritional deficiency among Americans. This is particularly true for younger Americans, who too often live on fast food that's devoid of vitamins.

These youngsters, if they remain deficient in folic acid for long, could be setting themselves up for trouble.

Researchers have long known that a diet short on folic acid can lead to anemia, fatigue, paleness and loss of appetite. "And newer studies suggest possible additional risks, including cancer, birth defects and even heart disease," says Howerde Sauberlich, Ph.D., professor of nutrition in the Department of Nutrition Sciences at the University of Alabama at Birmingham.

Cancer Cop

Folic acid helps cells in your body divide and multiply. In other words, it's essential for normal tissue growth and for the production of a cell's genetic material, DNA. When folic acid is missing, cell growth becomes abnormal and over time can progress to cancer, says Dr. Sauberlich.

On the other hand, folic acid supplementation may offer some protection against cancer. A study at the University of Alabama at Birmingham found that extremely large doses of folic acid and B_{12}

AT A GLANCE

FOLIC ACID

RDA: Men: 200 mcg. Women: 180 mcg.

Good food sources: Wheat germ, liver (although doctors recommend you limit your liver intake because of its high cholesterol content), oranges and orange juice, eggs, milk, lima beans, navy beans and green leafy vegetables such as spinach, asparagus and broccoli.

Who's at risk for deficiency: Pregnant or nursing women, the elderly, kids who eat a lot of junk food, drinkers, dieters, women taking oral contraceptives, people with intestinal absorption problems and people receiving kidney dialysis or taking certain drugs, such as cholesterol-lowering drugs, sulfasalazine and aspirin and other anti-inflammatories.

Possible signs of deficiency include: Fatigue, anemia, paleness, sore, reddened tongue, forgetfulness, confusion and irritability.

Advice for use: Folic acid is best taken as part of a multivitamin or a B-complex vitamin supplement. Megadoses of folic acid can interfere with the functioning of vitamin B_{12}.

helped reduce the severity of precancerous cell changes in the lungs. In that study, smokers with precancerous lung cells received 10 milligrams of supplemental folic acid and 500 micrograms of vitamin B_{12} for four months. At the end of that time, their cells appeared more normal compared with those of smokers who did not receive supplements.

Cervical cancer may also be linked to folic acid deficiency. "Adequate levels of folic acid appear to help protect women from infection with the papilloma virus. This virus is one of the primary causes of cervical dysplasia, which is the precursor of cervical cancer," Dr.

Sauberlich explains.

And if rectal cancer is a concern, you'll want to make sure you get enough folic acid, says Jo Freudenheim, Ph.D., associate professor of social and preventive medicine at the State University of New York at Buffalo.

When Dr. Freudenheim and her colleagues examined the folic acid intake of a group of women and men, they found that those with higher folic acid intakes had lower risk of rectal cancer.

And a study by researchers at the University of Chicago showed that people with ulcerative colitis who used folic acid supplements were half as likely to have precancerous cells in their colons. "Ulcerative colitis is a type of long-term inflammation of the large bowel," explains Bret Lashner, M.D., the study's main researcher. A drug used to treat this condition, sulfasalazine, inhibits absorption of folic acid and was probably responsible for the low folic acid levels, he adds. "I recommend that people with ulcerative colitis take at least 400 micrograms a day of supplemental folic acid." Many multivitamin supplements contain that amount.

Building Better Babies

Folic acid also plays an important role in a developing fetus, where rapidly dividing cells require its presence to grow normally. Low folic acid has been linked to neural tube defects—serious spinal cord and brain abnormalities.

The Centers for Disease Control and Prevention (CDC) in Atlanta recommend that *all* women capable of becoming pregnant should make sure they get 400 micrograms of folic acid daily—the RDA for pregnant women—to reduce the risk of having a baby with neural tube defects. To get 400 micrograms of folic acid, you may need to take supplements. Pregnant women, however, should not take any supplements without consulting their doctor.

The CDC also recommends that women who have had a baby with this sort of birth defect get four milligrams of folic acid daily one month before conception and during the first three months of pregnancy. The only way to get this high amount is with a prescription prenatal supplement, Dr. Sauberlich says.

A Balancing Act

Liver, eggs and milk contain a form of folic acid that is easiest to absorb, Dr. Sauberlich says. But only about half of the folic acid in most fruits and vegetables is absorbed and used by your body. "Orange juice, with 109 micrograms per cup, may be your best source for folic acid," he says. "Even though it has less than some sources, its folic acid is easily absorbed, it provides other important nutrients and it's low in fat and cholesterol."

Who's most likely to be low in folic acid? Dieters, heavy drinkers, youngsters, the elderly, people with intestinal absorption problems, pregnant or nursing women and women who use oral contraceptives. Also at risk are people getting kidney dialysis and those taking certain drugs.

Experts suggest that folic acid supplements be taken as part of a multivitamin or a B-complex vitamin. Most multivitamins contain about 400 micrograms of folic acid, which should be plenty for most of us, says Dr. Sauberlich.

Garlic Tablets

Guardians of Heart and Breath

POTENTIAL HEALING POWER

May help:
- Reduce cholesterol
- Lower blood pressure
- Inhibit blood platelet clumping
- Protect against heart disease
- Fight cancer

Joe, the guy at the desk next to you, can't shut up about the wonders of garlic. "Look at this," he exclaims, exhaling mightily as he waves a newspaper article under your nose. "Garlic can lower cholesterol and even prevent heart disease!"

At such close quarters it is all too apparent that Joe enthusiastically practices what he preaches, and it's all you can do not to recoil at the pungent aroma that envelops you as Joe leans near.

Maybe it's time to smuggle a bottle of garlic tablets onto Joe's desk and hope he takes the hint.

Tablets, Powder and Cloves

The thing is, you can't argue with Joe about the merits of this stuff: Garlic *does* have many healing qualities. For starters, people have long known that garlic can act as an antibiotic. Albert Schweitzer, the medical mis-

sionary, used it to treat amoebic dysentery, and in both world wars garlic was used to keep wounds from becoming infected.

More recently, researchers have learned that garlic can help reduce cholesterol levels and limit blood platelet clumping. Both of these effects protect you against heart disease. Other studies suggest garlic may also help lower blood pressure.

Garlic also inhibits cancer in animals, and two studies, one in China and the other in Italy, found that garlic apparently helped protect against stomach cancer in humans. There's also some evidence that garlic may help detoxify certain harmful substances in the body.

But does it work in the form of garlic tablets and powder?

Yes, at least in two regards, says Stephen Fulder, Ph.D., biochemist, researcher of natural and alternative medicine and author of *Garlic, Nature's Original Remedy*. Studies have specifically shown that garlic tablets can help lower cholesterol and reduce blood platelet clumping, he says.

In one four-month German study of 261 people with high blood fat and high cholesterol, cholesterol levels dropped 12 percent and blood fat levels dropped 17 percent in those who took 800 milligrams of dried garlic powder tablets a day. In another German study of 60 people having problems with blood platelet clumping, not only did the problems disappear but blood pressure dropped 9.5 percent, and blood flow in the small blood vessels improved nearly 50 percent.

The hitch, however, is that not all garlic preparations are created equal. To be effective, your garlic preparation must have a bit of an odor. Some brands might emit nary an odor before, during or after consumption—but you might as well be munching on cardboard for all the benefit you're getting. "If you want to check effectiveness, chew one of the tablets—there should be some garlic odor and taste," says Dr. Fulder.

You see, the *smell* is linked to many of the health benefits. One crucial ingredient is a rather smelly sulfur-containing compound called allicin. A raw, untouched garlic clove doesn't have allicin—at least not yet. That comes from the breakdown of another compound, alliin, when garlic is mashed or cut. No breakdown, no allicin. No allicin, no smell. No smell, no health benefits. (Or at least not *all* the health benefits: Some researchers think other, odorless ingredients in garlic also contribute to its effects.)

To be absolutely accurate, says Dr. Fulder, most commercial garlic preparations should be labeled "odor-controlled," not odor-free. Effective garlic preparations have a bit of a smell because the breakdown from alliin to allicin has al-

A EUROPEAN TRADITION

Step onto the Paris Metro in the morning rush hour and the heady aroma will quickly convince you that the ingestion of garlic is a long-standing European tradition.

So it's not surprising that overseas sales of garlic products have long outpaced domestic sales. In fact, garlic is one of the top-selling pills in Europe, claims Mike Moore, chief operating officer of garlic-product producer Lichtwer Pharma U.S., in Pittsburgh. As many as five million Europeans pop garlic pills.

ready begun. In theory, what happens next is that the coated tablets slide through your stomach and finish breaking down in your intestine. Though this hasn't yet been fully tested, says Dr. Fulder, judging from the effectiveness of garlic tablets in experiments, it's a likely bet.

The Pungent Question

Okay, but we really don't care if the tablets smell. The burning question is this: If Joe takes these tablets instead of munching on raw garlic daily, will *his* distinctive aroma be lessened?

Almost certainly. "There's very little smell after taking them," says Dr. Fulder. He personally prefers eating a clove of fresh, home-grown garlic daily—as he believes the raw variety is more effective—but he's not averse to popping a garlic tablet once in a while. "The fresh garlic is stronger," he says. "But sometimes I might have a pill instead—say if I were about to go to an important meeting."

Scientific studies suggest that some people may smell after eating dried garlic products, but not as much as with raw garlic—and not as badly. In the four-month German study, the aroma of garlic was detected in 21 percent of the people taking garlic pills (mostly by spouses) and in 9 percent of the people eating a look-alike powder with no garlic. In another three-month study where a dose of dried garlic caused a significant drop in blood pressure, only one of eight people reported a garlic smell.

How about side effects? "Fresh garlic can cause skin irritation and can be uncomfortable to digest. But I've never seen any reports of any side effects of garlic tablets," says Dr. Fulder. But considering garlic's ability to inhibit blood clotting, he recommends safety precautions for some people. You should consult a doctor before using garlic tablets if you're taking anti-clotting medication or are planning to have surgery.

Unfortunately, there's no standardization in either the size of garlic tablets or their content of allicin. But whichever brand you choose, says Dr. Fulder, you're generally safe with whatever dosage is recommended on the container.

Inositol

A Mother's Gift

> **POTENTIAL HEALING POWER**
>
> May help:
> - Protect premature babies from developmental problems
> - Prevent peripheral neuropathy, a complication of diabetes
> - Protect against cataracts in people with diabetes
> - Reduce cholesterol

Myra sits down to munch her way through her favorite breakfast: two slices of whole-wheat toast, half a cantaloupe and a big glass of orange juice. Down the hatch it goes: Without knowing it, Myra has blithely swallowed more than a gram of inositol.

No, Myra doesn't need to have her stomach pumped. Inositol, also called myoinositol, is a substance found in the tissues of many plants and animals—and that includes humans. Most of us eat about a gram of inositol a day, and we also make our own from glucose, producing about four grams daily in our kidneys and other tissues.

This nutrient keeps membranes healthy, carries messages in the body and helps transport fats from place to place. It also helps produce beneficial hormones called prostaglandins.

Although it's never been proved that we need to eat inositol, many researchers suspect we need at least some in our diet. But it's in so many foods that most of us get plenty without trying, says Bruce Holub, Ph.D., professor of nutrition in the Department of Nutritional

INOSITOL

RDA: None established.

Good food sources: Fresh fruits, nuts, beans, grains and seeds.

Who's at risk for deficiency: Premature infants and possibly people with diabetes.

Possible signs of deficiency include: There are no known signs of inositol deficiency.

Advice for use: Supplements are generally not recommended. Doses as high as 2 g a day have caused diarrhea. People with diabetes or kidney disease should use supplements only under a doctor's supervision.

Sciences at the University of Guelph in Ontario.

So why give inositol more than a passing thought? Well, for several reasons. Premature infants appear to benefit considerably from supplemental inositol, and it's possible that formula-fed babies need more as well. People with diabetes may also need more, and a few studies hint that extra inositol may help reduce cholesterol.

Protecting Babies

Inositol seems to be important to a baby's growth and development, says Dr. Holub. Why else would mother's milk contain 100 to 200 milligrams in every quart? Unfortunately, many commercial formulas offer much less. "It's disturbing when you have nutrients in breast milk that aren't present in the same amounts in formula," says Dr. Holub.

If you're unsure about the formula you're feeding your baby, check with your doctor.

It seems that preemies need inositol even more than most other babies. Doctors at Children's Hospital at the University of Helsinki in Finland looked at 221 premature babies who had respiratory distress syndrome, a condition that can sometimes cause fatal nervous system problems. About half of these babies were given daily supplements of inositol. Not only did more babies who received inositol survive, but they also had fewer developmental problems and less bronchopulmonary dysplasia, a chronic lung disease. In addition, they had fewer eye problems: Only 13 percent of those who got inositol had retina problems, compared to 26 percent of the other infants.

Sweet Returns

Babies may not be the only ones who need extra inositol. People with diabetes tend to have low levels of inositol in nerve tissue. Some researchers believe this lack of inositol may be one cause of peripheral neuropathy, a complication of diabetes that involves numbness, tingling and hot and cold feelings in the hands and feet. One study found that 500 milligrams of inositol twice a day for two weeks somewhat reduced the severity of these symptoms.

Inositol may also help protect people with diabetes against cataracts, concluded researchers at New Jersey Medical School in Newark. They found that daily doses of inositol for 14 weeks helped keep diabetic rats from developing cloudy lenses. This doesn't mean, however, that people with diabetes should rush out to buy supplements: Because inositol *could* alter sugar balance, it's crucial to check with a doctor first.

Other possible benefits? Some scientists have suggested that inositol supplements may help lower blood fats and cholesterol, but the effect is probably very small, says Dr. Holub.

There's still much to be learned about this nutrient. Until we know more, healthy adults should be content with the inositol they eat every day. "I don't think in healthy adults there's any evidence that we need inositol supplements," says Dr. Holub.

Iodine

The Purple Protector

The little girl skips along, toting her umbrella and spilling a stream of salt behind her. She's been featured on the outside of salt boxes for decades, changing a bit over the years to keep up with the times. And some-

POTENTIAL HEALING POWER
May help:
• Prevent goiter, a swelling in the neck
• Ward off cretinism, a serious disease that affects the body and mind

where on that box you will discover that the salt is iodized, meaning the contents have been fortified to supply you with iodine.

But times and dietary habits

have changed—just as the little girl's clothing and hairstyle have changed over the years—and today Americans may not need iodized salt to get enough iodine.

"We don't really need iodized salt in this country now," says John B. Stanbury, M.D., lecturer at Harvard Medical School and a physician at Massachusetts General Hospital in Boston. "We get plenty of iodine in our regular diet."

Statistics agree: A survey by the Food and Drug Administration found that women consume an average of 260 micrograms of iodine daily and men 410 micrograms—both well above the Recommended Dietary Allowance (RDA) of 150 micrograms. That's not including iodized salt, which researchers estimate would add about another 340 micrograms per day. Obviously, most of us don't need additional iodine, either from salt or supplements.

In isolated cases, however, a few people may be getting too little iodine, and a few may be getting too much.

A Crucial Messenger

Though most of us give it little thought, this purplish mineral, often used as an antiseptic, is also a busy and very necessary nutrient. It's part of a chemical messenger in your thyroid gland called thyroxin that regulates growth and development. Iodine also apparently helps you convert beta-carotene (the stuff that helps give carrots their orange color) to vitamin A, and it helps you use protein and carbohydrates as well.

When you don't get enough iodine, your thyroid gland swells to try to compensate. This swelling in the neck, one of the first signs of deficiency, is called goiter. The initial swelling is no health threat—it just *looks* bad—but eventually the growth can get so big it may put

---

A CAMPER'S FRIEND

Remember those little iodine tablets for purifying water that were in your Boy Scout or Girl Scout kit? It was comforting to know that if you needed them, they were always there. And—as any scout could tell you today—they are still available.

In fact, iodine may be a backcountry hiker's best friend: It's an easy and effective means of killing parasites such as *Giardia* that lurk in many a stream.

You should only use a form called tetraglycine hydroperiodide, available at camping supply stores.

AT A GLANCE

IODINE

RDA: 150 mcg.

Good food sources: Spinach, lobster, shrimp, oysters, milk and iodized salt.

Who's at risk for deficiency: Iodine deficiency is extremely rare in America. Minor deficiencies could exist among those who eat lots of foods containing goitrogens (cabbage, brussels sprouts, broccoli, cauliflower, peaches and almonds) without using iodized salt or eating seafood.

Early signs of deficiency: Fatigue, dry skin, intolerance to cold, weight gain and swelling in the neck.

Advice for use: Supplements are not recommended.

pressure on the trachea and interfere with breathing.

Worse yet, in some countries, such as India, serious and long-term iodine deficiency sometimes results in a condition called cretinism. The signs and symptoms include mental retardation, thickened skin, difficulty in walking and talking, and sometimes deafness.

Pumping In the Iodine

Seafood is laden with iodine, as is the drinking water in coastal areas. If you live by the sea, you can even absorb iodine from ocean mists. Inland, you may get iodine from plant and animal foods—if there's iodine in the soil. In some areas, mainly where soil comes from glaciers or where iodine has been washed from the soil by flooding or tropical rains, there just isn't enough iodine in the environment.

Goiter was once a problem in some areas of the United States, but in 1924 nutrition experts got the idea of increasing iodine intake by adding iodine to salt. (In some countries iodine has been added to bread, drinking water or candies.) It worked: The incidence of goiter plummeted, and no iodine deficiency has been found in the United States since 1970.

Today, both eating and food-processing habits in the United States have changed. No matter where you live, you're probably eating foods grown in various areas, so local low-iodine soils would not affect you as much. Iodine is also frequently used in bread-making and the processing of dairy products, so it's often in those foods as well.

You *might* need a bit more iodine if you eat lots of foods containing goitrogens. These foods, which can inhibit your body's use of iodine, include cabbage, brussels sprouts, broccoli, cauliflower, peaches and almonds. Experts don't recommend that you stop eating these foods—which are very healthy choices—but rather that you don't eat them exclusively.

The Other Side of the Coin

As mentioned, the RDA for iodine is 150 micrograms a day, and most of us get quite a bit more than this. A daily intake of up to 1,000 micrograms is considered safe, but if you get much over this level you may run into problems, says Nicholas Alexander, Ph.D., professor of pathology at the Uni-

versity of California–San Diego School of Medicine.

You could be loading up on extra iodine without realizing it. There's iodine in vitamin and mineral supplements, dietary supplements such as kelp extracts and certain drugs used for respiratory problems and heart problems. Some fast foods can be full of it. And the iodine in some antiseptics can be absorbed through the skin. Too much iodine, just like too little, can cause goiter, and possibly other problems such as rashes, asthma attacks or acne. Such problems, however, are rare.

Fortunately, most of us don't have to worry about either too much or too little iodine. "It's really no problem in this country," says Dr. Stanbury.

Iron

Forger of Blood Cells

You've been feeling weary and run-down lately. "Hmmm, must be low on iron," you say to yourself, envisioning shrunken, iron-starved blood cells as you reach for a supplement.

Hold it right there! Experts agree

POTENTIAL HEALING POWER
May help: • Prevent and treat iron-deficiency anemia • Stabilize mood • Improve depression • Boost stamina • Stimulate immunity

that you should never take iron supplements—even in a multivitamin/mineral supplement—unless your doctor has determined from a blood test that you need them.

What's the story? Iron *is* essential for your blood—and the hazards of iron deficiency are very real—but nutritionists agree that most people aren't deficient. In addition, some researchers say that extra iron, which is stored in your body, may put you at increased risk for heart problems (such as an irregular heartbeat), liver damage and cancer.

Who Needs Iron?

Most healthy men and post-menopausal women get plenty of iron through their diet. Those who *do* need to take special care to get enough iron are menstruating women—who lose iron when they lose blood—and people with bleeding conditions such as hemorrhoids and ulcers. Pregnancy and nursing also increase the need for iron, and children are at risk for mild deficiency when they have an increased iron need during two stages of rapid growth: up to age four and during early adolescence.

Iron is a vital component of hemoglobin, a key substance in red blood cells. Without hemoglobin, these cells couldn't pick up oxygen in the lungs and transport it throughout the body. Adequate iron prevents iron-deficiency anemia, which affects about 15 percent of the world's population but is less common in the United States. Normally you have extra iron stored in your spleen, liver and bone marrow, in addition to the iron in your blood. In anemia, however, intake of iron is so low or losses are so high that there isn't enough for daily needs, and the stored iron is exhausted as well. The result is weakness, fatigue and paleness. (Pernicious anemia, which is a different condition, is caused by a deficiency of folic acid or vitamin B_{12}.)

Low iron intake can apparently affect you before it progresses to anemia, however, and some studies suggest that as many as one-third to one-half of young American women are low in iron.

What Happens When You're Low

In adults, advanced deficiency can cause you to feel depressed and lethargic, says Ernesto Pollitt, Ph.D., professor of human development at the University of California, Davis. "If you're tired, listless and apathetic," he says, "you should have your iron levels checked."

In one Israeli study of 59 girls aged 16 and 17 who had complained of mood swings, fatigue and inability to concentrate, those who took iron supplements reported improvement in all three areas.

Iron deficiency can also reduce stamina and cause muscle weakness. In one study, active women with depleted iron stores had less endurance when tested on a sta-

AT A GLANCE

IRON

RDA: Men: 10 mg. Women: 15 mg; if postmenopausal, 10 mg.

Good food sources: Red meat, poultry, fish, shellfish, tofu, pumpkin seeds, dried apricots, potatoes, peas and beans.

Who's at risk for deficiency: Menstruating, pregnant and nursing women, infants, people with chronic bleeding conditions and people with poor diets.

Possible signs of deficiency include: Depression, lethargy, difficulty concentrating, weakness, fatigue, paleness, irritability and mood swings.

Advice for use: Supplements are not recommended unless prescribed by a doctor. They can cause abdominal pain, constipation or diarrhea. Doctors particularly advise against supplements for men and postmenopausal women, as excess iron may increase the risk of heart problems, liver damage and cancer. In children, illness from iron overdose can occur after taking supplements containing 200 mg.

tionary bicycle than those with normal levels. Lack of iron has also been linked to an increased risk of cataracts and a decrease in immune power.

In infants, iron deficiency tends to cause irritability and lack of responsiveness, according to Sheldon Saul Hendler, M.D., Ph.D., assistant clinical professor of medicine at the University of California, San Diego, and author of *The Doctor's Vitamin and Mineral Encyclopedia.*

The Possible Perils of Loading Up

No one doubts that too much iron can be dangerous. About 2,000 people become ill from overdosing on iron annually in the United States, mostly young children who swallow adult supplements.

But opinion differs about the effects of nontoxic amounts of iron above what you need for daily use. This extra iron is stored in the body.

Some experts think that this stored iron provides valuable insurance against illness or injury, when you might lose blood. Few people, they feel, need to worry about storing too much iron. "I believe people are still far more at risk for inadequate iron intake than for excessive iron intake," says Robert Hackman, Ph.D., associate professor of nutrition at the University of Oregon in Eugene.

Other researchers, however, believe iron stores not only delay the diagnosis of dangerous ailments such as gastrointestinal cancers—the stored iron prevents anemia, which could signal internal bleeding—but actually put you at higher risk for heart attack. "No one has proved that we need iron stores, and in fact the *reverse* may be true," says Jerome L. Sullivan, M.D., Ph.D., director of clinical laboratories at the Veterans Affairs Medical Center in Charleston, South Carolina.

After studying nearly 2,000 men for five years, Finnish researchers found that those with high stores of iron had a greater risk of heart attack (2.2 times higher) than that of those with low stores. They theorize that harmful substances called free radicals are released by the extra iron and damage the heart's arteries.

And the Framingham Heart Study, which chronicled heart disease in 4,000 people, found that women's risk for heart attack increased two years after menopause. Dr. Sullivan says this may be because menstruating women are "protected" by their periods, which deplete their iron stores. In the United States, women store around 300 milligrams of iron and men

---

How Much Iron Is in Your Cereal?

Trying to figure out if you get enough iron? Take a look at how much you're getting in your cereal bowl. Many breakfast cereals are fortified with iron.

Although iron in cereal is not as well absorbed as iron in meats, remember that the amounts given here are for a one-ounce serving of cereal. Many people can eat much more than one serving size per sitting.

Cereal (1 oz)	Iron (mg)	Cereal (1 oz)	Iron (mg)
Product 19	18.0	Cocoa Puffs	4.5
Total	18.0	Mueslix (Kellogg's)	4.5
Just Right	16.2	Raisin Nut Bran	4.5
Bran Flakes	8.1	Corn Flakes (Kellogg's)	1.8
Cheerios	8.1	Cracklin' Oat Bran	1.8
Grape-Nuts	8.1	Crispix	1.8
Oat Flakes	8.1	Frosted Flakes (Kellogg's)	1.8
Raisin Bran (Kellogg's)	8.1	Rice Krispies	1.8
Special K	8.1	Nutri-Grain	0.72
Wheaties	8.1	Quaker 100% Natural	0.72
All-Bran	4.5	Shredded Wheat (Nabisco)	0.72

WHEN HEREDITY DEALS A BAD HAND

Roberta suffers from anemia, constant respiratory infections and ever-increasing fatigue. She has hemochromatosis, a genetic condition that causes her body to store too much iron.

"Hemochromatosis may affect 1 in 300 people," says James Cook, M.D., professor of medicine and head of the Division of Hematology at the University of Kansas Medical Center in Kansas City.

Hemochromatosis can cause serious liver damage and heart problems. The extra iron could cause diabetes by damaging the cells that produce insulin, and iron deposits in the joints can cause arthritis.

Symptoms of hemochromatosis include weakness and fatigue, abdominal pain, impotence or amenorrhea (lack of menstruation). Some people also experience shortness of breath, depression or hearing loss and have a bronze skin color. If you suspect you have hemochromatosis, ask your doctor for a serum ferritin test, which will measure the amount of iron in your body.

Although serious, the disease is curable. Most often the doctor will suggest weekly blood donations for a year or two, which will deplete the excess iron.

store 1,000 milligrams in their spleen, liver and bone marrow.

Striking a Balance

The Recommended Dietary Allowance (RDA) of iron for women under 50 is 15 milligrams. For women over 50 and for men, the RDA is 10 milligrams. The most absorbable form of iron is heme iron, found in red meat, poultry, fish and shellfish. "You absorb up to 80 percent of the heme iron in one gram of meat," explains John Beard, Ph.D., professor of nutrition at Pennsylvania State University in University Park.

(The actual percentage is in proportion to how much you need.) Four or five ounces a day of meat, poultry or seafood would supply your daily need.

Nonheme iron, which is found mostly in plant products, is less available: Only about 10 percent of the iron in these foods is readily absorbable. You can improve the absorption of iron from plants, however, if you eat it with heme iron or with foods containing vitamin C. A meal of three ounces of lean meat, a medium baked potato and a serving of peas, for example, provides more than seven milligrams. Other iron-rich plant foods include tofu, lima beans and dried apricots.

We also get iron in bread, which is enriched with iron, and in many breakfast cereals. You can also boost intake by cooking in iron pots and skillets.

Because of the potential damage from too much iron, most doctors agree that no one should take iron in supplemental form unless a blood test confirms the need. If you are anemic, you should have a special blood test called a serum ferritin test to make sure that your anemia is caused by iron deficiency.

If a supplement is recommended, you'll absorb the iron best if you take it with food, especially food rich in vitamin C, such as citrus fruit. Calcium interferes with iron absorption, as do tea, coffee, eggs, lentils, beet greens and spinach, so postpone your supplement if you're eating these foods. Be aware that iron supplements can cause abdominal pain, constipation or diarrhea and may color your stool very dark.

But what if you're a man or postmenopausal woman who's concerned about getting *too much* iron? One way of easing your mind is by donating blood. Donating three to five times a year will clear the body of excess iron, says Dr. Sullivan. "That way you can eat meat and have iron-fortified foods every day and still not worry about getting too much," he says.

Vitamin K

The Clotting Component

POTENTIAL HEALING POWER
May help: • Control blood flow   • Prevent brain hemorrhage in premature babies

Want to know what vitamin K does? Just follow the thinking of the Danish researchers who discovered this nutrient. The "K" stands for *koagulation* to describe (in Danish, anyway) the important role of vitamin K in helping control blood flow. Without this nutrient, a simple cut or scrape would be a very serious matter.

This vitamin is also known to be involved in the production of numerous proteins. One is related to bone metabolism and another to kidney function. "Just how a vitamin K deficiency may affect these body parts, though, is not yet understood," says James Sadowski,

AT A GLANCE

VITAMIN K

RDA: Men: 80 mcg. Women: 65 mcg.

Good food sources: Parsley, spinach, broccoli, brussels sprouts, cabbage, lettuce, vegetable oils and dairy products.

Who's at risk for deficiency: Newborn infants, people on long-term tube feeding, people with intestinal malabsorption problems and people with low food intake who are recovering from serious illness, injury or surgery.

Possible signs of deficiency include: Gastrointestinal bleeding or hematoma (bleeding under the skin, characterized by a large, dark bruise).

Advice for use: Most people do not need supplements. Even though toxicity is low, experts say those with vitamin K deficiency should be treated by a doctor. In particular, people taking anti-clotting drugs should not take supplements that contain vitamin K without a doctor's consent.

Ph.D., chief of the Vitamin K Laboratory at Tufts University in Boston.

You're not alone if you haven't heard much about vitamin K. It was assigned a Recommended Dietary Allowance (RDA) only in 1989. You won't find signs at your local supermarket advertising certain foods as a "good source of vitamin K." You won't find doctors on midday talk shows urging people to "get more vitamin K." Chances are you won't even find vitamin K as a single-nutrient supplement, even at the biggest health food store in town, although you can find it in some of the higher-priced multivitamins (sometimes it's listed on the label as phylloquinone, a natural form).

Why so little hoopla? Because, apparently, very few people are deficient in this nutrient. "The RDA for vitamin K is very low—for men, 80 micrograms per day, the amount found in about ½ cup of cooked cabbage or less than ½ cup of broccoli," says John Suttie, Ph.D., professor of biochemistry and chairman of the Department of Nutritional Sciences at the University of Wisconsin in Madison.

Most of those who are at risk for vitamin K deficiency usually aren't in the best of health. They include people on long-term tube feeding, people with intestinal malabsorption problems and those recovering from serious illness, injury or surgery. They often require injections or dietary supplements of this nutrient and should be under a doctor's care.

Saving Newborns

There's another group that's often deficient in vitamin K, through no fault of their own. That's newborn babies. "Usually they're given a vitamin K shot soon after they reach the nursery," Dr. Sadowski says. "This has dramatically reduced deaths from brain hemorrhage after birth."

Premature babies lacking vitamin K run a high risk of brain hemorrhage during delivery, though. "These babies can't afford to wait to be born to get their K. Their blood vessels are too fragile to withstand the surges in blood pressure that occur during and immediately after delivery," says Walter J. Morales, M.D., Ph.D., director of maternal/fetal medicine at Arnold Palmer Hospital for Women and Children in Orlando, Florida.

In one study, Dr. Morales and his colleagues gave vitamin K to women who were expected to deliver prematurely. Of a group of 92 women, half received vitamin K injections every five days until delivery. The other half received no vitamin K.

Sixteen percent of the infants who received vitamin K through their mothers experienced internal bleeding in the head, compared with 36 percent of the babies whose moms got none. Not one of the vitamin K babies had severe bleeding, compared with 11 percent in the other group.

Dr. Morales says that large doses of vitamin K for expectant mothers should only be given under a doctor's care.

Go for the Green

Is there ever a time that a healthy adult (other than moms who may deliver early) should seek vitamin K supplements?

There's no reason to, says Dr. Suttie. "Lots of foods have vitamin K. Those who eat a balanced diet are sure to get enough."

Your best food sources include spinach, parsley, brussels sprouts and lettuce. Other good sources include cabbage, carrots, avocados, cucumbers, leeks and tomatoes. Some vegetable oils, such as olive, canola and soybean oil, also contain vitamin K, as do meats and cereals.

Lecithin (Choline)

An Unforgettable Supplement

Raphael Rat zoomed through the maze with ease. His brother, Randall, however, couldn't find his way through, no matter how hard he tried. Mama Rat couldn't understand how one of her sons could have such a better memory than the other.

The difference between them was that Raphael had received choline about two weeks after he was born, and Randall hadn't.

It may be a stretch to believe that a nutrient given to a baby rat can benefit its memory throughout its life. But that's exactly what researchers Warren Meck, Ph.D., and Christina Williams, Ph.D., found in their work at Columbia University and Barnard College in New York City.

Specifically, they found that when 16- to 30-day-old rats were given choline (or if their mothers received it before giving birth), they could remember how to get through a maze much better than choline-free rats. Even older rats that were given choline as infants showed improved memory.

But that's rats. The question is:

Can choline help improve memory in humans, too? Researchers suspect it can.

"If you'd asked me about this a decade ago, I might have told you these effects were too profound to believe," says top choline researcher Steven H. Zeisel, M.D., professor of nutrition at the University of North Carolina at Chapel Hill. But now researchers are beginning to study how choline can affect memory. "There is good science behind this research," says Dr. Zeisel.

Nothing Fishy Here

So what's choline? It's a building block for acetylcholine, a chemical found in your brain that transmits messages from one nerve cell to another. Choline is also important for making cell membranes. Your body produces a certain amount of choline on its own, but some believe more may be beneficial. For that, there are foods rich in choline and there are choline supplements. The problem with these supplements is that pure choline is broken down in the intestines to form a chemical with a fishy smell, so eating choline can make your breath smell likewise. For this reason, people who believe in choline supplementation prefer to get it in the form of lecithin, a substance that's rich in choline but causes no fishy odor.

Ever take a good look at the fine print on a chocolate bar? Lecithin is the substance that keeps the fat in the chocolate from separating. Don't count on chocolate as your primary source, however. Better sources include soybeans and oatmeal. You can also find lecithin and choline supplements for sale in health food stores.

The Brain Connection

Researchers have long suspected that choline levels affect the brain. Some people with Alzheimer's disease—which involves early loss of memory—have made modest, temporary improvements when given choline. Choline can also apparently influence mood, and daily supplements, in at least a few known cases, have helped control wild mood swings. Choline in the form of lecithin is also an experimental treatment for tardive dyskinesia, twitching and jerking that's a side effect of antipsychotic medicine.

A small study at Children's Hospital, affiliated with Harvard Medical School, indicates that supplemental choline can also help treat certain developmental problems in

---

AT A GLANCE

LECITHIN (CHOLINE)

RDA: None established.

Good food sources: Oatmeal, soybeans, cauliflower, kale, cabbage, peanuts, eggs, milk, seaweed and chocolate.

Who's at risk for deficiency: People who are being fed intravenously and possibly pregnant women.

Possible signs of deficiency include: There are no clear signs of choline deficiency.

Advice for use: Supplements are not recommended, although modest amounts are unlikely to be harmful. Doctors particularly suggest that people who have a history of depression avoid supplements, as lecithin can affect moods.

youngsters. Margarita M. Woodbury, M.D., a psychiatrist now in private practice in Walnut Creek, California, found significant improvement in two four-year-olds, who had numerous speech and learning problems, when they were given daily doses of choline. Four years later, they were still taking choline and continued to improve.

This was the first time choline was used to treat these types of problems in children. "I consider this a frontier of medicine," says Dr. Woodbury.

Full-Body Protection

Choline's effects seem to go far beyond the brain. For example, choline deficiency can actually trigger liver cancer in laboratory animals. Researchers believe that a lack of choline may disturb the cell signaling process and send a cancer-triggering message to the liver. "What we don't know," says Dr. Zeisel, "is whether giving extra choline would *lower* the cancer rate."

Other laboratory studies indicate that choline supplements may protect the liver from alcohol damage as well. Animals fed both alcohol and choline seem to be protected from liver scarring or cirrhosis, two common alcohol-related problems.

Other benefits? Choline seems to have a slight lowering effect on both blood pressure and cholesterol. Some studies suggest that choline prevents gallstones in ani-

mals, but there's no conclusive evidence that people eating choline have fewer gallstones.

Is It Essential?

While scientists have known for a long time that some animals need to eat choline, they aren't sure about humans, as we can make choline in our bodies. But one study at the Boston University School of Medicine indicates we may indeed require dietary choline. Men fed a choline-free diet for three weeks showed initial signs of liver problems. "They developed abnormalities that suggested that if we left them on the diet long term, they would have developed the same kinds of serious problems that laboratory rats do," says Dr. Zeisel.

Fortunately, many foods contain choline, and most of us take in from 400 to 900 milligrams a day. It's highly unlikely that any of us are actually deficient, says Dr. Zeisel.

Scientists are pretty sure, however, that certain groups of people need supplemental choline. People who are being fed intravenously should definitely have supplements, says Dr. Zeisel. Demand for choline is also high when an embryo is developing.

"In pregnancy the baby takes a lot of choline from the mother," says Dr. Zeisel. "We're now exploring whether during pregnancy there's an added need for choline. I suspect that's the case." (Pregnant women should not take choline or any supplements without approval from their doctor.)

What about the rest of us who might be eager to reap possible benefits from supplemental choline? Dr. Woodbury stresses that treating with choline is experimental and should always be supervised by a doctor, and Dr. Zeisel points out that there's still too

much we *don't* know about choline.

"Right now we can't be sure that there isn't some undesirable effect until we've studied it a little more," says Dr. Zeisel. "I don't feel I understand choline enough to take it myself or to recommend that people take it at this point." Instead, he recommends a balanced diet and waiting until more research appears.

Magnesium

The Patriot Mineral

POTENTIAL HEALING POWER

May help:
- Protect against heart disease
- Fight chronic fatigue syndrome
- Lower blood pressure
- Prevent recurrent kidney stones
- Ward off diabetes
- Slow bone loss
- Strengthen muscles

Ka-boooom! The night sky lights up with a soul-shattering explosion of red, white and blue. You watch as billions of colored sparkles fade into oblivion. And then . . . Ka-boooom! Another aerial burst. This one is so spectacular that you nearly drop your Fourth-of-July hot dog into your lap.

Part of what puts the spark into the sparkle of those fireworks is magnesium, a silver-white metallic powder that burns with a hot, bright light. It was also once used in photographers' flash bulbs and continues to be used by stage magicians to create special effects. But magnesium is also a mineral that's essential to your health—

and it's been known to create some very special effects right inside the human body!

As you'll see, there's evidence that additional magnesium—either in your diet or in the form of supplements—may help protect you against heart disease, fight chronic fatigue syndrome, lower blood pressure, prevent kidney stones, slow down bone loss, build muscles, and more.

Helping the Heart

Magnesium can befriend a heart in a number of ways. First, scientists suspect from animal studies that adequate magnesium may help fight atherosclerosis. Also known as "clogged arteries," atherosclerosis can lead to heart disease by slowing the flow of blood to the heart.

There's also evidence that magnesium can help control high blood pressure, another factor that puts you at risk for a heart attack. Research shows that some people with high blood pressure have more success controlling it when they're taking additional magnesium. Actually, it's magnesium working in harmony with other minerals, particularly calcium, that lowers blood pressure, says Karen S. Kubena, R.D., Ph.D., associate professor of nutrition at Texas A&M University in College Station. A four-year study of 58,000 women found that women who consumed 800 milligrams of calcium and 300 milligrams of magnesium reduced their chances of developing high blood pressure by *one-third!*

Given intravenously to people who have had heart attacks, magnesium can save lives. A survey of seven studies involving 1,301 patients found that only 3.8 percent of heart attack patients who received magnesium intravenously died, while 8.2 percent of the patients who were not given magnesium died. Doctors speculate that magnesium may help your arteries stay open for business.

A Fatigue Fighter?

Getting adequate magnesium may be a real boon to sufferers of chronic fatigue syndrome. Researchers at the University of Southampton and Southampton General Hospital in Great Britain noted that many of the symptoms of chronic fatigue syndrome are similar to those of magnesium deficiency. (These include fatigue, difficulty concentrating and muscle tenderness.) The researchers also found that people with chronic fatigue syndrome tend to have lower magnesium levels in their blood than people who don't have the condition.

In one experiment, the scientists divided 32 people with chronic fatigue syndrome into two groups. Members of one group received magnesium supplements for six weeks, while members of the other group received none. Twelve of the 15 in the magnesium group reported feeling better, while only 3 of the 17 who didn't receive magnesium felt better.

A Busy Mineral

Magnesium may come to the rescue in other cases as well. For example, magnesium supple-

AT A GLANCE

MAGNESIUM

RDA: Men: 350 mg. Women: 280 mg.

Good food sources: Nuts, wheat germ, sunflower seeds, whole grains, dark green leafy vegetables, seafood, dairy products and meats.

Who's at risk for deficiency: The elderly, people with diabetes, people on low-calorie diets, drinkers, people with fat malabsorption problems, people who engage in regular strenuous exercise and people taking regular doses of certain medications, including many heart drugs.

Possible signs of deficiency include: Diarrhea or constipation, muscle weakness, irritability, fatigue and muscle spasms.

Advice for use: People with kidney disease, certain heart problems or ileostomy (a surgical opening in the small intestine) should not take magnesium supplements. People taking the heart drugs digitalis or digoxin should talk to their doctor before taking supplements.

mentation has helped prevent recurring kidney stones. Swedish scientists found that daily supplementation with magnesium curtailed stone recurrence by nearly 90 percent in one group of people. Researchers speculate that magnesium works by bonding with oxalate, a prime ingredient in most kidney stones.

Another study found that magnesium supplements may help prevent diabetes. Italian researchers found that supplementation with 4,500 milligrams of magnesium a day for four weeks improved glucose tolerance in elderly people. Glucose tolerance is a measure of how well the body processes carbohydrates, and poor glucose toler-

ance often precedes the development of diabetes.

And a California study suggests that magnesium may help prevent bone loss in postmenopausal women. Nineteen women receiving a diet with twice the Recommended Dietary Allowance (RDA) of magnesium had approximately an 11 percent increase in bone density within a year, while the bone density of seven women who did not increase their magnesium intake increased less than 1 percent.

One other possible benefit to magnesium supplementation: stronger muscles. An experiment at the Exercise and Sport Science Laboratory in Seattle put 26 formerly inactive people on weight-lifting programs for seven weeks. The lifters were placed into two groups. Members of one group took in 507 milligrams of magnesium per day and increased their strength by an average of about 26 percent. Those in the other group consumed 246 milligrams of magnesium a day, and their strength increased by an average of only 11 percent. Researchers think the link between magnesium and muscles is magnesium's involvement in the synthesis of protein.

Balancing Your Intake

Although serious magnesium deficiency is rare, it's likely that many of us are marginally deficient. Studies have shown that three-fourths of the U.S. population may be taking in less than the RDA of 350 milligrams for men and 280 milligrams for women. And if you're low in magnesium, you won't know it right away: It can take a good while before you develop symptoms such as fatigue, muscle spasms, constipation or diarrhea, says Dr. Kubena.

You can boost your intake by eating more dark green leafy vegetables, whole grains, nuts and seeds. Some doctors also recommend supplementing with 200 to 400 milligrams daily in a multivitamin/mineral supplement.

Take heed, however. Taking too much magnesium can have unpleasant consequences. Researchers at Baylor University Medical Center in Dallas say that 5 percent of people with chronic diarrhea may actually suffer from *too much* magnesium.

You may be taking in too much magnesium without even knowing it: Magnesium is included in many over-the-counter remedies, including antacids, laxatives and pain relievers. (Some popular over-the-counter remedies that contain magnesium include Maalox, Mylanta, Phillips' Milk of Magnesia, Di-Gel, Bayer Plus and Bufferin.) If you're troubled by diarrhea, check the labels of your medications: Magnesium hydroxide or magnesium oxide can cause diarrhea, but magnesium gluconate shouldn't. People who have impaired kidney function should avoid using these products.

Manganese

A True Team Player

Manganese was just another trace element—needed for many biological processes in our bodies but with no claim to fame—until Bill Walton came along.

Bill was a standout center for the Portland Trail Blazers—when he wasn't on the bench. Unfortunately, he was consistently sidelined because of a broken bone in his foot. Doctors eventually discovered that low levels of manganese were partly to blame for the slow healing of the fractured bone.

So what does this mean to you, who presumably have little interest in spending much of your time hopping about a basketball court? It means that manganese (along with other minerals like calcium, zinc and copper) is important to the health of your bones—and, as you'll see, the health of some other important parts of your body as well.

Protecting Bones and Heart

Studies have shown that animals deficient in manganese have skeletal defects and bone problems similar to osteoporosis, plus reproductive problems possibly caused by bone problems in the fetuses.

How does this mineral work? "Manganese seems to be very influential in creating the framework on which bone is built," says Constance Kies, Ph.D., professor of nutritional science at the University of Nebraska in Lincoln. "And if a solid framework isn't there, no matter how much calcium you consume, there's no way for new bone to be deposited."

Preliminary research also indicates that manganese may help protect against degenerative diseases such as heart disease. Manganese acts as an antioxidant, a substance that neutralizes harmful free oxygen molecules that can cause wear and tear in our bodies, says Sheri Zidenberg-Cherr, Ph.D., nutrition science specialist at the University of California, Davis.

The Right Dose

The Estimated Safe and Adequate Daily Intake set for manganese by the Food and Nu-

AT A GLANCE

MANGANESE

Estimated Safe and Adequate Daily Intake: 2 to 5 mg.

Good food sources: Whole-grain cereals, nuts, fruits and green leafy vegetables.

Who's at risk for deficiency: People on extremely low-calorie diets and people being fed intravenously or by tube. People who have a high intake of iron, calcium, fiber and sugar may have decreased absorption of manganese.

Possible signs of deficiency include: There are no known signs of manganese deficiency in adults; in children, slow growth and development may signal deficiency.

trition Board of the National Research Council is two to five milligrams for adults, and some studies suggest that you may need the whole five milligrams. Women with osteoporosis in particular should eat plenty of manganese-rich foods.

While manganese is in a variety of foods—including whole-grain cereals, nuts and legumes—many factors affect how much of the manganese is actually available to your body. Iron, calcium, fiber and sugar can all interfere with manganese absorption or retention. There are no obvious symptoms of manganese deficiency—it can only be determined by a sophisticated blood analysis.

You can get at least the minimum recommended amount at breakfast: A cup of orange juice, a one-ounce serving of wheat bran

cereal and a banana contain just over 2.5 milligrams.

Dr. Kies advises caution in the use of supplements: Five milligrams in a multivitamin/mineral supplement is plenty, and you shouldn't take more than ten milligrams daily.

"You don't have to worry about overdosing on manganese from foods, but overdosing from other sources is possible," says Badi Boulos, M.D., Ph.D., associate professor of environmental and occupational health sciences at the University of Illinois in Chicago. Calcium supplements and over-the-counter antacids that contain calcium may also contain manganese.

"If your kidneys are in good health, a normal dose of these products won't hurt you," says Dr. Boulos. "What concerns me are women who are taking more than the recommended number of tablets a day." High blood levels of manganese could result in symptoms similar to those of Parkinson's disease, including trembling, shuffling and slow movements.

Manganese poisoning has also resulted from taking large doses of mineral supplements for four to five years—and from drinking well water contaminated from batteries buried in the ground. And mine workers exposed to manganese dust can actually experience "manganese intoxication," with a bizarre array of symptoms including laughter, delusions, hallucinations and increased sexuality, followed by deep depression and an inability to stay awake.

Molybdenum

Mo' Useful Than You Thought

You almost *never* beat your friend Martha at Scrabble, but for once you're ahead. Or so you think. Then Martha gets that horrible smug look, picks up all of her seven letters and plunks them down one at a time around your last word: Plop, plop, plop, spelling out MOLYBDENUM.

You don't know what the heck this is—but you do know that she's just scored a whopping 230 points and once again beaten you.

Don't feel bad: Not many people know what this mineral is, let alone how to pronounce it (it's *mo-LIB-duh-num*). And if you'd asked a nutritionist 30 years ago what it was good for, you probably would have gotten a blank look and a "Mo-*what*?"

Even now there's a lot of mystery surrounding this mineral, but scientists know it's essential and suspect that it may play such diverse roles as helping to fight cancer and reducing tooth decay.

The Catalyst Mineral

You may not realize it, but in some ways your body's like a roomful of chemistry experiments, with all kinds of ongoing reactions. Enzymes are the spark plugs that get these important reactions going, and molybdenum is an essential component of several important enzymes.

One of those enzymes (xanthine oxidase) helps us use iron, a mineral essential to the formation of

AT A GLANCE

MOLYBDENUM

Estimated Safe and Adequate Daily Intake: 75 to 250 mcg.

Good food sources: Legumes, breads, cereals, milk and milk products.

Who's at risk for deficiency: People on low-calorie diets and people being fed intravenously or by tube.

Possible signs of deficiency include: Physical signs of molybdenum deficiency are extremely rare. Urine testing may show high levels of sulfite, low levels of sulfate and low levels of uric acid.

Advice for use: Doses in excess of 500 mcg a day should not be taken without a doctor's okay. People who have gout or high levels of uric acid should consult a doctor before using supplements.

red blood cells. The same enzyme also helps our bodies produce uric acid. Uric acid, in excess, can cause a form of arthritis called gout. But scientists theorize that uric acid may also act as an antioxidant, a substance that helps fight off disease and slow down the aging process.

Another molybdenum-dependent enzyme may help detoxify sulfites, chemical preservatives that are used in some foods and drugs and to which some people are highly sensitive.

It's also possible that molybdenum somehow helps protect against cancer. Researchers have found that feeding animals molybdenum supplements helps ward off cancers of the esophagus and breast.

And molybdenum, according to one study, may help prevent tooth decay by encouraging the body to retain fluoride.

A Late Bloomer

One reason this mineral was ignored for so long is that deficiencies in humans are so rare that it took a long time to discover that we needed molybdenum at all. In 1967, however, scientists discovered in infants a rare genetic disease that prevents molybdenum from forming essential enzymes. The disease is always fatal.

"This showed that molybdenum is totally essential for normal development," says K. V. Rajagopalan, Ph.D., a professor in the Department of Biochemistry at Duke University Medical Center in Durham, North Carolina.

Laboratory studies have also linked diets low in molybdenum to abnormal growth and development in young animals. In one study, female goats low in molybdenum had difficulty getting pregnant, and mothers and their fetuses often didn't survive.

And in one case a hospital patient with a gastrointestinal disease who was being fed an intravenous solution without molybdenum slipped into a coma. When molybdenum was added to the IV solution, the patient improved.

Do You Need Mo'?

The Estimated Safe and Adequate Daily Intake for molybdenum established by the Food and Nutrition Board of the National Research Council is very small: 75 to 250 micrograms a day. Do you need supplements to get that amount? It's *very* unlikely, says Dr. Rajagopalan. The average American gets plenty of molybdenum in the normal diet, mostly from legumes, breads, cereals, milk and milk products.

Unless your doctor tells you that you need it, you should never take a supplement containing more than 500 micrograms of molybdenum, says Dr. Rajagopalan. Taking more may cause your body to lose copper, an important mineral.

And larger amounts of molybdenum can cause other problems. In one area of the former Soviet Union with unusually high levels of molybdenum in the soil and water, people were ingesting as much as 15,000 micrograms a day. Not surprisingly, because of the molybdenum/uric acid connection, many developed gout.

Multivitamin/ Mineral Supplements

POTENTIAL HEALING POWER
May help:
• Provide protection against vitamin or mineral deficiencies that could put you at risk for various diseases.

Your Most Basic Insurance Policy

You bolt down a bagel for breakfast. Your spouse works through lunch. The kids grab dinner on the way out the door. Are you and your family getting enough vitamins and minerals?

Maybe not. A survey of nearly 12,000 people found that only 9 percent of us eat the five or more daily servings of vegetables and fruits recommended for good health and protection against disease. While multivitamin/mineral supplements in no way make up for an unbalanced diet, they can provide you some nutritional peace of mind, says Robert E. Keith, Ph.D., professor in the Department of Nutrition and Food Science at Auburn University in Alabama.

But even for the 9 percent of Americans who eat healthy foods galore, a daily multiple may not be a bad idea. Some nutrients, such as folic acid, chromium and vitamin B_6, are tough to get even in a well-balanced diet.

The elderly in particular may benefit from a multiple supplement, as their intakes tend to be low in crucial nutrients such as beta-carotene, vitamins E and C, thiamin, riboflavin, folic acid, vitamin B_6, selenium and chromium. Among other things, extra nutrients may help protect their vision and improve their immunity. Other people who may especially benefit are athletes, those on reducing diets, pregnant and nursing women, adolescents, smokers and heavy drinkers.

In Search of a Perfect Pill

What you're looking for in a multi is a collection of most of the essential nutrients. A multi fallen from heaven would contain the following nutrients: beta-carotene, vitamin D, vitamin E, vitamin K, vitamin C, thiamin, riboflavin, niacin, vitamin B_6, folic acid, vitamin B_{12}, calcium, magnesium, zinc, selenium, biotin, pantothenic acid, copper, manganese, chromium and molybdenum.

Most experts agree that a multiple supplement should contain as close to 100 percent of the U.S. RDA as possible for each nutrient. When the U.S. RDA was set by the Food and Drug Administration in 1973, it was based on the highest recommended nutrient level for any age and sex group (excluding children under four and pregnant and lactating women). Supplement labels typically list each nutrient both as a percentage of the U.S. RDA and in specific units—either milligrams (mg), micrograms (mcg) or international units (IU).

Unfortunately, you're not likely to find the perfect multiple supplement: If one tablet or capsule contained 100 percent of everything, it would be too big to swallow. So manufacturers generally compromise by cutting down on two of the bulkiest minerals, calcium and magnesium.

But you needn't worry. If you want additional calcium, you can get it from low-fat dairy foods or calcium carbonate supplements. If you can't find enough magnesium in a supplement, you can pump up your intake of this mineral via lean meats, seafood, green vegetables or dairy products.

Besides low figures for calcium and magnesium, many supplements don't have a full 100 percent of the U.S. RDA for biotin, because it tends to be expensive. But biotin deficiency is rare, and the 30 micrograms in most supplements is adequate. You may also have trouble finding vitamin K in a multiple supplement. This vitamin is

---

STRESS FORMULAS: WORTH THE COST?

If your life is one hectic whirl and you feel tired all the time, you may be tempted to reach for supplements labeled "stress formula."

Don't waste your money. "There's no proof that mental stress increases your need for vitamins," says Jack M. Cooperman, Ph.D., former clinical professor of community and preventive medicine at the New York Medical College in Valhalla. These formulas often have extra B vitamins and vitamin C, which some manufacturers claim benefit people who suffer mental or emotional stress.

It's true that *physical* stress such as hard work or intense exercise increases the need for some nutrients, such as riboflavin and chromium. But, says Dr. Cooperman, there is no evidence that this is true of mental stress.

SHOULD KIDS TAKE SUPPLEMENTS?

Nutrition is important for everyone, but particularly for children, who are growing fast and need lots of nutrients to develop normally. Should they take supplements?

It's best to try to meet your growing child's needs through good food—but for a child over age three, a daily multiple supplement with no more than 100 percent of the U.S. RDA for each nutrient can provide insurance and a little peace of mind for parents, says Howerde E. Sauberlich, Ph.D., professor of nutrition in the Department of Nutritional Sciences at the University of Alabama at Birmingham.

"There's no harm in a daily supplement, and it may help," says Dr. Sauberlich. "Many kids just don't eat particularly well."

But parents should take care to keep all supplements out of the reach of children—especially flavored, chewable ones that might entice a child to down a whole bottle. Because of his small size, it's easier for a child to overdose on a nutrient than it is for an adult. Likewise, never give a child a single supplement (rather than a multiple) unless your physician has specifically recommended it.

available from vegetables and dairy products, and deficiency is rare.

One area where you want to make sure your multi doesn't fall short is in antioxidant nutrients, says Howerde E. Sauberlich, Ph.D., professor of nutrition in the Department of Nutrition Sciences at the University of Alabama at Birmingham. Many scientists believe that vitamins C and E and beta-carotene may help prevent disease and slow aging by latching onto harmful free oxygen molecules.

Your multi should give you *at least* 100 percent of the U.S. RDA for these nutrients, say most experts. There is some evidence that amounts of antioxidants higher than the U.S. RDA could help prevent some diseases. Research shows that antioxidants' protective powers are highest at daily intakes of 250 to 1,000 milligrams of vitamin C, 100 to 400 international units of vitamin E and 15 to 30 milligrams of beta-carotene.

What to Avoid

That's what you should look for in a multi—now for what you should avoid. Forget about timed-release supplements, says Dr. Sauberlich. These generally cost more, and for most people they just aren't necessary.

You also don't need sodium,

potassium, phosphorus and iodine. Yes, sodium, potassium and phosphorus are essential minerals, but you get plenty of them in your regular diet. (Many supplements list phosphorus, however, because it's in calcium phosphate, a common source of calcium.) And you don't need supplemental iodine, either, unless you never use iodized salt or eat seafood.

Doctors agree that men and postmenopausal women should avoid supplemental iron, because excess iron can be harmful. Menstruating and pregnant women may need iron, but they shouldn't take it unless it's recommended by a doctor.

"You don't need to spend a lot of money for extras," says John Erdman, Jr., Ph.D., director of the Division of Nutritional Sciences at the University of Illinois in Urbana. Ignore words such as natural, balanced, sustained, super-potency, therapeutic and geriatric. These are buzzwords with no specific meanings. And avoid multis that contain substances you don't recognize.

Finally, you want to avoid unbalanced supplements, cautions Dr. Sauberlich. Aside from the antioxidants discussed earlier, no one nutrient should exceed the U.S. RDA

by more than 50 percent. For example, you can buy a supplement with 5,000 percent of the U.S. RDA of pantothenic acid, but taking that much could be worse than taking in too little. (Huge amounts of pantothenic acid can cause you to lose niacin.)

Let the Buyer Beware

One additional thing to check before buying a multi is the expiration date, usually printed near the bottom of the label. It should be at least two years from the date of purchase.

And choose brand-name vitamins such as those bearing the name of a drugstore chain, which are likely to be made by reliable companies. Because the Food and Drug Administration regulates vitamins as foods—which require less exacting standards than do drugs—quality can vary.

Your last question about multiple supplements might be when to take them. The answer: Take them with food. "Nutrients taken with food are usually more efficiently utilized by the body than nutrients taken on an empty stomach," says Dr. Sauberlich.

Niacin

Prescription for High Cholesterol

POTENTIAL HEALING POWER
May help: • Reduce cholesterol • Lower triglycerides • Prevent cancer

The announcer takes the creamy white envelope and gently pulls it open. He removes the paper, reads it, looks up and clears his throat. "The winner of the Annual Nutrient Recognition Award is . . . "—*drum roll*—"NIACIN!"

If there really were an award for nutrients, niacin would be a likely recipient. While many nutrients are thought to help fight diseases, this particular vitamin has gone one step beyond that. It is the only vitamin that has actually achieved recognition by the medical community as a bona fide medicine: Taken in large doses by prescription, it's one of the most effective and cheapest ways of lowering cholesterol.

A Distinguished History

The first "miracle" that niacin accomplished was curing a disease called pellagra, a serious problem in the early 1900s in the southern United States. This devastating ailment was common among poor people whose diet consisted primarily of corn, with few milk or meat products. They came down with a skin inflammation called dermatitis, plus diarrhea and dementia (a progressive mental decline). Many sufferers died before it was discovered that the disease was caused by a niacin deficiency.

In the 1950s came the second miracle: Doctors found that large doses of niacin could cut high levels of cholesterol and harmful blood fats called triglycerides. A landmark study in 1975 showed conclusively that niacin can not only dramatically lower cholesterol levels but also reduce recurrences of heart attacks by nearly 30 percent.

More recently, scientists have begun to think that niacin may also battle another well-known killer. "We've gathered very convincing evidence that niacin may be one factor that helps prevent cancer," says Elaine L. Jacobson, Ph.D., professor of clinical sciences at the Markey Cancer Center at the University of Kentucky in Lexington.

Niacin Explained

Let's take a closer look at this B vitamin. Niacin helps form enzymes, or "spark plugs," that make many things happen in your body, including converting sugars into energy, using fats and keeping tissues healthy. There are two forms: nicotinic acid, which is the kind prescribed by doctors to treat cholesterol problems, and nicotinamide (also called niacinamide).

You can get niacin in foods such as whole grains and lean red meats. You can also get some of your niacin indirectly, from an amino acid called tryptophan. Tryptophan is present in protein-rich foods such as milk, meat and eggs, and it can convert to niacin in your body. You can't get *all* of your niacin this way, but you can get some of it.

So is niacin a nutrient or a drug? When you're chowing down on a chicken sandwich or taking a multiple supplement with a small amount of niacin, you're consuming niacin as a nutrient. When you're taking large doses of doctor-prescribed niacin to treat high cholesterol—or gulping high-dose supplements from the health food store—you're taking niacin as a drug.

The reason the distinction is so important is that, like most drugs, niacin as a drug can be dangerous and should *always* be prescribed and monitored by a physician.

Our Daily Needs

The Recommended Dietary Allowance (RDA) of niacin for adults is 15 milligrams for men and 13 milligrams for women. While few people in the United States are deficient to the point of developing pellagra, it's probable that many of us are marginally low, says Dr. Jacobson.

Preliminary results from a long-term study in Malmö, Sweden, found that about *one-fifth* of the city's population—mostly the middle-aged—were deficient in niacin. Similar tests haven't yet been performed on U.S. populations, but because the Swedish diet is much like our own, Dr. Jacobson suspects that similar deficiencies may occur in as many people in the United States.

Are you one of those who are likely to be low? Dr. Jacobson, who teaches nutrition to medical students, eats a well-balanced diet high in fruits, vegetables and grains as recommended by most nutritionists—and *she* has trouble getting the RDA. "I've analyzed my own diet, and unless I take a dietary supplement, I don't get adequate niacin," says Dr. Jacobson.

Those particularly at risk for being low in niacin include people who don't consume much meat, al-

AT A GLANCE

NIACIN

RDA: Men: 15 mg. Women: 13 mg.

Good food sources: Whole grains and lean meats. Milk and eggs are excellent sources of tryptophan, which converts to niacin.

Who's at risk for deficiency: The elderly, people on limited diets, alcoholics and people with eating disorders or absorption disorders.

Possible signs of deficiency include: Skin changes that may resemble sunburn; also anemia, anxiety, depression and fatigue.

Advice for use: Nicotinic acid (niacin) or timed-release niacin should be taken only with a doctor's supervision.

coholics, elderly people, and "youngsters who live on french fries," she says. It's also unclear if the currently recommended levels are adequate for optimal health, says Dr. Jacobson: She predicts that the RDAs will eventually be raised.

How Safe Is Niacin?

The niacin that's present in foods won't harm you. Supplemental niacin in the form of nicotinic acid, however, can have side effects. Some are fairly harmless—flushing, itchy and tingling skin, rash and headache—but others are potentially serious. High doses of nicotinic acid can cause or worsen liver damage, blood sugar problems, peptic ulcer and gout.

Yes, you can find nicotinic acid labeled as niacin on store shelves, but doctors agree you should *never* take these products unless they have been prescribed for you. Timed-release niacin, properly administered, is safe and effective. Improperly administered, however, it can be particularly dangerous. "There is definitely a problem with people self-medicating with slow-release niacin," says Jere P. Segrest, M.D., Ph.D., professor of medicine and biochemistry and director of the Atherosclerosis Research Unit at the University of Alabama at Birmingham.

"People think you don't get into trouble until you're on high doses for a long time," says Todd D. Miller, M.D., consultant in the Division of Cardiovascular Disease at the Mayo Clinic and assistant professor of medicine at the Mayo Medical School in Rochester, Minnesota. "With the timed-release form, however, you can develop liver problems at much lower doses after a relatively short time."

When doctors prescribe niacin, they often do routine tests to head off complications. Thomas G. Pickering, M.D., professor of medicine at Cornell Medical Center in New York City, tests liver function, blood sugar and uric acid in cholesterol patients who are being treated with niacin.

The other form of niacin, nicotinamide, won't cause flushing or liver damage, but in large doses it may cause other unpleasant symptoms, including headache, heartburn, nausea, hives, sore throat and fatigue. (And it does nothing for cholesterol or triglycerides.)

If you think you need to boost your niacin intake to reach the RDA, Dr. Jacobson suggests you take a daily multivitamin containing 15 to 20 milligrams of niacin in the form of niacinamide.

If you'd like to consider high doses of niacin for a cholesterol problem, talk to your doctor.

Pantothenic Acid

A Premature Debutante

> **POTENTIAL HEALING POWER**
>
> May help:
> • Speed wound healing
> • Ease arthritis pain
> • Lower cholesterol and triglycerides
> • Improve athletic performance

Talking about your career is a common conversational icebreaker. But when your life's work is studying a rather obscure vitamin, talking about it can be a real conversation killer.

"So what do you do for a living?"

"I study pantothenic acid." (Long pause.) "It's a vitamin." (Longer pause.) "Say, did you catch that last Wolverines game?"

But things have changed in recent years, says Won O. Song, R.D., Ph.D., associate professor at Michigan State University in East Lansing, who has been studying pantothenic acid for more than a decade. This B vitamin has not only clawed its way out of obscurity but has ascended to a prominent place on the shelves of health food stores. "This is all of a sudden a very popular vitamin for supplementation," says Dr. Song.

Which leaves Dr. Song with

mixed feelings. Sure, it's nice to have your favorite vitamin appreciated, but there's such a thing as "coming out" too soon. It's true that various studies hint tantalizingly at possible benefits waiting to be reaped from pantothenic acid— from helping arthritis to healing wounds to lowering cholesterol. But the research is still in its infancy.

"There are a lot of exciting prospects and exciting hypotheses," says Dr. Song. "But they are still just prospects."

An Inflated Reputation

Let's take a look at what pantothenic acid can or *may* do.

Many people pop pantothenic acid tablets in the hope that the nutrient will improve their ability to handle stress. This notion stemmed from a study conducted years ago that showed that pantothenic acid deficiency in rats caused failure of the adrenal gland, which pumps out the stimulant adrenaline. "From that, many people still associate a lack of pantothenic acid with stress, but making such a conclusion for humans based on rat studies is not sound thinking," says Dr. Song.

Others have the idea that pantothenic acid improves athletic ability. At least one study suggested this: Distance runners given large daily doses of pantothenic acid for two weeks outperformed other runners who didn't get pantothenic acid. Sounds great, right? But a similar study found no difference between runners who got the vitamin and ones who didn't. Conclusion: No one knows.

On a Promising Track

In several other areas, the research is a bit stronger. For instance, decades ago researchers found that people with rheumatoid arthritis have less pantothenic acid in their blood than other people. And when these people received 50 milligrams of pantothenic acid daily, in the form of calcium pantothenate, their blood levels became normal and many symptoms of arthritis improved. One study found that large daily doses of calcium pantothenate reduced stiffness and pain in people with rheumatoid arthritis. But other studies haven't yet confirmed this, says Dr. Song.

Moving down the list of possible benefits, you'll find triglycerides, a particularly harmful type of blood fat, and cholesterol. In several studies, a form of pantothenic acid called pantethine apparently lowered cholesterol around 15 percent and triglycerides about 30 percent in people with high cholesterol and high triglycerides. Once again, the research looks promising, but there's not enough of it to prove anything—at least not yet.

And finally, there's wound healing. Preliminary studies look good: In the laboratory, pantothenic acid has improved the skin

PANTOTHENIC ACID

Estimated Safe and Adequate Daily Intake: 4 to 7 mg.

Good food sources: Mushrooms, avocados, broccoli, baker's yeast, whole grains, peanuts, cashews, lentils, soybeans and eggs.

Who's at risk for deficiency: Alcoholics and elderly people on restricted diets.

Possible signs of deficiency include: Burning and tickling in the toes and soles of the feet, depression, fatigue, insomnia, vomiting and muscle weakness.

strength of scar tissue, and in another study a diet with no pantothenic acid apparently delayed healing. More recently, also in the laboratory, French researchers found that pantothenic acid caused increased skin cell growth and suggest that this vitamin may be useful in wound healing.

Just the Facts

The fact is that if you're deficient in pantothenic acid, you'll certainly benefit from taking in more of this nutrient, whether in supplement form or in foods such as whole grains, legumes and various vegetables. And pantothenic acid is readily available in many foods; *pantothen*, in fact, means "from all sides" in Greek.

But deficiency is nothing for you to worry about. It's only known to occur in the seriously malnourished. Poorly fed World War II prisoners in the Philippines, Japan and Burma, for example, suffered from something called burning foot syndrome, which improved with large doses of calcium pantothenate. Other symptoms of deficiency can include depression, fatigue, insomnia, muscle weakness and vomiting.

Few of us today are likely to be low in pantothenic acid, says Dr. Song. Alcoholics are at risk for a deficiency of this nutrient (as well as many other vitamins), and elderly people who eat a very limited diet also may be low.

There is no Recommended Dietary Allowance for this nutrient, but the Food and Nutrition Board of the National Research Council estimates that we need from four to seven milligrams a day. People in the United States generally take in about five to ten milligrams a day.

Pantothenic acid is a relatively harmless vitamin, and people have taken as much as 100 milligrams daily with no apparent harm. But Dr. Song doesn't recommend this. No one yet really knows how much pantothenic acid is too much and whether or not there may be bad effects from large doses, she says. In one study, rats receiving the equivalent of 10 to 20 times the recommended amount actually stored *less* of the vitamin than if they were taking in a reasonable amount!

Dr. Song recommends eating a balanced diet and leaving the pantothenic acid supplements on the shelf, at least until we know more.

Potassium

A Blood Pressure Tamer

POTENTIAL HEALING POWER

May help:
- Lower blood pressure
- Protect against stroke
- Thwart heart disease
- Prevent kidney problems
- Lower risk of cancer

Early man had lots to worry about—saber-toothed tigers, bears, marauding bands of wolves.

But, unlike modern man, one thing they most likely *didn't* have to worry about was high blood pressure and its deadly companions—stroke, heart disease and kidney failure.

Why? One reason is that the Stone Age diet of fruit, vegetables, roots, nuts and an occasional slab of woolly mammoth undoubtedly provided a huge amount of potassium.

Diets that include generous amounts of potassium-rich foods have been associated with lower blood pressure and fewer deaths from strokes. Some animal studies indicate that potassium may also protect against high cholesterol. And preliminary research suggests that a potassium-rich diet may even ward off cancer.

Dropping Blood Pressure

There's no doubt about it. In population studies from around the world, people who eat low-potassium diets have more heart disease, higher blood pressure and generally poorer health than those eating high-potassium diets. Groups whose potassium-poor diet puts them at highest risk include people in Scotland, Newfoundland and Tibet and blacks in the southeastern United States, says Louis Tobian, M.D., professor of medicine and head of the Hypertension Section of the University of Minnesota Hospital in Minneapolis.

"These people *don't* have what would be considered a classic potassium deficiency, with symptoms of muscle weakness, confusion and heart irregularities," Dr. Tobian says. "But there's no doubt that their marginal intake puts them at higher-than-normal risk for a variety of problems such as hypertension."

Several studies confirm the link between potassium and blood pressure. In one study, ten men with normal blood pressure were put on two experimental diets by researchers at Temple University School of Medicine and the University of Pennsylvania in Philadelphia. One diet provided normal amounts of potassium; the other was low in potassium. After nine days on the normal-potassium diet, the men showed no significant change in blood pressure. But after the same amount of time on the low-potassium diet, their blood pressure went up an average of five points. Similar results were observed in men with high blood pressure.

In another study, researchers in Italy found that when people with high blood pressure went on a potassium-rich diet that included beans, fruits and vegetables, within a year most were able to reduce their blood pressure medication to less than half the dosage they'd been using previously.

Sodium Check

Potassium helps to control blood pressure by interacting with sodium, or salt, to maintain a proper balance of fluid in the body, explains Gopal Krishna, M.D., attending physician with Central Coast Nephrology in Salinas, California.

Think of sodium as a kind of water magnet, Dr. Krishna suggests. "You do need some sodium in your body, but too much sodium makes your body retain water. In some people, that extra fluid ends up in the bloodstream and increases blood pressure."

Potassium helps the body to excrete sodium. Once you lose the sodium, you also lose the excess fluid that risks jacking up your blood pressure, Dr. Krishna explains.

Stopping Deaths from Stroke

If potassium protects against high blood pressure, it stands to reason that it would also help to protect against stroke, a potentially fatal brain hemorrhage that occurs much more frequently in people with high blood pressure.

As yet, the link between potassium and the risk of stroke has not been studied enough for scientists to make any firm conclusions. But a study by researchers at the University of California, San Diego, shows that getting about an extra banana's worth of potassium in your diet each day may save your life if you have a stroke. And that protection works whether your blood pressure is high or normal, researchers say.

The researchers spent 12 years looking at people who lived in a large retirement community. At the end of that time, they found that those who ate the least potassium had the highest incidence of stroke-associated death. "The more potassium these people ate, the less their risk of death from stroke," Dr. Krishna explains.

And those in the study who ate the most potassium had *no* deaths from stroke. How much were they eating? About 3,000 milligrams a day. That's an amount that can be achieved in a diet that includes five to six servings each day of fresh fruits and vegetables, such as bananas and potatoes. One baked potato, for example, has about 850 milligrams of potassium.

How might the potassium work in this case? Dr. Tobian has found that, besides helping to keep blood pressure normal, potassium may also protect blood vessel walls from the ravaging effects of salt and cholesterol. In one laboratory study, says Dr. Tobian, a high-potassium diet reduced the buildup of artery-

---

AT A GLANCE

POTASSIUM

RDA: None established. Researchers suggest 3,000 to 4,000 mg a day.

Good food sources: Prune juice, carrot juice, low-sodium tomato juice, orange juice, baked potatoes, avocados, bananas, clams, nonfat yogurt and many fruits and vegetables (as long as they're steamed, not boiled).

Who's at risk for deficiency: People taking potassium-depleting diuretics, digitalis (a heart drug) or steroids, people who don't eat fruits or vegetables, heavy drinkers, people who have prolonged vomiting or chronic diarrhea or abuse laxatives.

Possible signs of deficiency include: Weakness, confusion, loss of appetite, nausea, listlessness, apprehension, drowsiness and irrational behavior. Severe deficiency can cause heart irregularities.

Advice for use: Supplements are not recommended except when prescribed by a doctor. Too much potassium can upset the balance of other minerals in the body and cause heart and kidney problems.

clogging cholesterol deposits in animals by 64 percent.

In another animal study, a diet rich in potassium helped to prevent the microscopic thickening and splitting of artery walls that invites cholesterol deposits, Dr. Tobian adds.

KO'ing Cancer?

Studies also have found that laboratory animals that are fed a potassium-poor diet are more likely to develop cancerous tumors than animals fed a high-potassium diet. And several population studies suggest there might be a role for potassium in cancer prevention for humans as well.

"Potassium, counteracting sodium, seems to help regulate cell growth," says researcher Birger Jansson, Ph.D., professor of biomathematics at the M. D. Anderson Cancer Center in Houston.

"In the presence of excess sodium, cells can grow abnormally," Dr. Jansson explains. "Their chances of becoming cancerous increase. But adequate amounts of potassium help reduce the harmful effects of sodium and so normalize cell growth and reduce the likelihood of cancer."

Upping Your Intake

Although serious potassium deficiency is rare, it's likely that many of us aren't getting enough potassium to fully benefit from its protective effects, Dr. Tobian says.

How much potassium do you need each day to get maximum benefits? No one knows for sure. "An ideal amount has yet to be determined," Dr. Krishna says.

There is no Recommended Dietary Allowance for potassium. Both Dr. Krishna and Dr. Tobian suggest you aim for 3,000 to 4,000 milligrams of potassium a day. Studies show that intake varies widely. (The incidence of serious kidney damage caused by high blood pressure is 18 times higher among blacks than whites and correlates with differences in potassium intake.)

Besides eating more fruits and vegetables, Dr. Tobian suggests you trade in your favorite diet soda for orange juice (with 500 milligrams per eight-ounce glass) or grapefruit juice (with 375 milligrams for the same amount). Low-sodium tomato juice (525 milligrams), prune juice and carrot juice (700 milligrams each) are also top-notch sources.

Are potassium supplements necessary or desirable? They may be, for some people.

Potassium supplements are routinely prescribed for people taking a potassium-depleting diuretic (a drug that promotes urine excretion and is used to reduce high blood pressure). "They lose so much potassium through their kidneys that they simply can't make up for it in their diet," Dr. Tobian explains. Their blood levels of potassium are monitored by their doctor.

And Dr. Tobian may add potassium supplements to a potassium-rich diet for someone who's at high risk for stroke. "I have some patients with a horrible family history for stroke. They are scared to death, and I want to do everything I can for them, so they get potassium supplements."

These people may get 5,000 milligrams or more a day of potassium, through diet and supplements. Again, their blood levels of potassium are carefully monitored. "That's important," Dr. Tobian says. "People with diabetes or kidney problems, people who are taking a potassium-sparing diuretic called spironolactone and people taking

an ACE inhibitor (a heart drug) may all retain potassium and build up dangerous levels in their blood. They need to be careful."

Potassium supplements are sold over the counter. Because of possible stomach irritation caused by some forms of potassium and the risks associated with overdose, they are available only in small dosages. The Food and Drug Administration allows no formula to offer more than 99 milligrams per tablet. That's about as much potassium as in one or two bites of potato. Most doctors agree you'd be better off eating the potato. Supplements containing larger amounts of potassium are available only with a doctor's prescription.

Primrose Oil (GLA)

Promise or Puffery?

You're leafing through a magazine and there at the back—sandwiched between an offer for mail-order toupees and one for a secret muscle formula—is an ad that jumps out at you. PRIMROSE OIL: Cures eczema! Relieves breast pain! Helps with diabetes! Treats arthritis! Fights cancer!

POTENTIAL HEALING POWER

May help:
- Treat rheumatoid arthritis
- Control atopic dermatitis
- Relieve some symptoms of diabetes
- Inhibit cancer
- Relieve breast pain

Sounds like just the thing for your family. The stuff's kind of pricey but hey, what price health, right?

The problem is that no one has proved that primrose oil accomplishes any of these things, says Robert Chapkin, Ph.D., assistant professor of molecular and cell biology at Texas A & M University in College Station. "I've done possibly more studies on this than almost anyone in the world," he says, "and I'm hesitant to tell you to take primrose oil."

It's true that studies, mostly with animals, have turned up some promising results—and Dr. Chapkin is quick to point out that he may change his tune a few years down the road—but currently there's no strong evidence that primrose oil offers any benefit to humans.

The Special Ingredient

What is primrose oil, and what's in it that makes scientists pay attention? If you've strolled around after dinner and noticed yellow-petaled flowers that open in the evening, you've seen evening primroses, whose seeds are the source of primrose oil. In turn, primrose oil is a source of something called gamma-linolenic acid (GLA). It's GLA that buyers of primrose oil are *really* after.

What's so great about GLA? In your body it turns into a hormone called a prostaglandin. Among other things, prostaglandin helps keep your blood vessels healthy, your gastrointestinal tract functioning and your blood sugar stable.

You can get GLA in two ways.

Your body can make it from another fat, linoleic acid, which you can eat every day in oils, fish, nuts and other foods. Or you can take a primrose oil supplement, available at many health food stores. (Borage oil, a supplement made from the borage plant, and black currant oil are also potential sources of GLA.)

Taking GLA directly from a supplement *may* have beneficial effects, says Dr. Chapkin. One promising area of GLA research concerns arthritis. A 1988 study at the Centre for Rheumatic Diseases in Glasgow, Scotland, showed that people with rheumatoid arthritis who took GLA daily in the form of primrose oil showed definite improvement.

"GLA is converted to a prostaglandin that appears to have anti-inflammatory properties under certain conditions," says Dr. Chapkin. The unanswered question, he says, is whether taking GLA in supplement form will cause significant, consistent improvement in people with arthritis.

Down the Road

How about all those other claims?

"There's some evidence, albeit inconsistent, that an appropriate dose of GLA over several weeks can be of some moderate benefit in controlling an inflammatory skin condition known as atopic dermatitis," says Bruce Holub, Ph.D., professor in the Department of Nutritional Sciences at the University of Guelph in Ontario. As yet, however, GLA as taken in primrose oil is not a standard treatment for this condition.

There's also evidence that GLA from primrose oil may help those with diabetes. In a Tokyo study, children with diabetes who were given GLA supplements over eight months could metabolize fats and prostaglandins better than other children with diabetes. Researchers suggest that GLA supplementation might help prevent the kinds of blood vessel problems common among people with diabetes. But, here again, the results are speculative.

And researchers at the University Hospital of South Manchester in Great Britain report that women with breast pain who took primrose oil daily for four months reported that they had less breast pain and tenderness.

How about cancer? A study at Rhodes University in Grahamstown, South Africa, found that GLA inhibited the growth of cancer cells in laboratory mice. But this doesn't necessarily mean that GLA has any effect on cancer in humans, says Dr. Chapkin.

The bottom line on primrose oil? "We just don't know yet," says Dr. Chapkin. If you want to try it, it probably won't hurt you. But don't expect miracles, he says. And do consult your doctor first.

AT A GLANCE

PRIMROSE OIL (GLA)

RDA: None established.

Good food sources: None.

Who's at risk for deficiency: Primrose oil is not considered essential, so deficiency is unlikely.

Possible signs of deficiency include: There are no known signs of primrose oil deficiency.

Advice for use: Suggested dosages of primrose oil pose little risk to healthy people. But those with temporal lobe epilepsy or manic-depressive disorder should avoid it, because supplements have been reported to aggravate these conditions.

Riboflavin

The Exerciser's Ally

POTENTIAL HEALING POWER

May help:
- Improve memory
- Combat certain cancers
- Prevent cataracts, particularly among smokers
- Foster wound healing

Josephine, who's nearly 70, just doesn't have the appetite she did when she was younger. Hank, a teenager, probably eats more junk food than he should. Paula, a marathon runner, trains daily.

Who's likely to be deficient in riboflavin?

You're right if you picked Josephine . . . or Hank . . . or Paula. People likely to be marginally deficient in this vitamin include the elderly, people who don't consume dairy products and those who are physically very active.

Those in Need

We get riboflavin (also known as vitamin B$_2$) primarily from foods such as milk, eggs, meat and green leafy vegetables. Statistics tell us that most people get at least the Recommended Dietary Allowance (RDA): U.S. Department of Agriculture (USDA) studies showed that in 1985 men consumed an average of 2.1 milligrams and women 1.3 milligrams. That's above the RDA of 1.7 milligrams for men and right on the money for women whose RDA is 1.3. But some people do fall short.

The elderly tend to be low because they eat fewer riboflavin-rich foods. And anyone who avoids dairy products may also be low in riboflavin. A study of 431 high school students, for example, found that 16 percent of the girls and 6 percent of the boys had inadequate riboflavin intakes. The less milk they drank, the more likely they were to have a deficiency.

The third group of people who may be short on riboflavin are the physically active.

"If you're an athlete, you may need as much as 50 percent more riboflavin," says Jack M. Cooperman, Ph.D., former clinical professor of community and preventive medicine at New York Medical College in Valhalla. Exercise increases the need for riboflavin, apparently because it increases the rate at which you excrete this vitamin.

When You Run Low

Riboflavin is a "helper" nutrient that makes many reactions in the body happen, including reactions that "release" other nutrients. Riboflavin helps change vitamin B_6 and folic acid into forms the body can use. It also helps to change the amino acid tryptophan (found in protein) into yet *another* essential B vitamin, niacin. Translated, this means that if you're low in riboflavin, you're likely to end up low in B_6, folic acid and possibly niacin as well.

Early riboflavin deficiency can cause symptoms such as cracks at the corners of the mouth, inflamed lips and a reddened tongue, although these symptoms can take several months to appear. Riboflavin deficiency can also slow growth and cause scaling of the mouth, nose and genitals.

Marginally low levels of riboflavin also may affect short-term memory, according to research at the USDA's Human Nutrition Research Center at Grand Forks, North Dakota. In a study of 28 healthy people over the age of 60, the ones with higher levels of riboflavin showed better performance on tasks that emphasized memory.

AT A GLANCE

RIBOFLAVIN

RDA: Men: 1.7 mg. Women: 1.3 mg.

Good food sources: Milk, yogurt, cheese, cottage cheese, egg whites, beef, pork, lamb, chicken, broccoli and asparagus.

Who's at risk for deficiency: People on poorly balanced or low-calorie diets, people who don't consume dairy products, eggs or meat, alcoholics and possibly people who are very physically active.

Possible signs of deficiency include: Cracks at the corners of the mouth, inflamed lips and reddened tongue. Later symptoms include slowed growth (in children) and scaling of the mouth, nose and genitals.

Advice for use: It's best to get riboflavin from foods or in a balanced supplement. Supplemental riboflavin is safe up to 100 mg daily, but in larger doses it could possibly cause kidney stones.

The Twilight Zone

Some of the claims you might hear about riboflavin are still being debated by scientists.

The evidence for cancer prevention, for example, is spotty. In laboratory studies, a lack of riboflavin enhances the growth of some cancers, while it *slows* other types. Some research does show that a riboflavin deficiency in animals can cause changes similar to early esophageal cancer in humans.

Some people believe that you need more riboflavin in times of stress. While hard work, heat stress and exercise may cause riboflavin to be excreted, there's no good evidence that mental stress increases the need for riboflavin, says Dr. Cooperman.

And there's some suggestion that riboflavin may help prevent cataracts. In a study of 1,380 adults, intakes of riboflavin, along with the vitamins C and E and carotene, were linked with lower risk of cataracts. It's also possible—but by no means proven—that people who smoke may need higher levels of riboflavin to help prevent cataracts.

Pumping In the Riboflavin

Wondering how much is enough? Two cups of skim milk a day provide about half your daily requirement. Meat and eggs are also good sources, and one serving of most fortified breakfast cereals contains about 25 percent of the U.S. RDA.

But if you suspect you don't get adequate riboflavin via foods—either because you consume little meat, milk, eggs or cereal or because you exercise strenuously—go ahead and take a daily balanced multivitamin containing riboflavin. You can also find riboflavin in single supplements up to 100 milligrams. Although that's far, far more than you can use, it probably won't harm you. But beware, says Dr. Cooperman—very high levels could put you at a higher risk for kidney stones.

Selenium

Cure of the Future?

The year is 2020, and you're at the doctor's office with an arthritic knee. The guy next to you has a heart condition, and the woman next to him is there for a precancerous growth. The doctor sees each of you in turn and hands out individual prescriptions. Each prescription is for the same thing: selenium tablets.

Farfetched? Gerhard Schrauzer, Ph.D., chemistry professor at the University of California, San Diego, firmly believes that selenium will someday be widely used as a preventive for cancer. Other experts say this mineral may increase immunity, help fight arthritis and reduce the incidence of heart attack.

But some other researchers pooh-pooh the whole idea that supplements of selenium can help fight disease. "There's a lot of 'wishful thinking' with selenium," says Raymond Burk, M.D., director of the Division of Gastroenterology at the Vanderbilt University School of Medicine in Nashville, Tennessee. "I don't think there's any convincing evidence that supplemental selenium will improve your health." Who's right? Let's take a look at what scientists have discovered so far.

The Cancer Connection

You've probably heard of "free radicals." These are by-products of normal chemical reactions in your body, and they can weaken a cell enough to make it susceptible to cancer. Luckily, your body produces certain enzymes that help keep these developments from happening. Selenium just happens to be essential in the formation of these enzymes. That's the first piece of evidence that selenium is a cancer fighter.

The second piece of evidence can be seen on a map. People with the highest cancer rates live in areas with the *least* selenium in the soil. And there are fewer cancers of the lung, rectum, bladder, esophagus, cervix and uterus in areas with *lots* of selenium.

Scientists also know that selenium protects against liver, skin, mammary and colon cancer in animals. In one study of mice likely to develop cancer, only 10 percent of the mice receiving selenium developed cancer, while *82 percent* of the other mice did.

Helping Circulation

How about your heart and arteries? Pick up that map again. Stretching from Georgia through the Carolinas there's a "stroke belt," an area that has high rates of stroke and heart disease—and little selenium in the soil. In China, there's a large selenium-poor area that runs from the north-

east to the southwest, where selenium-deficient women and children are prone to a disease that damages heart muscle.

More evidence of the heart/selenium connection comes from Finland, where a study of 11,000 people found that three-fourths of the people who died from heart attacks had low blood levels of selenium.

These population studies do not prove that selenium is a heart protector, but they certainly point in that direction.

Promising Possibilities

Selenium may help fight arthritis and other inflammatory diseases. Take another look at China, where millions of people—usually children—develop Kashin-Beck

---

AT A GLANCE

SELENIUM

RDA: Men: 70 mcg. Women: 55 mcg.

Good food sources: Fish, shellfish, whole-grain cereals, bagels and breads, mushrooms, Brazil nuts and dairy products.

Who's at risk for deficiency: Possibly people who live in areas where the soil is low in selenium.

Possible signs of deficiency include: Muscle pain and weakness, disease of the heart muscle and abnormal fingernails.

Advice for use: Selenium yeast and selenomethionine are the preferred forms of supplements. Individual supplements of sodium selenite should be avoided. Doses in excess of 200 mcg a day in any form should not be taken.

WHERE DO YOUR FOODS RANK?

Wondering whether the asparagus you're dining on is high or low in selenium? It depends on where it was grown. These ten states (listed alphabetically) have the highest soil content of selenium, and foods grown there tend to have the highest selenium content.

Arizona	New Mexico
Colorado	North Dakota
Kansas	South Dakota
Montana	Utah
Nebraska	Wyoming

disease, with enlarged joints, a deformed spinal column and atrophied muscles. Once again, selenium deficiency appears to be a culprit: One study found that supplementation with selenium and vitamin E helped 83 percent of these people. Another study in Brussels, Belgium, showed promising improvement in 40 percent of people with rheumatoid arthritis who took selenium supplements.

Other studies suggest that selenium may help boost your immune power, which could help you fight off anything from a cold to the flu to a sinus infection. A study of people being fed intravenously found their immune system improved when they were given 200 micrograms of selenium daily for two months. In animals, selenium increases the production of antibodies that fight infection.

And at least one study suggests that selenium may affect your mood as well as your health. Researchers at the University College in Swansea, Wales, found that when dietary intakes of selenium went down, people reported feeling anxious, depressed and tired more often. A daily supplement of 100 micrograms improved mood and anxiety levels.

The Perils of Selenium

Despite these bright promises, selenium does have a dark side: It *can* be toxic. In 1984 one woman experienced hair loss, infected fingernails, fatigue, nausea and vomiting. Puzzled doctors at first blamed her symptoms on emotional stress from the death of her husband. But it turned out that she was taking a selenium supplement containing over 200 times the amount it should have. Each tablet had about 31,000 micrograms of selenium—while the current Recommended Dietary Allowance (RDA) for women is 55 micrograms. At least 12 other people also experienced problems from the incorrectly formulated supplements.

In other cases, people who took in 5,000 micrograms a day from foods grown in high-selenium soils in China (yes, some parts of China have more than enough selenium) experienced hair loss and fingernail changes, and one person who took 1,000 micrograms of selenium daily for more than two years had thickened, fragile nails and a garlicky odor.

Finding the exact point where selenium becomes dangerous is difficult, says Orville A. Levander, Ph.D., research chemist with the U.S. Department of Agriculture's Human Nutrition Research Center in Beltsville, Maryland. "You have to rely on your hair falling out," he says, "which is way beyond the point people want to be." One U.S. study, however, found no problems when people were taking in as much as 724 micrograms a day.

Finding a Balance

In 1980 the Food and Nutrition Board of the National Research Council suggested that 50 to 200 micrograms a day was a safe and adequate intake, but in 1989 the board set RDAs of 70 micrograms

daily for men and 55 micrograms for women. Most of us easily get this much. Statistics show that the average daily intake is over 100 micrograms. Have you had a tuna sandwich lately? You just downed 95 micrograms of selenium. Other everyday sources of selenium include bagels (32 micrograms), cottage cheese (23 micrograms) and mushrooms (13 micrograms).

But what about taking selenium to stave off disease? There's no official stance on this, but Dr. Schrauzer recommends 150 to 200 micrograms daily in addition to the selenium you get in foods. Sheldon Saul Hendler, M.D., Ph.D., assistant clinical professor of medicine at the University of California, San Diego, and author of *The Doctor's Vitamin and Mineral Encyclopedia*, suggests supplementing your daily diet with 50 to 200 micrograms.

If you're shopping for a selenium supplement, experts agree you should look for one marked either "selenomethionine" or "selenium yeast." Avoid those marked "sodium selenite." This form can not only react with vitamin C to block selenium absorption, points out Dr. Hendler, but is also more likely to cause side effects such as nausea, blackened nails and a garlicky odor. Many multivitamin/mineral supplements that contain selenium offer it in the form of sodium selenite. The amount in these supplements, however—usually 25 micrograms—is too small to cause problems.

Silicon

A Calcium Crony

What's the most common element on earth? Okay, that's easy—you probably correctly guessed oxygen. But what's the *second* most common?

Unless you remember your chemistry classes better than most of us do, you won't get this one right. The answer is silicon, which is also the most abundant mineral in the earth's crust.

Yes, this is the same element used to make glass, semiconductors and those controversial breast implants. It's also a mineral that researchers suspect may be essential to strong, healthy bodies.

Good to the Bone

Based on animal studies, nutritionists believe that silicon plays a role in forming and maintaining bones, skin, fingernails and connective tissue. Certain silicon-deficient animals, for example, show poorly formed joints and abnormal bones, including abnormally shaped skulls. Part of silicon's power seems to be its role in helping bones to use calcium.

Some researchers think silicon also plays a role in preventing atherosclerosis—plaque deposits in the arteries. "In aging there is a decrease in silicon content in the heart's aorta," says Edith M. Carlisle, Ph.D., professor in the Environmental and Nutritional Sciences Department in the School of Public Health at the University of California, Los Angeles. "Silicon could be involved in maintaining the health of the cardiovascular system," she says.

Taking Out Insurance

How much silicon do we need? Nobody knows for sure—there's no Recommended Dietary Allowance or Estimated Safe and Adequate Daily Intake. It's not even proven that silicon is essential to humans, even though scientists believe that animals require it.

It's been suggested that an adequate intake for humans is five to ten milligrams a day, and according to Forrest H. Nielsen, di-

AT A GLANCE

SILICON

RDA: None established.

Good food sources: Unrefined grains and cereals, and root vegetables such as carrots, potatoes and beets.

Who's at risk for deficiency: Possibly the elderly.

Possible signs of deficiency include: In animals, deficiency causes slowed or stunted growth and abnormalities in bones and joints. There are no known signs of silicon deficiency in humans.

Advice for use: Supplements are not recommended.

rector of the U.S. Department of Agriculture's Human Nutrition Research Center in Grand Forks, North Dakota, most of us consume this amount.

If you're low in silicon, you won't know it: Scientists have never seen silicon deficiency in humans, and they don't know what the symptoms are.

Where do you get silicon? It's present in foods such as unrefined grains and cereals, root vegetables, and of course dietary supplements. It's also in many antacids, in the form of magnesium trisilicate.

So do you need a supplement?

"If your diet is rich in high-fiber grains and cereal, or if your multivitamin contains silicon, there is little need, if any, for separate silicon supplements," says Dr. Carlisle.

Thiamin

The Balancing B Vitamin

Signing up for the Japanese navy was once a risky business. In the four years from 1880 through 1883 alone, more than 6,000 sailors died—nearly *one-third* of those who had set sail.

No, they didn't die in battle. The deaths were caused by the lack of one little nutrient. The sailors' diet of primarily rice contained virtually no thiamin, and they died from a disease called beriberi. When thiamin-rich foods were added to the sailors' diet, beriberi disappeared.

A Debilitating Disease

The word *beriberi* means "I cannot" in Sinhalese, a language of Sri Lanka, and probably refers to the lack of muscle coordination caused by the disease. It occurs most often in certain Asian countries like Myamos (formerly Burma), where some people practically live on processed white rice. This unbalanced diet creates a double whammy: Not only does it contain little thiamin (also known as vitamin B_1), but the high amount of refined carbohydrate increases the need for this vitamin.

Alcoholics are also vulnerable to thiamin deficiency. Not only do they often eat unbalanced diets, but alcohol interferes directly with thiamin. It partially blocks thiamin's absorption in the intestine, keeps other tissues from storing it and interferes with its conversion into a form the body can use.

Many alcoholics, in fact, show symptoms of early beriberi, including confusion, vision problems and staggering. Other early symptoms of thiamin deficiency include irritability, nausea, loss of appetite and numbness in the legs. Full-blown beriberi takes on two forms—"wet" and "dry." With dry beriberi, sufferers become thin and emaciated. With wet beriberi, the limbs swell and fluid accumulates in the heart muscle, eventually causing heart failure.

Flirting with Deficiency

Full-blown thiamin deficiency seldom occurs in the United States, except in some alcoholics. But a few other groups may be at risk for *marginal* deficiency, particularly the elderly, says Robert E. Keith, Ph.D., professor in the Department of Nutrition and Food Science at Auburn University in Alabama. "Some groups of the elderly are deficient in several vitamins," he says. "Frequently they just don't eat enough."

Who else is at risk? Say you've gotten tired of those extra pounds around your middle, and you've gone on a strict diet and added an hour of daily exercise.

This could produce marginal thiamin deficiency, says Dr. Keith. You're probably decreasing your thiamin intake as you eat less food, and the increased physical activity is burning up more as well. Ironically, it's possible that very active athletes who take in *too many* calories—particularly in the form of refined carbohydrates—may also be low in thiamin.

Therapy with Thiamin

It's modern folklore that thiamin cures depression, and there may be a bit of truth to this—at least when there's a mild deficiency involved. In one study, researchers from the University of California, Davis, fed thiamin supplements to 80 older Irish women who had moderate thiamin deficiency. The supplements improved the women's sleep patterns, decreased fatigue and restored appetite and general

---

AT A GLANCE

THIAMIN

RDA: Men: 1.5 mg. Women: 1.1 mg.

Good food sources: Pork, whole-grain wheat and rye products, oatmeal, brown rice, green peas, brewer's yeast and eggs.

Who's at risk for deficiency: Chronic alcoholics and people on low-calorie diets.

Possible signs of deficiency include: Confusion, vision problems, staggering, irritability, nausea, loss of appetite and numbness in the legs.

Advice for use: It's best to take thiamin in a balanced multivitamin/mineral supplement. Single supplements should not exceed 10 mg daily.

well-being. The researchers suggested that people over 65 with symptoms of depression consider having their thiamin status checked.

Another use of thiamin has never been scientifically validated, but some folks swear by it: They believe it repels biting insects such as mosquitoes and fleas. The theory is that the vitamin releases an odor in your sweat that repels the invaders. While there's no proof, experts say that it can't hurt to try moderate doses.

To Supplement or Not to Supplement?

Once again, few of us have to worry about serious deficiency: You probably get enough thiamin in your daily diet. For example, a breakfast of orange juice, toast and cereal with milk, topped by a banana, provides more than half your daily requirement.

But marginal deficiencies do exist. So what's an athlete or dieter or elderly person to do? You could get enough thiamin by very carefully selecting foods high in this vitamin—such as whole grains and eggs—but it wouldn't hurt to also take a balanced multivitamin/mineral supplement containing a milligram or so of thiamin, says Dr. Keith. "It's sort of the shotgun approach," he says. "It won't hurt, and it may help."

For most of us, there's not much point in taking enormous doses of this vitamin, which you can find on health food store shelves in amounts as high as 500 milligrams. Most of us require a bit over 1 milligram a day, and you wouldn't be able to use much more, says Dr. Keith. Thiamin has to attach to an enzyme to work, and you only have a limited number of these enzymes. "If you take in 50 milligrams of thiamin, you may have 48 milligrams with no place to go but into your urine."

Dr. Keith advises against such high doses. "We just don't know much about thiamin in huge doses," he says.

Zinc

An Immune Assistant

POTENTIAL HEALING POWER

May help:
- Maintain sense of taste
- Foster wound healing
- Protect sexual health
- Combat some vision problems
- Prevent premature delivery
- Maintain memory
- Shorten duration of cold symptoms

After taking a nibble of peas and mashed potatoes, Aunt Mimi pushes her roast beef around on her plate, her fork wavering in her thin hand.

"Come on, Mom," urges Cousin George, worried that your elderly aunt is becoming too gaunt. "You need to eat to keep your strength up." Aunt Mimi, however, puts her fork down. Nothing seems to taste good anymore.

Aunt Mimi's lack of appetite isn't necessarily an unavoidable part of growing older—it could be caused by not getting enough zinc. "The first sign of zinc deficiency is lack of taste, and you see this frequently in older people," says Jack M. Cooperman, Ph.D., former clinical professor of community and preventive medicine at New York Medical College in Valhalla. Studies show that many elderly people probably aren't getting enough of this mineral.

Elderly people often don't eat enough foods high in zinc, such as beef and chicken, says Ranjit Kumar Chandra, M.D., research professor and director of immunology at Memorial University of Newfoundland in St. John's. And it's also possible that they don't absorb zinc as well as they did when they were younger.

But older people aren't the only ones who may be deficient. "Most people don't get enough zinc," says Robert Hackman, Ph.D., associate professor of nutrition at the University of Oregon in Eugene. Pregnant women are at risk for deficiency, and many men, who lose zinc in sweat and in semen, get only about two-thirds of the zinc they need. Vegetarians are particularly at risk, not only because they don't eat meat but also because fiber and another substance in plant foods called phytate interfere with the absorption of zinc. Drugs such as tetracycline, cortisone and diuretics can also interfere with the absorption of zinc, as can lots of iodine.

Why should anyone care about zinc? Because besides maintaining your sense of taste, it helps to fight diseases, heal wounds and keep men sexually potent and their sperm healthy. Severe deficiency can stunt growth and sexual development.

Researchers are also turning up exciting new possible therapeutic uses for zinc. Zinc may help fight colds, improve memory, protect vision and even prevent pregnancy complications and premature births.

Keeping You Healthy

Of all the minerals, zinc is probably the most important for maintaining immunity," says Terry M. Phillips, Ph.D., D.Sc., director of the Immunogenetics and Immunochemistry Laboratories at George Washington University Medical Center in Washington D.C. Too little zinc can lead to a drop in infection-fighting white blood cells. Many other parts of your immune system need zinc, and people with low zinc may be more susceptible to many diseases.

For folks who bemoan the lack of a cure for the common cold, there's hope yet. Zinc can help cut suffering time by more than half. In a study at Dartmouth College in Hanover, New Hampshire, cold-suffering students who sucked on zinc gluconate lozenges at regular intervals got well in about four days, while cold sufferers who took no zinc required nine days to get well. These lozenges particularly helped coughing, nasal drainage and congestion.

Your Brain Needs It

Experiments at the U.S. Department of Agriculture's (USDA) Human Nutrition Research Center in Grand Forks, North Dakota, and elsewhere suggest that zinc is also important to your mind.

When 11 young, healthy men were fed diets very low in zinc, Grand Forks researchers found that their short-term memory, spatial skills and attention span were less than when they were taking in about ten milligrams of zinc a day. In another experiment, zinc and iron supplements helped improve the short-term memory and attention span in 34 young women who had been low in these nutrients.

And when patients at the Lexington, Kentucky, Veterans Administration Medical Center who had suffered head injuries were given large doses of zinc for a month, they showed faster recovery in their mental functioning than those who didn't receive zinc.

"We know zinc is involved in enzyme reactions in the brain," says James Penland, Ph.D., research psychologist with the USDA. "This could influence our brain's ability to function," he says.

AT A GLANCE

ZINC

RDA: Men: 15 mg. Women: 12 mg.

Good food sources: Oysters, crab, lean beef, poultry, milk and whole grains.

Who's at risk for deficiency: The elderly, pregnant women and vegetarians.

Possible signs of deficiency include: Loss of appetite and sense of taste, slowed growth (in children and adolescents), decreased immunity and skin inflammation.

Advice for use: Doses in excess of 15 mg daily should not be taken regularly unless prescribed by a doctor. Too much could adversely affect the immune system, cause stomach irritation and vomiting and prevent the absorption of copper, iron and calcium. Higher doses can also affect taste and smell. If zinc is taken, copper supplements (one-tenth of the zinc dosage) should be taken as well.

Sexual Health

Folklore links eating oysters with fertility and sexual potency, and with good reason, says Dr. Cooperman. Oysters are loaded with zinc, which is important to men's sexual health.

Mild zinc deficiency causes low sperm count, and moderate and severe deficiency can cause a loss of interest in sex. Supplementing with zinc can help increase not only sperm count but also the amount of the male sex hormone testosterone in the blood. A study at the Grand Forks research center showed that men receiving less than 10.4 milligrams of zinc a day had less semen and less testosterone.

And Still More

Zinc may also help maintain good vision. In a study of 151 people with macular degeneration—a progressive eye condition that can eventually lead to near blindness—those who took zinc supplements had better vision than those who didn't take them.

Zinc is also necessary for wound healing. In one study, ten people who took zinc daily required only 46 days for their surgical wounds to heal, while a nonzinc group took 80 days. And another study showed that ulcers healed three times faster in people who took zinc than in those who didn't.

Getting enough zinc may also help prevent premature births. In

295 pregnant teenagers in New Orleans, daily zinc supplements cut the rate of premature birth by nearly a third. In another study, women who took supplements had fewer complications giving birth.

Supplemental zinc also has helped treat acne in people with severe zinc deficiency. Zinc applied on the skin can also help treat acne, especially when combined with the antibiotic erythromycin.

Regulating Your Intake

A woman needs about 12 milligrams of zinc a day; a man needs 15 milligrams. Oysters have a whopping 78 milligrams per three-ounce serving! Three ounces of crab provides more than 6 milligrams; beef supplies about 4.5 milligrams; and dark-meat chicken has more than 2 milligrams.

If you eat little meat (or crab or oysters), you may not be getting enough zinc. Vegetarian fare doesn't dish up much. (A cup of milk, a cup of cooked oatmeal or two slices of wheat bread provide about 1 milligram of zinc each.) What's the answer? A multivitamin/mineral supplement that provides no more than 15 milligrams of zinc.

With all the great potential benefits from zinc, you may be tempted to take more. But regular doses above 15 milligrams carry the risk of side effects, including nausea, diarrhea and vomiting. And in one

study, young men who took 80 to 150 milligrams of zinc daily for several weeks lowered "good" cholesterol levels. More important, too much zinc can *suppress* your immune system, says Dr. Chandra. He found that daily doses of 150 milligrams for six weeks weakened the immune system of healthy young adults.

The bottom line? Most experts agree that you should take no more than 15 milligrams daily on a regular basis—but that *short-term* higher doses can be safe. If you're worried about sucking on zinc lozenges while you're fighting a cold, put your mind at rest. Although these lozenges have about 23 milligrams of zinc, four or five a day for three days won't harm you. "The evidence so far is that up to about 25 milligrams daily is probably safe for up to a few months," says Dr. Chandra.

One final caveat: Zinc competes with the essential mineral copper for absorption in your body, and taking supplemental zinc without copper can cause a copper deficiency. So if you're taking zinc, you should also take copper—about one-tenth as much, says Dr. Chandra. (Example: 1.5 milligrams of copper for 15 milligrams of zinc.) Your best bet is a multiple supplement that contains all essential vitamins and trace minerals, including zinc and copper in the right proportions, he says.

PART

III

HERBAL
REMEDIES

Herbal Remedies

Nature's Practical Wisdom

Since the dawn of time, people have turned to plants for medicine. In fact, until this century, plant medicine, mingled with faith and luck, was just about the *only* medicine. Then came laboratories, scientists in white smocks and a host of powerful tablets and injections that grabbed the spotlight from leaves, roots, bark and berries. As dreaded diseases were conquered, many gentle and time-honored natural remedies were all but forgotten.

Now things seem to be coming full circle. Many people, seeking alternatives to the cost and side effects of synthetic medications, are turning back to herbs for all kinds of ailments.

But the revival of herbal medicine has brewed up a controversy hotter than a cup of chamomile tea. Are herbs an unexplored treasure trove of natural cures? Or are they a snake oil salesman's dream come true?

There is no easy answer to that question. Recent research shows that some herbs do, in fact, offer powerful medicinal benefits. Chances are there are many beneficial herbs as yet unresearched and not yet recognized by American medical authorities. But there are also a lot of extravagant claims made for herbs. And diagnosing and dosing yourself with herbs can be a dangerous game. In this section, we'll show you how to explore the potential benefits of herbs while steering clear of possible risks.

Plant Power

The simplest description of an herb is a "useful plant." Even in this day of high-tech drugs, plants continue to serve as potent and powerful healing agents. In the United States, about a quarter of all prescriptions contain active ingredients from plants, says Norman R. Farnsworth, Ph.D., director of the Program for Collaborative Research in the Pharmaceutical Sciences at the University of Illinois at Chicago.

For decades, plant-based medications such as digitalis (from the herb foxglove) for the heart and quinine (from the bark of the cinchona tree) for malaria have been saving lives. Joining them are newer drugs such as taxol, a potent cancer therapy derived from the Pacific yew, says John Beutler, Ph.D., a chemist with the National Cancer Institute. Dr. Beutler screens thousands of exotic plants each year for their cancer-fighting potential. "Plant medicines are not hokum," he says. "They offer real promise, but first scientists have to take a good, critical look at them."

Even the corner drugstore holds an herbal bouquet of familiar remedies. A wide variety of nonprescription products—from mentholated cough drops (derived from mint) to psyllium laxatives and witch hazel—contain real or synthesized plant substances. Technically, even a cup of coffee is a

---

AN HERBAL GLOSSARY

Astringent: An agent that diminishes internal or external secretions or causes soft tissues to pucker.

Bitter: A substance that stimulates secretion of saliva and increases appetite.

Decoction: A water extract of herbs made by boiling or simmering; stronger than a tea.

Demulcent: A substance that soothes inflamed mucous membranes.

Digestive: Improving digestion.

Diuretic: Increasing flow of urine.

Elixir: An alcohol-based medication, usually sweetened.

Essential oil: A volatile (easily vaporized) and scented plant oil found in many herbal medications.

Expectorant: Easing the coughing up of mucus.

Infusion: A medication made by combining plants or plant extracts with boiling water; similar to a tea.

Mucilage: A sticky substance found in plants, used to soothe inflammation.

Poultice: A moist, hot compress applied externally to the body.

Simple: A medicinal herb without strong effects.

Tea: A dried substance, usually from a plant, steeped in hot water for drinking.

Tincture: A medication with its active agent dissolved in alcohol.

Tonic: An agent to maintain or restore health in one organ system or the whole body.

CAUTION: PLANTS CAN BE DANGEROUS

Some people believe that all herbal products are safe. This is far from true. Although the following is not a complete list of unsafe plants, those listed here deserve special attention.

The herbs in this list are dangerous and should not be used as remedies.

Plant	Potential Danger
Borage	Harmful in large doses; may cause liver damage and cancer
Broom	Toxic; powerful laxative
Chapparal	May cause illness; banned in the U.S.
Coltsfoot	May cause cancer
Comfrey	May cause liver damage and cancer (but not through external use)
Foxglove	Potent heart toxin
Pennyroyal	The essential oil may cause convulsions in large doses; possibly harmful to pregnant women
Pokeweed	Poisonous
Rue	Dangerous to pregnant women
Sassafras	May cause cancer
Sweet woodruff	Large doses may cause dizziness and vomiting

These herbs are potentially dangerous and should be used with caution.

Plant	Potential Danger
Aloe	Used internally, a powerful laxative
Buckthorn	Powerful laxative
Goldenseal	Poisonous in large doses
Juniper	Should not be used by pregnant women or people with kidney disease
Licorice	Excessive amounts may cause fluid retention and high blood pressure

mild herbal stimulant.

For most of us, though, a mention of "herbs" conjures up plants with quaint names like feverfew and goldenseal, brewed up in teas and used in tinctures. Many of these plants have a long history of use, described in folklore of various cultures. It's possible that your own grandmothers used them.

In some cases, research has proved that the old-time herbalists were on the right track. "A fairly high percentage of useful plant-derived drugs were discovered as a result of scientific follow-up of well-known plants used in traditional medicine," says Dr. Farnsworth. Not all traditional herb uses stand up under strict scientific scrutiny, however. Some of them have proven to be ineffective or even toxic. And many simply haven't been thoroughly studied yet.

What Labels Don't Tell

If you have ever shopped for herbal products in a health food store, you may have noticed something odd: The labels almost never tell the potential medical benefits of the herb. And unlike standard medicines such as aspirin, most herbal remedies come without directions or precautions for use.

The reason? The Food and Drug Administration (FDA) prohibits manufacturers from making claims that any product will treat or prevent a disease until that product has been exhaustively tested.

Many herbs have long histories as safe healers—in Asia, for example, angelica has long been used to treat arthritis. But to claim this on the package, the manufacturer would have to get the FDA to approve angelica as a new drug—a lengthy process that costs more

than $200 million, experts estimate.

Since natural substances such as herbs cannot be patented, it would never be profitable to go through the approval process, says Daniel B. Mowrey, Ph.D., director of the American Phytotherapy Research Laboratory in Salt Lake City, Utah, and author of *The Scientific Validation of Herbal Medicine.* This is also the reason that big drug companies have little interest in exploring even the most promising herbal remedies.

To sidestep the problem of FDA regulation, herb purveyors have simply sold their products as food supplements, without therapeutic claims. Unfortunately, that leaves the consumer without a clue as to a product's uses or possible risks and with no assurance of its potency or quality, says Varro E. Tyler, Ph.D., professor of pharmacognosy at Purdue University School of Pharmacy in West Lafayette, Indiana, and author of *The Honest Herbal.* According to some studies of expensive herbal products, he says, "consumers have less than a 50 percent chance of actually getting what the label says they're buying."

As Dr. Farnsworth warns, "When it comes to herbal products, it's 'buyer beware.'"

Out of the Maze

Given this confusion, here are a few ways to help you pick safely from nature's garden of healing plants.

BUYING HERBAL PRODUCTS

Using herbs is simple. You just pick some up in your local health food store and . . . Whoa! Stop! Halt! The fantasy of the no-fuss, no-trouble use of herbs is all too frequently just that—a fantasy. You may do quite well buying bulk herbs locally, but the fact of the matter is that the quality of commercially sold herbs varies widely.

Dried herbs may lose their potency quickly if not stored properly. More expensive herbs are often adulterated or otherwise tampered with. Even packaged products are not sacrosanct. Investigators have found, for example, that often products labeled "ginseng" contain either an inexpensive substitute or none whatsoever of the costly herb.

Herbal products are not subject to government regulation for quality, potency or authenticity. What's a person who wants to use herbs to do?

In general, beware of products that are accompanied by extravagant health claims or that are exorbitantly expensive. Herbal experts advise purchasing herbs only from reputable companies with a name and reputation to protect.

The following firms are well-known suppliers to naturopathic physicians. All sell directly to the public, either through retailers such as health food stores or by mail order.

Cardiovascular Research/
 Ecological Formulas
c/o L&H Vitamins
37-10 Crescent Street
Long Island City, NY 11101

Eclectic Institute
14385 S.E. Lusted Road
Sandy, OR 97055

Herb and Spice Collection
3021 78th Street
P.O. Box 118
Norway, IA 52318-0118

Herb Pharm
Box 116
Williams, OR 97544

Nature's Herb Company
1010 46th Street
Emeryville, CA 94608

Nature's Way
P.O. Box 4000
Springville, UT 84663

Penn Herb Company
603 North 2nd Street
Philadelphia, PA 19123

Pharmacists Nutrition Center
9775 SW Commerce Circle,
 Suite CS
Portland, OR 97070

Educate yourself. Read up on herbs, but be skeptical. Today's self-styled herbalists seldom have a good background in chemistry and botany, says Dr. Tyler, and many rely on outdated or inaccurate information. As long as it's not part of the labeling, they may make outrageous claims for an herb's healing powers, he says. Look for experts with credentials in medicine or pharmacognosy—the science of discovering medicinal products in nature.

Don't play doctor. Never diagnose yourself or use any "alternative" therapy instead of a proven medical treatment without telling your doctor first, says Alan R. Gaby, M.D., a Baltimore physician who practices nutritional and natural medicine and is president of the American Holistic Medical Association. "In some cases, you can use herbs and other natural treatments as a substitute for conventional medicine," he says, "but there are also curative treatments you'll miss if you don't go for a checkup." Unless you're absolutely sure what's wrong, he advises, don't try to self-medicate.

If you wish to try herbal remedies, says Dr. Farnsworth, use them for conditions that you know are not serious and will eventually clear up by themselves—for example, colds or minor arthritis pain. If a chronic condition persists or gets worse, see your doctor.

And when it comes to such life-threatening diseases as cancer or AIDS, beware of peddlers or practitioners who prey on desperate people, says Dr. Beutler. If a so-called cure sounds too good to be true, it probably is.

Don't presume that "natural" equals "safe." According to Dr. Farnsworth, "People often presume that just because an herb is a plant, it's safe to use. That's not necessarily true. Some of the most virulent toxins known come from plants."

Many herbs have been used by thousands of people for hundreds of years with virtually no ill effects and possibly much benefit. But occasionally there are reports of herbal remedies causing sickness or even a rare death. Often, says Dr. Farnsworth, the herbs may have been misidentified or adulterated with other plants or toxic substances. He advises buying herbs and herbal products only from reputable growers and manufacturers.

Start low and go slow. If you try a new herbal product, start with the lowest dose, and if you experience no benefit after a week or so, increase it gradually, recommends Dr. Farnsworth. Don't take more than the recommended amount, however, and don't take high doses of any remedy for months or years unless the long-term effects have been well studied. For most herbs, he adds, the active ingredients and long-term effects are poorly understood or unknown.

If you feel worse after taking an herbal remedy, stop taking it. Allergies or other adverse reactions to any plant substance are always a

FINDING EXPERT HELP

For referrals to practitioners of herbal medicine in your area, write to the Institute for Traditional Medicine, 2017 S.E. Hawthorne, Portland, OR 97214 or send a self-addressed, stamped envelope to the American Association of Naturopathic Physicians, 2366 Eastlake Avenue East, Suite 322, Seattle, WA 98102.

possibility. If an herb disagrees with you or if you develop any new symptoms after taking it, discontinue use.

Avoid herbal remedies if you are pregnant, nursing or taking other medication. Little is known about the effects of herbs or their active ingredients on an unborn child or on a baby through breast milk. It's best to err on the side of caution, says Dr. Farnsworth. He also advises against mixing herbal remedies with prescription or over-the-counter drugs—an herb may make the action of another medication weaker or stronger.

How to Use Herbs

It's easy to take aspirin: Just read the label, which says something like "take every four hours." But what about herbs? Whether you grow your own herbs or buy them from a health food store, you're faced with a challenge. Sometimes—as with many herbal teas—there's a label to help you. But some herbs come in many forms. Echinacea, for example, can be pur-chased in the form of capsules, tinctures or tea; alone or combined with other herbs; in a concentrated extract or in a preparation made from the fresh roots and flowers. Which one do you choose?

Here again, there are no easy answers. Some herbalists believe that products made from the whole plant are superior to preparations containing only the "active ingredients." Mother Nature, they reason, knows best what subtle combination of compounds will deliver the most benefits with the fewest side effects. Other herbalists prefer standardized extracts.

Herbalism remains an inexact science. A plant's therapeutic activity in the human body may vary with its time of harvest, the methods of storage and cultivation, the dosage and what else is going on in the body. Like the medicine men and wise women of old, today's herb user must rely to a great extent on trial and error to discover which products seem to work best.

"People often ask about the right dose, but we may not need to get that technical," says Steven Dentali, Ph.D., quality assurance director and natural products chemist for Trout Lake Farm and Flora Laboratories in Trout Lake, Washington, and a private herbal consultant. "Take an herb with a history of safe use, for a self-limiting condition, and find out what it does for you."

Back to the Future

Herbal medicine has become big business in the United States, although it is still just a sprout compared to the giant pharmaceutical industry. This herbal renaissance has grown out of consumer demand: People are beginning to try herbs, and they like what they are finding.

Don't look for herbs to take the place of wonder drugs any time soon. But some scientists, like Dr. Farnsworth, see real hope for herbs to help bolster the body's immune response and ease chronic conditions like asthma and arthritis.

And then there's all that research that's looking into the potential of plant-derived substances as cancer treatments. "I can't say there's another taxol ready to emerge from

the research pipeline, but we're encouraged. We see some very interesting things ahead," says Dr. Beutler.

More research is, in fact, the key to unlocking the age-old potential of healing herbs for treating a wide variety of human ills. Herb enthusiasts are heartened, for example, by the fact that the prestigious National Institutes of Health in 1991 established an Office of Alternative Medicine to evaluate the scientific merit of herbalism and other nonstandard healing methods. And a small but growing number of medical doctors are already combining so-called alternative techniques such as herbalism and acupuncture with standard medical practice.

In the end, though, ordinary people—not doctors and scientists—are the ones bringing nature and medicine together again. "Herbs are people medicine," says Dr. Dentali. And if people use them appropriately, he says, they can be effective medicine indeed, readily available to anyone.

"Herbs are a reminder that our lives depend absolutely on plants. Grow them, use them, enjoy them," he says.

Allspice

A Blend of Flavors and Benefits

Allspice owes its name to its unique flavor: a zesty blend of cinnamon, pepper, juniper and clove. Thanks to its oil, it also has mild but significant healing powers as a digestive aid and topical anesthetic.

Aromatic allspice berries have a long history in Caribbean folk healing. Jamaicans drink hot allspice tea for colds, menstrual cramps and upset stomach. Costa Ricans use it to treat indigestion, flatulence and diabetes. Cubans consider it a refreshing tonic. And Guatemalans apply crushed berries to bruises and joint and muscle pains. Most of these uses have been confirmed by modern science.

"Allspice owes its medicinal actions to eugenol, a chemical constituent of its oil," says Daniel B. Mowrey, Ph.D., director of the American Phytotherapy Research Laboratory in Salt Lake City, Utah, and author of *The Scientific Validation of Herbal Medicine*. "Eugenol promotes digestion by enhancing the activity of the digestive enzyme trypsin. It's also an effective pain reliever and anesthetic."

Dentists use eugenol as a local anesthetic for teeth and gums, and the chemical is an ingredient in the over-the-counter toothache remedies Numzident and Benzodent.

"Allspice oil is not as rich in eugenol as clove oil," says James A. Duke, Ph.D., a botanist retired from the U.S. Department of Agriculture and author of *The CRC Handbook of Medicinal Herbs*. That's why dentists favor clove oil. But allspice oil has similar anesthetic action and may be applied directly to painful teeth as first aid until professional care can be obtained.

Putting the Herb to Work

For toothache, apply allspice oil directly to the tooth, one drop at a time, using a cotton swab. Take care not to swallow it. Powdered allspice adds a warm, rich flavor to foods, but its highly concentrated oil should never be swallowed. As little as one teaspoon can cause nausea, vomiting and even convulsions.

Allspice is on the Food and Drug Administration's list of herbs generally regarded as safe. But in people with sensitive skin, particularly those with eczema, allspice oil may cause inflammation. If inflammation develops, stop using it.

For a medicinal tea, use one to two teaspoons of allspice powder per cup of boiling water. Steep for 10 to 20 minutes and strain. Drink up to three cups a day. When using commercial preparations, follow the package directions.

Aloe

Herbal First Aid

POTENTIAL HEALING POWER
May help: • Heal burns and scalds • Relieve sunburn • Treat minor wounds

As a healing plant, aloe is something of a celebrity. Across America, the spiky plant sits on untold numbers of kitchen windowsills, just waiting. Waiting for what? A spattered bit of grease, a careless moment at the oven, and the inner gel of the aloe leaves gets called into service as a burn salve. Even scientists take advantage of this simple home remedy.

"To treat minor burns, scalds and cuts, I keep a potted aloe on the windowsill of my kitchen," says Daniel B. Mowrey, Ph.D., director of the American Phytotherapy Research Laboratory in Salt Lake City, Utah, and author of *The Scientific Validation of Herbal Medicine.* "Everyone should."

Most household burns and scalds, and many other minor mishaps, occur in the kitchen. With an aloe plant close by, it's easy to snip off one of the thick, fleshy leaves, slit it open and squeeze the clear gel onto the injury. "Aloe gel dries into a natural bandage," Dr. Mowrey explains. "It also promotes healing and helps keep burns from becoming infected."

Aloe has a long history as a healer. Around 1500 B.C., the ancient Egyptians began using aloe as a powerful laxative and a treatment for skin problems. When Alexander the Great conquered Egypt, he learned that an island off Somalia teemed with aloes. He immediately seized it to guarantee a supply of the wound treatment for his troops, while keeping the herb from his enemies. Arab traders carried aloe from Spain to Asia around the sixth century. Traditional Indian Ayurvedic doctors and Chinese physicians quickly adopted it as a laxative and skin treatment. American pioneers used aloe gel to treat wounds, burns, hemorrhoids and rashes.

Scientific validation of aloe's wound-healing power dates from the 1930s, when radiologists noticed that aloe gel scooped straight from the cut leaves of the plant hastened the healing of x-ray burns. Since then, many studies have confirmed the herb's ability to promote healing of cuts, frostbite and first- and second-degree burns.

"Aloe contains allantoin, a substance that speeds wound healing," says Alan R. Gaby, M.D., a Baltimore physician who practices nutritional and natural medicine and is president of the American Holistic Medical Association.

One chemical in this herb—aloe-emodin—"has anti-tumor activity," according to James A. Duke, Ph.D., a botanist retired from the U.S. Department of Agriculture and author of *The CRC Handbook of Medicinal Herbs*. Aloe is not currently used to treat cancer, but one day it might be. And some derivatives of aloe are also being studied for both anti-AIDS and anti-cancer potential.

Squeeze a Leaf for Relief

Before applying aloe to burns or cuts, wash them thoroughly with soap and water. For minor burns, scalds, sunburns or cuts, select a lower (older) leaf, cut off several inches and slice it lengthwise. Scoop out the gel, apply it liberally to the affected area and allow it to dry. (The injured aloe leaf quickly closes its own wound. Periodic leaf-snipping does not harm the plant.)

Aloe gel is safe for external use by anyone who does not develop an allergic reaction. If your skin shows signs of redness or irritation after using aloe, discontinue use. And if a burn or cut does not heal significantly within two weeks, consult a physician.

Even if you have a brown thumb, you can grow aloes. They need little water and no care other than good drainage and a temperature above 40°F. They prefer sun but tolerate shade, and they don't mind poor soil. Aloes periodically produce offshoots, which may be removed and replanted when they are a few inches tall. Simply uproot or unpot the plant, work the soil gently to separate the offshoot and return the parent plant to its bed or pot.

Angelica

Regaining Popularity as *Dang-qui*

POTENTIAL HEALING POWER

May help:
- Relieve menstrual discomfort
- Minimize symptoms of menopause
- Treat colds and other respiratory problems
- Prevent arthritis
- Combat certain cancers

In the West, Chinese angelica's time came and largely went. But now, after more than a century as a minor healer, this eight-foot plant, once called wild celery, has returned to popularity, thanks to its place of honor in Chinese medicine.

Chinese angelica, also known as *dang-qui* or *tang-kuei*, "is the leading Chinese herb for gynecological health," says Pi-Kwang Tsung, Ph.D., former assistant professor of pathology at the University of Connecticut Medical School in Farmington and currently editor of *The East-West Medical Digest*.

Treatment of gynecological problems is a far cry from angelica's uses in medieval Europe, where peasants made necklaces from the leaves of European angelica (*Angelica archangelica*) to protect their children from illness and witchcraft.

The herb became medically prominent because of an epidemic of bubonic plague in 1665. Legend has it that a monk dreamed an angel told him that wild celery could cure the dread disease. The monk renamed the plant "angelica" in honor of his dream-visitor, and not long afterward, the British Royal College of Physicians incorporated the herb into its official plague treatment, The King's Excellent Plague Recipe. Despite the recipe's supposed excellence, plague killed tens of thousands, and faith in angelica's healing abilities plummeted.

By the 18th century, European herbalists had relegated angelica to the relatively insignificant role of treating minor respiratory complaints, cold symptoms and coughs. These uses appear to be scientifically based. "In German animal studies, the oil in angelica has shown a relaxing effect on the trachea (windpipe)," says Bernie Olin, Pharm.D., editor of *The Lawrence Review of Natural Products*, a St. Louis–based newsletter that summarizes scientific research on medicinal herbs.

Women's Healer from China

Asian physicians maintain that Chinese angelica (*A. sinensis*) is considerably more valuable than the European variety. For thousands of years, Chinese and traditional Indian Ayurvedic physicians have prescribed it as *the* tonic for gynecological problems.

"Studies show that dang-qui increases red blood cell counts," Dr. Tsung explains. "That's why Chinese physicians give it to women who have just given birth. Childbirth involves blood loss, and dang-qui helps the body replace lost red blood cells."

Angelica also helps relax the uterus, and combined with other Chinese herbs it can stimulate secretion of the female sex hormone estrogen. Low estrogen levels can cause menstrual problems and are responsible for many menopausal complaints. Dang-qui helps minimize them.

But Chinese angelica is not just for women, according to Dr. Tsung. Dang-qui's ability to boost the production of red blood cells explains why it is used for treating weakness and fatigue in both men and women. Red blood cells carry oxygen to the tissues. As red blood cells proliferate, oxygenation of the blood increases, enabling the body to function more efficiently.

Also, "an immune-stimulating substance has been identified in dang-qui," Dr. Tsung says, "which can help both men and women stay healthy." In particular, he says, it may help prevent chronic diseases such as cancer and arthritis.

On the other hand, Varro E. Tyler, Ph.D., professor of pharmacognosy at Purdue University School of Pharmacy in West Lafayette, Indiana, and author of *The Honest Herbal*, remains skeptical of claims for dang-qui: "Chinese research is not always as rigorous as it ought to be, so I don't consider this herb to have proven benefit."

Calling on the Angel

Herbal experts recommend using European angelica for respiratory complaints and dang-qui for gynecological health and stimulating the immune system. To make a medicinal tea, use one teaspoon of crushed root per cup of boiling water. Steep for 10 to 20 minutes.

Angelica has a fragrant aroma and a warm, vaguely sweet taste reminiscent of juniper, followed by a bitter aftertaste. When using a commercial preparation, follow package directions.

Anise

Licorice-Flavored Gas Reliever

Anise is a flavor appreciated by connoisseurs of fine liquors around the world—the Greeks have their ouzo and the French their pastis. But aside from its use as a flavoring agent, aniseed is valued for other reasons as well.

As far back as the days of the ancient Greeks and Romans, the licorice-flavored herb was used for various medicinal purposes, including freshening the breath, relieving gas, promoting milk production in nursing mothers and helping expel excess phlegm.

And there just may be something to a few of these ancient claims. Today, herb experts particularly tout anise's ability as a digestive aid and gas reliever. Anise is quite safe—anyone who has an upset stomach or gas can give it a try, according to James A. Duke, Ph.D., a botanist retired from the U.S. Department of Agriculture and author of *The CRC Handbook of Medicinal Herbs*.

Calming Colic

Anise can also be effective in relieving colic in infants, says Dr. Duke. "People tend to use dill and fennel more, but they all have the same properties," he says.

To make anise tea to calm the stomach or relieve gas, crush one teaspoon of aniseed and mix it in one cup of boiling water. Steep for 10 to 20 minutes. Drink up to three cups a day. For additional digestive relief, Dr. Duke recommends adding fresh or dried peppermint leaf. You can also chew a handful of the seeds to freshen your breath.

To give anise tea to an infant, dilute ½ cup of tea with ½ cup of water. And make sure you allow it to cool sufficiently.

Astragalus

Chinese Immune System Booster

Astragalus, used as a tonic in traditional Chinese medicine since antiquity, is now finding its way to the shelves of American health food stores. Also called milk vetch, astragalus is a member of the legume, or bean, family. The sweet-tasting roots, which are the parts used medicinally, are black with a pale yellow core. In Chinese, the herb is called *Huang-qi,* or "yellow leader." Researchers in both the United States and China have found clues that it may well live up to its 2,000-year-old reputation as an immune system booster.

"Astragalus is one of the most commonly used herbs in all of Chinese medicine," according to Subhuti Dharmananda, Ph.D., director of the Institute for Traditional Medicine in Portland, Oregon. Chinese herbalists prescribe it to build up the vital energy, or *qi* (pronounced *key*), of a weakened person, he explains, and include it in many combination remedies to promote the action of other herbs. It's used to promote urination, speed healing of burns and abscesses and generally bolster the body's resistance to disease.

Chinese healers also use astragalus to treat the common cold, arthritis, weakness, diarrhea, asthma and nervousness. Sometimes they pan-roast the roots in honey or use them as an ingredient in soup.

Cancer Therapy Helper

In Chinese hospitals, astragalus is used to help people with cancer recover from the immune system wipeout caused by chemotherapy.

In research conducted at the M. D. Anderson Cancer Center in Houston, a team of Chinese and American scientists studied the effects of compounds taken from astragalus roots on immune system cells taken from people with cancer and AIDS. The results: The researchers noted an increase in the functioning of T-cells, which are key fighters in the body's immune defense network. These were test-tube studies, though, and there's no proof yet that people with cancer who take astragalus preparations will benefit.

Cancer isn't the only ill for which astragalus may hold promise. In Shanghai, doctors have shown that compounds from the root can protect heart cells from damage caused by the Coxsackie B virus, which can scar the hearts of both adults and infants. In one experiment, people suffering from this viral infection not only improved but showed enhanced resistance to the common cold.

Putting Astragalus to Work

Astragalus preparations are available at many health food stores in the form of capsules, teas and tinctures. To prepare them, simply follow the directions on the package. The herb has not been reported to cause dangerous side effects, according to Dr. Dharmananda, but some people report loose stools or abdominal bloating. If you experience any unpleasant symptoms, cut back your dose or discontinue use.

An important note: There are many flowering plants in the astragalus family, including native American species that are toxic when eaten by cattle. (Ranchers call the plant locoweed because of its effect on their herds' behavior.) The particular herb known as astragalus in Chinese medicine is a species called *Astragalus membranaceus*.

For the maximum benefit from astragalus, Dr. Dharmananda recommends consulting a Chinese herbalist or other practitioner trained in traditional Chinese medicine. Like other Chinese herbs, "yellow leader" is often prescribed with a complex blend of other herbs and foods for maximum effect.

Astragalus itself is not a cancer cure; as with any traditional therapy, don't add it to a treatment regimen without discussing it with your doctor.

Balm

All-Purpose Soother

Stomach comforter, blues banisher, herpes fighter, even bug repellent: The reputed uses of balm are so varied that it's no wonder this lemon-scented herb

POTENTIAL HEALING POWER

May help:
- Heal minor wounds
- Ease indigestion
- Relieve menstrual cramps
- Treat cold sores
- Relax nerves
- Aid sleep
- Repel insects

has been nicknamed "cure-all."

Although its therapeutic usefulness is little known in this country, balm (sometimes referred to as lemon balm but officially called *Melissa officinalis*) is widely used and highly valued by legitimate herbal practitioners in Western Europe.

The leaves of this pungent member of the mint family have been used medicinally for some 2,000 years. The 11th-century Arab physician Avicenna believed it "causeth the mind and heart to become merry" and recommended it to dispel melancholy.

Balm was considered a must-have plant for Elizabethan herb gardens, and over the centuries it seems to have been a popular home remedy for a host of common ailments. "Let a syrup made with the juice of it and sugar . . . be kept in every gentlewoman's house to relieve the weak stomachs and sick bodies of their poor sickly neighbours," wrote English physician Nicholas Culpeper in *The Complete Herbal* of 1653.

Modern research has suggested that there may be some truth to some, if not all, of these folk uses. There's no proof that balm makes you merry, but various small-scale laboratory studies in Germany have demonstrated that balm leaves contain compounds with sedative, digestive and anti-spasmodic effects, says Varro E. Tyler, Ph.D., professor of pharmacognosy at Purdue University School of Pharmacy in West

Lafayette, Indiana, and author of *The Honest Herbal*. Culpeper's crude recipe, then, may indeed help relieve tummy troubles.

Help for Herpes?

Recent research has shown another use for balm that the Elizabethans never dreamed of: battling herpes simplex, the virus that causes cold sores. "That's pretty well documented," says Dr. Tyler, adding that a cream containing highly concentrated balm compounds, sold in Europe but unavailable in the United States, has been shown to speed the healing of herpes lesions and lengthen the time between outbreaks.

Can you heal herpes by drinking balm tea? Don't bet on it. "You can't kill the herpes virus by taking it internally," says Norman R. Farnsworth, Ph.D., director of the Program for Collaborative Research in the Pharmaceutical Sciences at the University of Illinois at Chicago. "The studies showing antiviral activity are probably due to the tannins in balm; applied externally, they may act as an astringent and kill some surface viruses." Even applied externally, balm leaves or home brews probably aren't strong enough to be effective, says Dr. Tyler: "The tea would contain the tannins, but not in the same concentration as a commercial preparation."

Balm causes no documented safety problems, although it has

been shown to inhibit certain thyroid hormones. For this reason, people with Graves' disease or other thyroid-related problems should use this herb cautiously, if at all.

Balm has another potential virtue: While bees may love it, mosquitoes reportedly hate it.

Using Balm

Modern herbalists recommend a balm tea made from fresh or dried leaves to calm the nerves, aid sleep, ease menstrual cramps and reduce fever. Use about two teaspoons of chopped leaves (preferably fresh, not dried) to one cup of boiling water. Steep 10 to 20 minutes and drink while hot. Balm tincture is another option, with the usual dose being a teaspoon or less as needed.

Balm leaves are a fragrant and soothing addition to herbal baths or pillows. You can also apply a poultice of the crushed leaves to soothe insect bites and stings and help heal wounds, according to Dr. Farnsworth. Balm's properties as an insect repellent are unproven, but you might try rubbing balm oil, or the pleasantly scented leaves themselves, over your skin on a summer night, just in case.

Black Haw

Menstrual Pain Reliever

POTENTIAL HEALING POWER
May help: • Relieve menstrual cramps

In the 19th century, women with menstrual cramps couldn't reach into a medicine cabinet for Midol. Instead they drank a tea made from black haw bark. The "uterine tonic," first written about in 1857, was reputed to relieve menstrual pain, prevent miscarriage and ease the pain that follows childbirth.

Women have been using it ever since to relieve menstrual cramps. "I used to work in a drugstore in Massachusetts when I was in college, and a product called Hayden's Viburnum Compound was sold," recalls Norman R. Farnsworth, Ph.D., director of the Program for Collaborative Research in the Pharmaceutical Sciences at the University of Illinois at Chicago. "It was the worst-smelling and -tasting thing. But women would come in and swear that when they had menstrual cramps, it worked." (*Viburnum prunifolium* is the scientific name for the herb.)

Can women today turn to black haw bark tea as an alternative to their over-the-counter medications? It may, in fact, be helpful.

The bark contains substances that appear to affect smooth muscle, says Glenn S. Rothfeld, M.D., clinical instructor in the Department of Community Health at Tufts University School of Medicine in Boston. "These substances have been shown to work actively on the uterus, particularly to relax it," he says.

"I would not encourage women to use black haw or other herbs to prevent miscarriage unless they are under someone's care who has expertise in treating with herbs," says Dr. Rothfeld. But the herb may be used for relieving menstrual cramps, he says. Pregnant women shouldn't take any herb for health or healing without the consent of an obstetrician.

To make a decoction or tea from black haw bark, says Dr. Rothfeld, use one ounce of herb to a pint of freshly boiled distilled water. Steep for 10 to 15 minutes and strain. Drink one cup two to three times a day to relieve cramping, he says.

Black Walnut

Fungus Terminator

Expert gardeners know better than to plant under the black walnut tree.

"Have you ever seen what grows under a black walnut tree? Nothing. There's a reason for that: It contains a chemical that kills anything that it comes in contact with," says Christopher W. W. Beecher, Ph.D., associate professor of pharmacognosy in the Department of Medicinal Chemistry and

Pharmacognosy at the University of Illinois at Chicago.

Some American Indian tribes apparently recognized black walnut bark's destructive power and turned it against conditions like ringworm, a fungal skin infection. "For something like ringworm, a topical application of this chemical is going to

POTENTIAL HEALING POWER

May help:
- Cure ringworm
- Treat athlete's foot
- Fight jock itch
- Prevent certain cancers

go right in there and bind to the infected cells. And that should be the end of the fungus," says Dr. Beecher. Black walnut's active component may also be effective against stubborn fungal problems like athlete's foot and jock itch.

And what's bad for your fungal infections, investigators say, may also be bad for cancer. During a study conducted in the 1960s, researchers injected two of the chemicals found in the hull of the black walnut into tumors in laboratory animals. The result: Both the size and the weight of the tumors decreased dramatically. Researchers investigating the same effect obtained a German patent in 1990 for this anti-cancer treatment.

Black walnut fruit, on the other hand, also seems to show promise in the fight against deadly disease. Although much more research needs to be done, preliminary studies conducted during the 1960s revealed that large doses of the chemicals in the nut could help lower blood pressure. And perhaps even different walnuts don't fall too far from the tree: More recent studies of the English walnut have documented its effectiveness in helping lower cholesterol as part of a heart-healthy diet.

Kiss Fungus Good-Bye

If you'd like to try black walnut's potent fungus-fighting power for yourself, you can purchase a liquid extract at many health food stores. Follow the package instructions before applying it to your skin.

Black walnut extract capsules are also available at health food stores, but, in view of their toxicity, Dr. Beecher suggests consulting a health professional before using them.

Buckthorn

Possible Cancer Treatment

POTENTIAL HEALING POWER
May help:
• Relieve constipation
• Treat certain cancers

Buckthorn became popular in European herbal medicine about 1,000 years ago. At the time, little was known about the body. Doctors believed the key to curing disease lay in purging "foul humours." Not surprisingly, strong laxatives were prescribed for dozens of ailments. Buckthorn was a favorite because it produced reliable results, although it sometimes caused severe gastrointestinal irritation and cramping when people took too much.

Buckthorn's laxative action is the result of chemicals in the plant called anthraquinones. They stimulate the colonic muscle contractions we experience as "the urge." Several other laxative herbs—aloe, cascara sagrada and senna—also contain anthraquinones.

"Buckthorn is about as powerful as cascara sagrada," says Daniel B. Mowrey, Ph.D., director of the American Phytotherapy Research Laboratory in Salt Lake City, Utah, and author of *The Scientific Validation of Herbal Medicine*, "and less potent than aloe and senna." (Some experts feel that aloe and senna are too powerful to use as laxatives.)

Buckthorn has also been used fairly extensively around the world among traditional herbalists as a cancer treatment. And there is apparently something to this use for the herb.

"Buckthorn has shown some anti-tumor action," says James A. Duke, Ph.D., a botanist retired from the U.S. Department of Agriculture and author of *The CRC Handbook of Medicinal Herbs*. "It deserves more research."

Harnessing Powerful Laxative Action

In Germany, where herbal healing is more mainstream than it is in the United States, some physicians prescribe a laxative tea containing ½ teaspoon each of buckthorn, fennel seed and chamomile flowers (fennel and chamomile soothe the stomach) per cup of boiling water, steeped for ten minutes. If you try this, drink no more than one cup. It's best to take it before bed.

If you gather your own buckthorn, make sure it has been dried thoroughly before you use it as a laxative. Poorly dried buckthorn can cause vomiting, severe abdominal pain and violent diarrhea.

If you're constipated, you should consider anthraquinone laxatives only as a last resort. Doctors recommend eating a high-fiber diet and getting more exercise as the first line of treatment for constipation. If that doesn't work, the next thing to try, they say, is a bulk-forming laxative, such as psyllium (Metamucil). Only after you've given all these a shot should you move on to an anthraquinone laxative such as buckthorn.

Buckthorn should not be used by those with chronic gastrointestinal problems such as ulcers, colitis or hemorrhoids. Pregnant women should also avoid it.

Buckthorn should never be used for more than two weeks, because over time it can cause "lazy bowel syndrome," an inability to move stool without chemical stimulation.

Buckthorn is still a long way from being an accepted cancer treatment. If you have cancer and would like to try this herb in addition to standard therapy, discuss it with your physician.

Burdock

The Tenacious Tonic

Burdock's name is a combination of *bur*, for its spiked seed covers, or burrs, that grab onto anything that touches them, and *dock*, Old English for "plant." Many scientists dismiss burdock as useless, but like its seeds, its reputation clings tenaciously as an herbal healing agent because of its subtle tonic benefits and its intriguing potential as a treatment for cancer.

Throughout history, burdock has been recommended for an astonishing number of illnesses. Ancient Chinese physicians used it to treat colds, coughs, tonsillitis, measles, skin infections and snakebite. Traditional European and American herbalists and homeopaths prescribed it for colds, arthritis, gout, stomach problems, fever, canker sores, leprosy, boils, gonorrhea, ringworm and infertility. They also considered it an excellent diuretic and prescribed it for urinary tract infections, kidney problems and painful urination.

Many of these traditional recommendations still echo through contemporary herb guides. But several herb experts scoff at burdock. Among them is Bernie Olin, Pharm.D., editor of *The Lawrence Review of Natural Products*, a St. Louis-based newsletter that summarizes scientific research on medicinal herbs. Some therapeutic activity has been associated with burdock, he notes, "but there is little evidence to suggest that it is useful in the treatment of any human disease."

True, burdock is not powerfully therapeutic, but Daniel B. Mowrey, Ph.D., director of the American Phytotherapy Research Laboratory in Salt Lake City, Utah, and author of *The Scientific Validation of Herbal Medicine*, insists that it deserves its enduring place in herbal healing because of its value as a tonic—a subtle strengthener with cumulatively helpful effects.

"Burdock's action is mild but real," Dr. Mowrey explains. "It has antibacterial and antiviral powers, and it reduces blood sugar, which helps prevent diabetes. I recommend using a little every day. And when you're ill, use it in addition to standard therapies."

A Potential Cancer Fighter

And after all is said and done, burdock may one day prove valuable as a cancer fighter. Burdock's use against cancer goes way back. The 12th-century German abbess and herbalist Hildegard of Bingen used burdock to treat cancerous tumors, and down through the centuries it has been used as a tumor treatment in Russia, China, India and the Americas. In the United States, it was an ingredient in the popular but highly controversial Hoxsey Cancer Formula, an alternative therapy marketed from the 1930s to the 1950s by ex-coal-miner Harry Hoxsey.

"Five good foreign studies show intriguing anti-tumor or anti-mutation activity," says Dr. Mowrey. (Most substances that cause genetic mutations also cause cancer.) "Recently," says James A. Duke, Ph.D., a botanist retired from the U.S. Department of Agriculture and author of *The CRC Handbook of Medicinal Herbs*, "the National Cancer Institute became interested in burdock as part of its Designer Foods Program, an effort to use biotechnology to introduce cancer-preventive chemicals into common food crops."

To brew a pleasantly sweet-tasting tonic tea, boil one teaspoon of crushed, dried burdock root in three cups of water for 30 minutes. Drink up to three cups a day. Dr. Duke enjoys eating a soup made from the leaf stalks of fresh burdock, which resemble celery when cooked and taste even better, he says.

When using commercial preparations, follow the package directions.

Of course, cancer requires professional care. If you're being treated for cancer and would like to try burdock in addition to standard therapies, discuss it with your physician.

The Toxicology of Botanical Medicines identifies burdock as a uterine stimulant. Pregnant women should not use it.

Butcher's Broom

Sweep Away Circulatory Problems

POTENTIAL HEALING POWER
May help: • Relieve hemorrhoids   • Treat leg vein problems

Herbal medicine has no shortage of plants called broom. In addition to butcher's broom, there is broom, dyer's broom, Spanish broom and corn broom, among others. They all have tough stems and rigid leaves that make them useful for sweeping. They also are often confused with one another. To prevent mix-ups, it's a good idea to learn the Latin name for butcher's broom—*Ruscus aculeatus.*

Butcher's broom is closely related to asparagus, and its young shoots can be prepared and eaten just like the familiar vegetable. If the shoots go unharvested, this herb becomes a low-growing evergreen shrub.

Ancient Greek physicians recommended butcher's broom as a laxative and diuretic, but this herb did not become widely used in healing until the 1950s, when French scientists isolated two chemicals from butcher's broom rhizomes (underground stems). These chemicals have therapeutic value in that they cause blood vessels to narrow and help reduce inflammation.

Following this research, herbalists immediately began recommending butcher's broom for treatment of hemorrhoids, which result from distended veins in the anal area. The final word isn't in yet on whether or not it works. Over time, however, anecdotal reports accumulated that the herb helped treat a lower-leg condition called venous insufficiency or chronic phlebopathy, meaning that the veins there don't function properly, causing swelling, itching, tingling, cramping and a feeling of heaviness.

Studies of butcher's broom for leg vein problems have produced intriguing results. A scientifically rigorous 1988 study showed that a combination of butcher's broom, vitamin C and another chemical found in citrus fruits improved symptoms. "The swelling, itching and tingling improved greatly," says Bernie Olin, Pharm.D., editor of *The Lawrence Review of Natural Products,* a St. Louis–based newsletter that summarizes scientific research on medicinal herbs. Cramping and heaviness were also relieved to a small extent.

Brewing Up the Broom

Although questions remain about this herb's effectiveness, Daniel B. Mowrey, Ph.D., director of the American Phytotherapy Research Laboratory in Salt Lake City, Utah, and author of *The Scientific Validation of Herbal Medicine,* recommends it for venous insufficiency. "Just make sure you use a guaranteed potency extract with 10 percent total saponins (the active elements in butcher's broom). Several herb companies market them through health food stores," he says. When using a commercial preparation, follow the package directions.

To make a less potent medicinal tea, use two to four teaspoons of twigs or one to two teaspoons of fresh rhizome per cup of boiling water. Steep 10 to 20 minutes. Drink up to three cups a day.

Taking butcher's broom requires some caution. If this herb does indeed constrict the leg veins, it might also raise blood pressure, which may increase the risk of heart attack and stroke. Circulatory problems require professional care.

Before using butcher's broom for swelling or cramping in the legs, consult your physician.

Camphor

Moth Repellent and Muscle Soother

Who'd ever think that the same odoriferous herb that repels wool-eating moths also soothes muscle aches and pains?

It's true. And the herb is camphor, a white crystalline substance that's distilled from the wood and roots of the camphor tree—a large evergreen that grows in Asia, South America, Florida and California—and has a smell akin to turpentine. You may not be as familiar with this particular herb as you think—these days most commercial products said to contain camphor actually contain a synthetic version of it.

Until it was replaced by more effective repellents such as naphthalene, camphor was an insect-banishing blessing. "People would put cakes or pellets of camphor on their closet shelves or between wool blankets or sweaters," explains Varro E. Tyler, Ph.D., professor of pharmacognosy at Purdue Univer-

sity School of Pharmacy in West Lafayette, Indiana, and author of *The Honest Herbal*. The camphor would vaporize, and its pungent fumes would ward off bugs with a taste for cashmere.

Medically, camphor has a long and varied history, although many of its uses have fallen out of favor because of potential toxicity problems. Camphor in alcohol, for example, which was once popular as a "pick-me-up," can actually cause liver damage.

Easing Muscle Aches

External uses, however, have stood the test of time.

"For years, one of its most popular uses was as a rub-on oil, called camphor liniment, which consisted of cottonseed oil containing enough dissolved camphor to make a strong 20 percent solution," Dr. Tyler explains.

Camphorated oil was banned by the Food and Drug Administration (FDA) in 1980 after reports of poisoning through accidental ingestion and, less commonly, through skin absorption. But topical creams such as Ben-Gay and Aurum Gold Analgesic, containing up to 11 percent camphor, are available and are considered safe by the FDA. These creams produce a sensation of warmth that helps to counter pain. They also increase blood flow to the area to which they are applied, making your skin rosy-pink.

Vicks VapoRub and Vicks Vapo-Steam also contain camphor, and there is some evidence that inhaling fumes from a vaporizing camphor ointment rubbed on the chest can help to ease coughing.

You can buy cakes of pure camphor—usually by special order—at a pharmacy and make your own camphorated oil. But you may want to think twice before experimenting with this potentially harmful substance. "I believe you are much better off simply buying an over-the-counter product that contains camphor in safe amounts than fooling around with it on your own," Dr. Tyler says. "Ingesting amounts as small as a teaspoonful can be fatal."

Cascara Sagrada

Heavy-Duty Laxative

In Spanish, *cascara sagrada* means "sacred bark," perhaps because this woody shrub has provided blessed relief for more than a few constipated souls. The reddish-brown bark of this herb is harvested, dried, aged and used as a laxative, either as a powder or a liquid extract.

POTENTIAL HEALING POWER
May help:
• Relieve constipation
• Treat cold sores

Cascara sagrada's purgative power has earned it a reputation as the world's most widely used laxative and made it the main ingredient in several over-the-counter laxatives.

"The active ingredients in cascara sagrada—anthraquinones—probably act by irritating the intestines to produce wavelike contractions of the muscles of the intestinal wall," explains Norman R. Farnsworth, Ph.D., director of the Program for Collaborative Research in the Pharmaceutical Sciences at the University of Illinois at Chicago. "Most people see results within eight hours."

Even though laxative products containing cascara sagrada are sometimes marketed as "nature's remedy" or "all-natural," or said to "restore bowel tone," they present the same risks as all stimulant laxatives. If you use them on a regular basis, you can develop a condition known as lazy bowel syndrome—you can't go without chemical stimulation! "A bulk laxative, such as psyllium, is a better choice for long-term chronic constipation," Dr. Farnsworth says.

Some anthraquinones, including some of those found in cascara sagrada, have the ability to kill herpes simplex, the virus that causes cold sores, reports Heinz Rosler, Ph.D., associate professor of medicinal chemistry at the University of Maryland School of Pharmacy in Baltimore.

Another ingredient in cascarda sagrada—aloe-emodin—has an anti-leukemia action in laboratory animals, lending some support to the herb's traditional use as an alternative cancer treatment. Unfortunately, aloe-emodin is also quite toxic, and scientists say more research is needed before it can be used to treat leukemia.

Use with Caution

Your best bet for taking cascara sagrada safely is to purchase a product that contains this herb as its active ingredient and to follow the product directions for use, Dr. Farnsworth says. If you are using the bark of this shrub, make sure it has been aged for at least a year before use. As long as the product is labeled "Cascara Sagrada Bark U.S.P.," you can be sure this has been done. Bark that has not been aged correctly contains chemicals that can cause violent diarrhea and severe intestinal cramps.

To make a laxative tea, boil one teaspoon of well-dried bark in three cups of water for 30 minutes. Drink the tea at room temperature, taking one to two cups a day before bed.

Avoid using cascara sagrada if you are pregnant or have ulcers, ulcerative colitis, irritable bowel syndrome, hemorrhoids or other gastrointestinal conditions.

Cayenne (Red Pepper)

The Hottest Healer

The fiery taste and bright red appearance of cayenne pepper make it one of the world's most noticeable spices. Recently, this herb has become as hot in healing as it is on the tongue. Cayenne has proved remarkably effective at relieving certain types of severe, chronic pain. It also aids digestion and may help prevent heart disease.

Cayenne comes from the Caribbean Indian word *kian*. Today Cayenne is the capital of French Guiana. But ironically, only a tiny fraction of the U.S. red pepper supply comes from South America or the Caribbean; most comes from India and Africa. Tabasco (Louisiana pepper), a close cousin of cayenne with all the same health benefits, grows along the Gulf Coast of the United States.

In India, the East Indies, Africa, Mexico and the Caribbean, red pepper enjoys a long history as a stomach-settling digestive aid. "I believe it works," says Varro E. Tyler, Ph.D., professor of pharmacognosy at Purdue University School of Pharmacy in West Lafayette, Indiana, and author of *The Honest Herbal.* Cayenne assists digestion by stimulating the flow of both saliva and stomach secretions. Saliva contains enzymes that begin the breakdown of carbohydrates, and stomach secretions contain acids and other substances that help digest food.

But most Americans doubt the digestive benefits of cayenne, believing instead that the fiery spice can cause ulcers. It doesn't. In one study, researchers used a tiny video camera to examine subjects' stomach linings after both bland meals and meals liberally spiced with jalapeño peppers, another close cousin of cayenne. Their conclusion: There was no difference. Eating highly spiced meals causes no damage whatsoever to the stomach, they reported. However, this finding relates only to people with normal gastrointestinal tracts. "I wouldn't recommend red pepper to anyone with an ulcer," Dr. Tyler says.

What about the burning sensation in your mouth from eating too much red pepper? The best treatment is a glass of milk. The milk protein washes away capsaicin, the chemical in red pepper that's responsible for its heat.

The Heat That Heals

For centuries, herbalists have recommended rubbing red pepper onto sore muscles and joints. Medically, this is known as a counterirritant, a treatment that causes minor superficial discomfort but distracts the person from the more severe, deeper pain. Heet is one brand of capsaicin counterirritant available over the counter.

Recently, however, red pepper has been shown to provide more compelling relief for certain kinds of chronic pain. For reasons still not completely understood, capsaicin interferes with the action of substance P—a nerve chemical that sends pain messages to the brain.

"Capsaicin has proved so effective at relieving pain that it's the active ingredient in the over-the-counter cream, Zostrix," says James A. Duke, Ph.D., a botanist retired from the U.S. Department of Agriculture and author of *The CRC Handbook of Medicinal Herbs.*

Doctors now recommend Zostrix for arthritis, diabetic foot pain and the pain of shingles. Shingles is an adult disease caused by the same virus that causes chicken pox in children. The virus remains dormant in the body until later in life when, for unknown reasons, it reappears in some people as shingles, causing a rash on one side of the body that progresses from red bumps to blisters to crusty pox resembling chicken pox. In most adults, shingles clears up by itself within a few weeks. But many experience lingering, sometimes severe, pain.

Research suggests that capsaicin can also help relieve the awful pain of cluster headaches. In one study, people who regularly experienced cluster headaches rubbed a capsaicin preparation inside their nostrils and outside their noses on the same side of the head as the headache pain. Within five days, 75 percent reported less pain and fewer headaches. They also reported burning nostrils and runny noses, but these side effects subsided within a week.

Finally, red pepper may help the heart. "It cuts cholesterol levels and reduces the risk of the internal blood clots which trigger heart attack," says Daniel B. Mowrey, Ph.D., director of the American Phytotherapy Research Laboratory in Salt Lake City, Utah, and author of *The Scientific Validation of Herbal Medicine.*

Harnessing Cayenne's Healing Power

Perhaps the most enjoyable way to enjoy cayenne's medicinal benefits is to simply season your food to taste. Even these small amounts of red pepper are therapeutic.

Remember to wash your hands thoroughly after using either cayenne or Zostrix. Cayenne may be kind to your stomach lining, but you definitely don't want to get any in your eyes.

To aid digestion and possibly reduce the risk of heart disease, experts recommend cayenne in capsules, which are available from most herbal suppliers. Follow the directions on the package.

Celery Seed

A Health-Giving Spice

POTENTIAL HEALING POWER

May help:
- Prevent certain cancers
- Regulate blood pressure
- Reduce cholesterol

Celery seed adds a distinctive bite to sauerkraut, a fine-edged sharpness to coleslaw and a tangy zip to soups, stews and salad dressings.

Yet along with its refreshing flavor, scientists have found that celery seed may also be adding protection against cancer, high blood pressure and high cholesterol.

In a study for the National Cancer Institute, Luke Lam, Ph.D., and his colleagues at LKT Laboratories in St. Paul, Minnesota, have been analyzing the chemical constituents of celery seed oil and their effect on living beings.

"We isolated five compounds of interest," says Dr. Lam, who was formerly a researcher at the University of Minnesota. "Then we took three of those compounds and looked for their ability to prevent tumor formation in animals."

The result? "The compound sedanolide was the most active," says Dr. Lam. It and a related compound—butyl phthalide—reduced the incidence of tumors in laboratory animals anywhere from 38 to 57 percent. Whether celery can help prevent cancer in people as well as in animals is not yet known.

Studies also suggest that celery seed may give people an edge on another health front: lower blood pressure. So reports William Keller, Ph.D., professor and head of the Division of Medicinal Chemistry and Pharmaceutics at the Northeast Louisiana University School of Pharmacy in Monroe.

In one study at the University of Chicago, laboratory animals given a daily dose of butyl phthalide experienced a 12 percent reduction in their systolic (the top number) blood pressure over a four-week period.

What's more, laboratory studies also indicate that butyl phthalide may help reduce high cholesterol.

If you'd like to try celery seed for yourself, you can prepare a tea by pouring boiling water over one teaspoon of freshly crushed seeds. Let it steep for 10 to 20 minutes before drinking.

Chamomile

Calming Comfort

Centuries-old folklore holds that the chamomile flower is both an internal and external healer. Recent research suggests that much of this folklore is based on fact. More than just a popular and fragrant tea, chamomile can help quiet an upset stomach, quench the fires of inflammation and bring a restful night's sleep.

The two species of plant, the Roman and German varieties, both belong to the same family as asters and daisies. The secrets of chamomile's healing power lie in a complex blend of substances found in the flowerheads, which resemble miniature daisies and yield an azure-blue volatile oil when distilled. Various compounds in this oil, with names such as chamazulene, bisabolol and flavonoids, are

POTENTIAL HEALING POWER

May help:
- Reduce inflammation
- Soothe skin irritation and diaper rash
- Lessen toothache and teething pain
- Ease earache
- Combat indigestion and colic
- Calm nerves
- Lessen cold symptoms
- Relieve menstrual cramps
- Prevent stomach ulcers

believed to hold the key to the herb's medicinal properties.

Centuries of Use

Chamomile is one of those herbs with a reputation for being "good for what ails you." Over 400 years ago, herbalists noted that drinking chamomile tea helped indigestion, and bathing in an infusion of the flowers seemed to relieve strained muscles and aching joints. Wherever the body felt hot, sore or itchy, chamomile has been there to provide gentle relief.

In shampoos and rinses, chamomile is alleged to keep blonde hair at its golden best. The herb is also traditionally recommended for redness, heat or swelling associated with burns, arthritis and sprains. Due to its mildness, it is favored for children's ailments, including colic and teething.

Out of the Blue

Today's herbalists still use chamomile for much the same bouquet of remedies. "Chamomile is a very mild sedative, and it probably relieves itching when applied externally," says Norman R. Farnsworth, Ph.D., director of the Program for Collaborative Research in the Pharmaceutical Sciences at the University of Illinois at Chicago. "And in the best restaurants all over the world, you can get chamomile tea after a big meal. It seems to relax the stomach."

Moreover, "chamomile is one of the few medicinal plants that still have a prominent role in traditional medicine," says Daniel B. Mowrey, Ph.D., director of the American Phytotherapy Research Laboratory in Salt Lake City, Utah, and author of *The Scientific Valida-* *tion of Herbal Medicine.* European researchers have found that the essential oil of this tiny daisy has anti-inflammatory, anti-spasmodic and analgesic properties, reports Dr. Mowrey.

Some studies, performed on animals, have shown that substances in chamomile oil or extract help prevent stomach ulcers and soothe burned or irritated skin. The herb's sedative power was also observed in tests on mice, adds Dr. Mowrey—although anyone who has ever curled up with a cup of chamomile tea on a cold afternoon may not need a cageful of calm mice to be convinced. So far, however, there's no scientific study on whether chamomile-rinsed blondes have more fun.

Rx: Using Chamomile

In Europe, chamomile is an ingredient in dozens of remedies. Some of these are available from American herbal and health food suppliers, reports Dr. Mowrey. They include:

Chamomile tincture. Take 10 to 20 drops in water three or four times a day for nervousness, indigestion and menstrual cramps.

Chamomile lotion. Apply to irritated skin, aching teeth and ears.

Chamomile-containing ointment or cream. Use for wounds and diaper rash.

Chamomile extract. This is a concentrated essence to be used only as directed. A German study showed that home steam inhalation with chamomile extract eased the sniffly miseries of the common cold; the stronger the infusion, the greater the relief.

Take Tea and See

Of course, the simplest way to take chamomile is in the form of tea. A cup of chamomile tea delivers a much more diluted dose of active ingredients than commercial products like tinctures or extracts. Even strong tea contains only about 10 to 15 percent of the volatile oil contained in the flowers themselves. However, some experts believe that a daily cup of chamomile tea may have healthful benefits over months or years.

If you would like something stronger than what you would get from a typical chamomile tea bag, brew about a tablespoon of flowerheads per cup of water, then sip. When cooled, the solution can also be used as a refreshing rinse for hair and body. You can also make your own body oil by steeping an ounce of flowers in olive oil for several days, then straining the oil.

Allergy Sufferers, Beware

Chamomile is considered one of the safest herbs, even for children and pregnant women. It is drunk daily by many thousands of people around the world with no problem, points out Varro E. Tyler, Ph.D., professor of pharmacognosy at Purdue University School of Pharmacy in West Lafayette, Indiana, and author of *The Honest Herbal.* But for a few people, he warns, the pollen-rich flowerheads used to brew the tea can provoke an allergic reaction—in rare cases, a serious one, especially if the person is exposed to other allergens at the same time (for example, during hay fever season).

"If you are allergic to ragweed and other members of the daisy and aster family, such as chrysanthemums, you should be cautious about drinking chamomile tea," says Dr. Tyler. Although chamomile is used in some skin-care products, there have been scattered reports of skin irritation after contact with it. If a chamomile-containing product for external use seems to cause or worsen redness or irritation, he advises, discontinue use.

Cilantro and Coriander

Two Herbs in One

POTENTIAL HEALING POWER

May help:
- Promote digestion
- Ease colic
- Relieve arthritis
- Prevent infection in minor wounds

Cilantro and coriander are twin herbs that come from the same plant. Cilantro, sometimes called Chinese parsley, refers to the leaves. Coriander is the name for the seeds. Historically, the seeds were more popular, but today both the leaves and seeds are widely used. And both have the same medicinal benefits in helping to soothe digestion and control infection.

Coriander tastes like a warm combination of sage and citrus. Cilantro has a similar but milder taste. The seeds apparently stimulate the imagination as well as the taste buds, because around the eighth century, the mythical Arabian princess Scheherazade described coriander as an aphrodisiac in the stories later collected as *The Thousand and One Arabian Nights*. (Science is so far silent concerning this use for the seeds.)

Coriander was used as a digestive aid for thousands of years from China to Europe. In Egypt, the seeds were found in pharaohs' tombs, presumably to prevent indigestion in the afterlife. While the Hebrews were slaves in Egypt, they adopted coriander. According to the Bible, God fed them manna, which the holy book says was "like coriander." If manna did what coriander does, the Hebrews did not suffer indigestion. "Cilantro/coriander helps settle the stomach," says James A. Duke, Ph.D., a botanist retired from the U.S. Department of Agriculture and author of *The CRC Handbook of Medicinal Herbs*.

The ancient Romans used both the leaves and the seeds to preserve meats. And modern Russian researchers have discovered why: The herb is an antioxidant. Antioxidants are chemicals that, among other things, help prevent animal fats from turning rancid. Cilantro and coriander also contain substances that kill meat-spoiling bacteria, fungi and insect larvae. The same microorganisms can cause infections in wounds.

Finally, some studies suggest that cilantro/coriander has anti-inflammatory action, suggesting it might help relieve arthritis.

Try a Spot of Curry

I've never heard of any problems with cilantro or coriander," says Daniel B. Mowrey, Ph.D., director of the American Phytotherapy Research Laboratory in Salt Lake City, Utah, and author of *The Scientific Validation of Herbal Medicine*. "But some people just don't like it. Quite often when people don't like curry, what they object to is the coriander in it. But curry spices are very healthful."

If you'd rather sip a tea than eat curry, use one teaspoon of dried leaves or crushed seeds (or ½ teaspoon of powdered seeds) per cup of boiling water. Steep for five minutes. Drink up to three cups a day before or after meals.

Weak coriander tea may be given to children under two for colic.

You can also sprinkle the powdered seeds on minor cuts and scrapes. Before you do, thoroughly wash the wound with soap and water.

Cinnamon

Good and Good for You

Hot apple cider tastes flat without a cinnamon stick, and toast, cookies, candies and fruit salads all benefit from a generous sprinkle of cinnamon powder. But cinnamon is more than just a kitchen spice. It's been used medicinally for thousands of years. Modern science has confirmed its value for preventing infection and indigestion and has also discovered a couple of new therapeutic uses for the herb.

Cinnamon comes from the bark of an Asian tree. (The sticks are actually pieces of bark.) Ancient Chi-

POTENTIAL HEALING POWER

May help:

- Soothe indigestion
- Control blood sugar in people with diabetes
- Prevent stomach ulcers
- Ward off urinary tract infections
- Fight tooth decay and gum disease
- Prevent vaginal yeast infections

nese herbals mention it as early as 2700 B.C., and Chinese herbalists still recommend it for fever, diarrhea and menstrual problems. Cinnamon was an ingredient in ancient Egyptian embalming mixtures. In the Bible, Moses used it in holy anointing oil.

After the fall of Rome, trade between Europe and Asia became difficult, but cinnamon was so prized that it still found its way west. The 12th-century German abbess and herbalist Hildegard of Bingen recommended it as "the universal spice for sinuses," and to treat colds, flu, cancer and "inner decay and slime," whatever that means.

Boastful Benefits

Several toothpastes are flavored with cinnamon, and for good reason. "Like all the spices used in curries," says Daniel B. Mowrey, Ph.D., director of the American Phytotherapy Research Laboratory in Salt Lake City, Utah, and author of *The Scientific Validation of Herbal Medicine*, "cinnamon is an antiseptic that helps kill the bacteria that cause tooth decay and gum disease." Cinnamon also kills many disease-causing fungi and viruses.

One German study showed it "suppresses completely" the cause of most urinary tract infections (*Escherichia coli* bacteria) and the fungus responsible for vaginal yeast infections (*Candida albicans*).

Like many culinary spices, cinnamon helps soothe the stomach. But a Japanese animal study revealed that it also may help prevent ulcers.

It also appears to help people with diabetes metabolize sugar. In one form of diabetes (Type II, or non-insulin-dependent), the pancreas produces insulin, but the body cannot use it efficiently to break down glucose—the simple sugar that fuels body functions. U.S. Department of Agriculture (USDA) researchers discovered that cinnamon reduces the amount of insulin necessary for glucose metabolism.

Spicing Up Your Health

"One-eighth of a teaspoon of cinnamon triples insulin efficiency," says James A. Duke, Ph.D., a botanist retired from the USDA and author of *The CRC Handbook of Medicinal Herbs*. Dr. Duke suggests that people with Type II diabetes discuss cinnamon's benefits with their doctor.

In foods, simply season to taste. For people with diabetes, ⅛ to ¼ teaspoon of ground cinnamon per meal may help control blood sugar levels.

To brew a stomach-soothing tea, use ½ to ¾ teaspoon of powdered herb per cup of boiling water. Steep 10 to 20 minutes. Drink up to three cups a day.

In powdered form, culinary amounts of cinnamon are non-toxic, although allergic reactions are possible. Cinnamon oil, however, is a different story. On the skin, it may cause redness and burning. Taken internally, it can cause nausea, vomiting and possibly even kidney damage. Don't ingest cinnamon oil.

Clove

Painkilling Preservative

When you were a kid, ham wasn't your favorite food, particularly when Mom studded it with cloves. You tried to pick the little devils out, but one would always slip by and set your entire mouth on fire.

It may have seemed like torture then, but Mom used cloves for a reason. "In addition to providing flavor, cloves are a preservative," says Ara H. DerMarderosian, Ph.D., professor of pharmacognosy and medicinal chemistry at the Philadelphia College of Pharmacy and Science. "You put cloves in ham and it will last several days longer in the refrigerator."

In addition to their preservative powers, cloves are reputed to have health benefits as well.

Spicy Digestive Relief

In South America, cloves are used to fight digestive disorders; people in Uruguay use tea and liquor made from the spice for relief. The aromatic seeds come from small evergreen trees that grow there, as well as in northeastern Brazil.

The herb's usefulness in combating intestinal problems has yet to be fully tested in humans, but laboratory studies indicate it may be effective. The main component of cloves is eugenol, which has been known for some time to help kill bacteria and viruses, says Gary Elmer, Ph.D., associate professor of medicinal chemistry at the University of Washington School of Pharmacy in Seattle. So drinking clove tea for intestinal problems may be worth a try, he says.

Cloves may even help get your system back on track after travel. Cloves fight a type of bacteria, *Escherichia coli*, which play a role in traveler's diarrhea, says Dr. Elmer. "If you have traveler's diarrhea, you could try clove tea."

The eugenol in cloves also makes the herb effective as an antiseptic and painkiller, says Dr. DerMarderosian. You may have encountered the sweet/hot taste of clove oil in over-the-counter toothache medicines. And while not generally used in the United States, poultices of clove can be used on the skin for cuts and bites. "Indonesians put it on top of wounds, on top of bites, that sort of thing. It has an anti-septic quality," says Dr. DerMar-derosian.

Using a poultice of cloves for cuts and bites may be very effec-tive, says Dr. Elmer. Studies show that clove oil can help kill several strains of staphylococcus bacteria and one strain of pseudomonas—organisms that can cause infection in the skin.

Putting Cloves to Work

Clove tea for intestinal problems can be made using one tea-spoon of powdered cloves per cup of boiling water. Steep for 10 to 20 minutes before drinking.

To make a poultice for a cut or bite, grind up several cloves, mix them with water and apply the paste to the skin. Cover it with a warm towel.

Coffee

Surprising Benefits from Caffeine

Although most people don't think of it as such, coffee is America's most popular herbal beverage. It helps a sleepy nation wake up in the morning. It also has therapeutic value. It can act as a decongestant for colds. It may help prevent asthma attacks. It may boost athletic performance. And it increases the pain-relieving power of aspirin.

Of course, coffee can also cause problems—jitters and insomnia. But despite scare headlines that have linked coffee to many serious diseases, the latest medical review concludes: "Coffee appears to pose

POTENTIAL HEALING POWER

May help:

- Combat drowsiness
- Temporarily boost athletic performance
- Ease congestion due to colds and flu
- Prevent asthma attacks
- Enhance the pain-relieving effects of aspirin

no particular threat in most people if consumed in moderation."

Coffee has been around for a long time. Our word *coffee* comes from Caffa, the region of Ethiopia where the fabled beans were first discovered. The beverage we know as coffee emerged around A.D. 1000, when Arabians began roasting and grinding coffee beans and drinking the hot beverage as we do today. Until the 17th century, Arabia supplied all the world's coffee through the port of Mocha, which became one of coffee's names. Then the Dutch introduced the plant into Java, and the island quickly became synonymous with coffee.

The medically important constituent of coffee is, of course, caffeine, but coffee's caffeine content depends on how it's prepared. A cup of instant contains about 60 milligrams of caffeine. Drip or percolated coffee has about 100. A cup of espresso contains about 100 milligrams, too, but this is in a 2½-ounce cup—the traditional serving size for espresso.

Boosting Performance

Coffee is best known as the powerful stimulant that helps people stay awake during night drives and cramming before final exams. It does not, however, help anyone sober up after overindulging in alcohol. In fact, it can upset hung-over stomachs.

Some over-the-counter cold formulas contain caffeine, partly to counteract the sedative effects of the antihistamines they contain. Caffeine may also help open the bronchial tubes, relieving the congestion of colds and flu. Coffee's action as a bronchodilator can also help prevent asthma attacks.

If you take aspirin for pain relief, perhaps you should take it with a cup of coffee. Several studies show that, compared with plain aspirin, the combination of aspirin and caffeine relieves pain significantly better than aspirin alone.

Coffee may also improve physical stamina, according to a report published in the journal *The Physician and Sportsmedicine.* The International Olympic Committee forbids "caffeine loading" and tests urine for illegal amounts. To reach illegal levels, an endurance athlete would have to drink four or five cups in 30 minutes. Athletes who want coffee's benefits without risking disqualification typically drink three or four cups during the hour or two before an event.

How Much Is Too Much?

Caffeine is such an integral part of our culture, we seldom realize how much of a drug it is. The fact is, caffeine is classically addictive. Regular users develop a tolerance and require more to obtain the expected effect. Deprived of caffeine, regular users usually develop withdrawal symptoms, primarily a headache, which can last several days.

Coffee is most notorious for causing insomnia and increasing anxiety, irritability and nervousness. It can also aggravate panic attacks. Coffee increases the secretion of stomach acids and can upset the stomach. Doctors say that people with ulcers or other gastrointestinal conditions should use it cautiously, if at all. Contrary to popular mythology, coffee does not cause ulcers. It can, however, make ulcers worse in people who already have them.

Coffee also raises blood pressure in those who are not accustomed to drinking it. But once java junkies have developed a caffeine tolerance, the body adjusts, and normal consumption no longer affects blood pressure.

But coffee's worst press has concerned its association with heart disease. The subject is extremely controversial, with evidence supporting both sides of the argument. Most studies indicate that coffee can increase cholesterol levels. Oddly, decaffeinated coffee has the same cholesterol-boosting effect as regular, suggesting that caffeine is not the culprit. For reasons that remain a mystery, filtered coffee raises cholesterol less than boiled coffee. If your cholesterol is high, discuss your coffee consumption with your physician.

Independent of coffee's action on cholesterol and blood pressure, it may increase the risk of heart attack. The danger level is more than four cups a day.

There are also reports that coffee aggravates premenstrual syndrome in many women. And coffee has been accused of contributing to infertility, birth defects, gallstones, immune impairment and many forms of cancer. To date, none of these allegations has been proven.

"I'd advise limiting caffeine intake to 250 milligrams a day," says Varro E. Tyler, Ph.D., professor of pharmacognosy at Purdue University School of Pharmacy in West Lafayette, Indiana, and author of *The Honest Herbal*. "That's about two cups of brewed coffee."

"Personally, I drink five or six cups a day," says James A. Duke, Ph.D., a botanist retired from the U.S. Department of Agriculture and author of *The CRC Handbook of Medicinal Herbs*. "But I don't recommend drinking more than two."

Not everyone who quits or cuts back develops withdrawal symptoms, but most people do. The throbbing headache usually begins within 18 to 24 hours and lasts a few days. Constipation is also possible for a day or two.

Dill

From Pickles to Colic

Ever wonder how dill got into dill pickles? Flavor enhancement is only part of the reason. The herb is also a natural preservative, and in the days before refrigeration, vegetables were often pickled in vinegar or brine to preserve them. With dill added, they lasted even longer. Dill also helped settle the stomach, because the herb is a digestive aid.

In fact, the ancient Egyptians, Greeks, Romans and Chinese all used dill to soothe the stomach. The Vikings also appreciated dill's digestive benefits. Our word *dill* comes from the Old Norse *dilla,* to lull or soothe. During the Middle Ages, dill was used to protect against witchcraft, and throughout history, cooled dill tea, or "dillwater," has been a popular folk remedy for infant colic.

"Dillwater works," says Daniel B. Mowrey, Ph.D., director of the American Phytotherapy Research Laboratory in Salt Lake City, Utah, and author of *The Scientific Validation of Herbal Medicine.* "It's gentle enough for infants."

"For colic, many herbalists recommend a combination of dill and fennel," says James A. Duke, Ph.D., a botanist retired from the U.S. Department of Agriculture and author of *The CRC Handbook of Medicinal Herbs.* "Both herbs contain stomach-soothing oils."

Dill owes its preservative action to its ability to inhibit the growth of several bacteria (staphylococcus, streptococcus, pseudomonas and *Escherichia coli*). This effect suggests that it might help prevent another common early childhood gastrointestinal illness—infectious diarrhea caused by these same microorganisms.

Traditional herbalists also recommended dill for prevention of flatulence, and perhaps there was something to this. The herb has anti-foaming action, suggesting that it might help break up gas bubbles.

How to Do Dill

To brew a stomach-soothing tea, use two teaspoons of mashed seeds per cup of boiling water. Steep for ten minutes. Drink up to three cups a day. In a tincture, take ½ to 1 teaspoon up to three times a day.

To treat colic or gas in children under two, give small amounts of a weak tea.

In sensitive individuals, ingesting dill might cause skin rash, but the leaves, seeds and seed oil are generally considered nontoxic. If any skin irritation develops, discontinue use.

Echinacea

Nature's Immunity Booster

Looking at echinacea's reputation through history is like riding a roller coaster. It's up, it's down, it's up again. Before European colonists showed up, the Plains Indians were using this native North American wildflower as a healing herb. The colonists started using it, too, and in the 1870s, a Nebraska doctor popularized it as a "blood purifier" and snakebite remedy.

For years most households in this country kept tincture of echinacea (*ek-i-NAY-see-uh*) on hand as an infection fighter. With the advent of antibiotics, however, the herb fell from favor.

Now, thanks to modern medical science, echinacea is once again receiving favorable attention. Although it's no substitute for antibiotics, this herb holds some promise

POTENTIAL HEALING POWER
May help:
• Fight infections
• Reduce symptoms of colds and flu
• Stimulate the immune system
• Heal minor wounds and burns

as an immune system booster after all. In order to reestablish its reputation as a healer, however, this American herb had to do a little traveling. In Germany, extensive research over the past few decades has uncovered a host of infection-fighting properties.

"The herb normalizes the number of white blood cells in the blood and helps them surround and destroy bacteria and viruses," says Daniel B. Mowrey, Ph.D., director of the American Phytotherapy Research Laboratory in Salt Lake City, Utah, and author of *The Scientific Validation of Herbal*

Medicine. It also slows the spread of infection to surrounding tissues and helps flush toxins away from infected areas, he says.

In several studies, injections of concentrated compounds derived from echinacea caused people's immune systems to activate macrophages. These germ-gobbling cells are crucial to beating infection, and they may have anti-tumor activity as well. Echinacea may even play a role in curbing the misery of colds and flu. In one study done in Germany, liquid echinacea extract was shown to help ease the symptoms of influenza and speed recovery.

Applied externally as a poultice to wounds, sores and burns, echinacea may also protect against infection and stimulate tissue repair and healing.

Make Sure It's the Real Thing

To battle a cold or the flu, take echinacea at the first sign of symptoms, says Varro E. Tyler, Ph.D., professor of pharmacognosy at Purdue University School of Pharmacy in West Lafayette, Indiana, and author of *The Honest Herbal.* He recommends taking about a teaspoonful of alcohol-based tincture a day to duplicate the effective dose in the German flu study.

A tea made from echinacea provides a tasty but somewhat less potent alternative. To make a tea, pour boiling water over two to three tablespoons of dried, fresh or powdered herb and steep for five minutes. Sip over a period of 30 to 90 minutes and repeat six to eight hours later.

Dr. Tyler warns, however, that the lack of standardization in American herbal products makes it hard to guarantee even an approximate dosage of a particular compound. There have also been reports of echinacea products being adulterated with other herbs. His advice: Purchase herbal products only from well-established, reputable suppliers. Echinacea is generally considered safe, says Dr. Tyler, although an allergic reaction is always a possibility. Discontinue use if you experience any adverse effects.

Ephedra

The World's Original Healer

Ask most people if they've ever heard of Sudafed and they'll say, "Sure, the drugstore decongestant." But ask if they're familiar with the plant it comes from—ephedra—and all they'll say is "Huh?"

Ephedra is one of the world's oldest medicines. Few people who take over-the-counter decongestants containing a component of this herb—pseudoephedrine—have any idea they are participating in an herbal healing tradition that dates back 5,000 years.

The origins of Chinese medicine are lost in legend, but authorities say that Chinese physicians began prescribing Chinese ephedra (*Ephedra sinica*), or *ma huang*, for colds, asthma and hay fever around 3000 B.C.

"Ma huang is the herb for chest congestion and asthma," says Pi-Kwang Tsung, Ph.D., former assistant professor of pathology at the University of Connecticut Medical School in Farmington and currently editor of *The East-West Medical Digest*. "Studies show that its major active constituents are ephedrine and psuedoephedrine."

Unfortunately, not all plants called ephedra have the decongestant benefits of the Chinese variety. American ephedra (*E. nevadensis*), also called Mormon tea, is a pleasant, piney-tasting beverage. "But many studies have shown that it contains no decongestant chemicals," says Bernie Olin, Pharm.D., editor of *The Lawrence Review of Natural Products*, a St. Louis–based newsletter that summarizes scientific research on medicinal herbs.

Weight Loss, Chinese-Style

The decongestants in Chinese ephedra can also increase basal metabolic rate (BMR)—the speed at which the body burns calories. A few studies have shown that ephedrine-induced increases in BMR can help obese women shed pounds in medically supervised weight-loss programs. The catch is that it only helps those who are seriously obese, not those who want to drop a few extra pounds.

Ephedra can increase heart rate and raise blood pressure, so don't use it if you have high blood pressure, heart disease, diabetes or glaucoma. You should also not take ephedra if you have thyroid problems. In fact, ephedra can be harmful when taken improperly and should not be used by anyone with health problems. If you want to take ephedra or any product containing it, you should discuss it with your doctor.

To brew a medicinal tea, mix 1 teaspoon of dried ma huang per cup of water, bring it to a boil, then simmer for 10 to 15 minutes. Drink up to two cups a day. In a tincture, take ¼ to 1 teaspoon up to three times a day. When using commercial preparations, follow package directions.

Eucalyptus

The Australian Antiseptic

If you've ever used Listerine, Vicks VapoRub, Dristan Nasal Decongestant Spray or Hall's Mentho-Lyptus Cough Suppressants, you're undoubtedly familiar with the unique, refreshing scent of eucalyptus. And if you've ever seen a koala, you've also seen a eucalyptus tree, because its long, scythe-shaped leaves are the sole food source for the cute, furry critter.

Australia's aborigines used eucalyptus to treat fever, cough and asthma—and European settlers quickly adopted it as medicine. For a time, doctors thought eucalyptus could cure malaria, and they called it the Australian fever tree. Alas, that use didn't pan out, but eucalyptus leaf oil does contain a chemical, eucalyptol, that has decongestant and antiseptic action.

"Eucalyptol is a very effective decongestant," says Varro E. Tyler, Ph.D., professor of pharmacognosy at Purdue University School of Pharmacy in West Lafayette, Indiana, and author of *The Honest Herbal*. "It loosens phlegm in the chest, making it easier to cough up. That's why so many decongestants, cough lozenges and chest rubs contain it."

"Eucalyptol also kills several types of bacteria and viruses," says Daniel B. Mowrey, Ph.D., director of the American Phytotherapy Research Laboratory in Salt Lake City, Utah, and author of *The Sci-*

entific Validation of Herbal Medicine. After minor wounds have been washed, eucalyptus oil or clean crushed leaves can be applied to help prevent infection.

Recently, a new eucalyptus product, Eucalyptamint, has been promoted as a treatment for muscle soreness. Researchers at the University of California at Irvine tested the ointment and discovered that it increases blood flow to muscle tissue, lending credence to the product's claims.

Using the Australian Healer

To brew a pleasant-tasting medicinal tea, use one to two teaspoons of dried, crushed leaves per cup of boiling water. Steep ten minutes. Drink up to two cups a day. When using commercial products, follow the package directions.

If you live in the South or on the West Coast and have access to eucalyptus leaves, place a handful in boiling water and inhale the steamy vapor. For an herbal bath, wrap a handful of leaves in a cloth and run bathwater over it.

You can use a few drops of eucalyptus oil in boiling water or in the bath as an inhalant, but never ingest the oil. When the oil is taken internally, it is highly poisonous. Fatalities have been reported from ingestion of as little as a teaspoonful.

Eucalyptus oil is considered nonirritating to the skin, but sensitive individuals may develop a rash. If your skin gets red or irritated from the oil, discontinue use.

Fennel

Comfort for New Parents

POTENTIAL HEALING POWER

May help:
- Alleviate gas
- Relieve colic

You're at an Indian restaurant waiting to be seated when you notice a small bowl of fennel seeds on a table by the door. You wonder what they're for, and before you know it, you're entertaining yourself with possibilities: An air freshener? Seasoning for the mango chutney? Something to be tossed over your shoulder for good luck?

The answer: The seeds are meant to be chewed in order to relieve gas, says Ara H. DerMarderosian, Ph.D., professor of pharmacognosy and medicinal chemistry at Philadelphia College of Pharmacy and Science. Through the ages, as far back as the ancient Romans, fennel has had a reputation as a flatulence reliever.

Historically, fennel has also been used to strengthen eyesight, relieve stomach upset, stimulate milk production in nursing mothers and promote menstruation. And those were just a few of its uses. It was reputed to be so effective, in fact, that an old Welsh doctor once proclaimed that "He who sees fennel and gathers it not, is not a man, but a devil!"

Yet few of the historical uses of fennel have been scientifically substantiated. Its reputation as an aid for expelling gas is probably the most sound claim to date.

Possible Cure for Colic

A 1993 study conducted in Israel provides some support for the traditional use of fennel to relieve colic in infants. Researchers gave an herbal tea preparation containing fennel to 33 colicky babies and a nontherapeutic (placebo) drink to 35 other colicky infants for seven days. The researchers concluded that colic was eliminated in more of the babies who received herbal tea than in those who received the placebo drink.

Although the study is far from conclusive, it can't hurt to try giving fennel tea to a colicky baby. "It's worth a try, because colic is such a complex thing," says Dr. DerMarderosian.

To make fennel tea, steep ⅓ teaspoon of crushed fennel seed in a cup of boiling water.

Make sure you let the tea cool sufficiently before giving it to an infant. And, of course, if *you're* feeling a little gassy, you might want to try the tea yourself. Or you can do as the Indians do and nibble on a handful of fennel seeds—they have a pleasant, licorice-like flavor.

Fenugreek

Help for High Cholesterol

From ancient times through the late 19th century, fenugreek played a major role in herbal healing. Then it fell by the wayside. Now things are once again looking up for the herb whose taste is an odd combination of bitter celery and maple syrup. Modern scientific research has found that fenugreek can help reduce cholesterol levels, control diabetes and minimize the symptoms of menopause.

The ancient Greeks fed this herb to horses and cattle. The Romans then started using it, too, calling it "Greek hay." (In Latin, "Greek hay" is *foenum-graecum,* and that evolved into "fenugreek.") As fenugreek spread around the ancient Mediterranean, physicians learned that its seeds, like many seeds, contain a gummy substance called mucilage. Mixed with water, mucilage expands and becomes a gelatinous soother for irritated tissues.

In India, the herb was incorporated into curry blends. India's traditional Ayurvedic physicians prescribed it to nursing mothers to increase their milk. In American folk medicine, fenugreek was considered a potent menstruation pro-

---

POTENTIAL HEALING POWER

May help:

- Minimize symptoms of menopause
- Relieve constipation
- Control diabetes
- Reduce cholesterol
- Soothe sore throat pain and coughs
- Ease minor indigestion
- Relieve diarrhea

---

moter. It became a key ingredient in Lydia E. Pinkham's Vegetable Compound—one of 19th-century America's most popular patent medicines for "female weakness" (menstrual discomforts). Today, fenugreek is most widely used in the United States as a source of imitation maple flavor. But this may change as its medicinal value becomes better known.

Almost a century after Lydia Pinkham's death, scientists have confirmed that fenugreek seeds contain chemicals (diosgenin and estrogenic isoflavones) similar to the female sex hormone estrogen. Loss of estrogen causes menopausal symptoms, so adding fenugreek to the diet might help minimize them. Estrogen can also cause breast swelling. "One woman told me her breasts grew larger after she started eating fenugreek sprouts," says James A. Duke,

Ph.D., a botanist retired from the U.S. Department of Agriculture and author of *The CRC Handbook of Medicinal Herbs.*

Cholesterol Buster . . . and More

Several studies have shown that fenugreek reduces cholesterol in laboratory animals, and Indian researchers have shown the same effect in people with high cholesterol levels. The people in one Indian study added about four ounces a day of powdered fenugreek seeds to their diet for 20 days. During that time their total cholesterol levels and their levels of low-density lipoprotein (LDL, or "bad") cholesterol fell significantly. At the same time their high-density lipoprotein (HDL, or "good") cholesterol levels remained unaffected. "There's no question that fenugreek reduces cholesterol," says Daniel B. Mowrey, Ph.D., director of the American Phytotherapy Research Laboratory in Salt Lake City, Utah, and author of *The Scientific Validation of Herbal Medicine.*

Fenugreek also "has great promise in alleviating Type II (non-insulin-dependent) diabetes," says Dr. Duke. And according to one study, it may also help people with Type I (insulin-dependent) diabetes. For ten days, Indian re-searchers added about four ounces of powdered fenugreek seeds a day to the diets of people with Type I diabetes, which requires daily insulin injections. The injections, however, did not entirely eliminate a key sign of the illness, sugar in their urine. With fenugreek added to their diet, their urinary sugar levels fell by 54 percent.

Fenugreek's soothing mucilage can also help relieve sore throat pain, cough and minor indigestion. "Because its mucilage expands in the gut, it also adds bulk to the stool," says Bernie Olin, Pharm.D., editor of *The Lawrence Review of Natural Products,* a St. Louis–based newsletter that summarizes scientific research on the medicinal value of herbs. "As a result, it can help treat constipation and diarrhea."

To make a medicinal tea, gently boil two teaspoons of mashed seeds per cup of water, then simmer for ten minutes. Drink up to three cups a day. To improve the flavor, you can add sugar, honey, lemon, anise or peppermint.

Fenugreek is considered safe. But several of the conditions it helps—diabetes, elevated cholesterol and menopausal symptoms—require professional care. If you'd like to use this herb in addition to standard therapies, consult your physician.

Feverfew

Powerful Migraine Mauler

POTENTIAL HEALING POWER

May help:
- Prevent migraine headaches
- Relieve arthritis
- Ease menstrual cramps

Despite its name, feverfew won't get rid of a fever. In fact, if today's scientists could rename this plant, they might want to dub it migraine-few.

In the 1980s, several studies done in the United Kingdom showed that people who regularly suffer from migraine headaches often find relief with feverfew. In the studies, migraine sufferers who chewed fresh feverfew leaves or took capsules of dried, ground leaves experienced fewer and less severe headaches.

The key to this effect, researchers believe, is parthenolide, a compound in feverfew that helps control the expansion and contraction of blood vessels in the brain. The unpleasant symptoms of migraine—nausea, throbbing head pain and sensitivity to light—apparently occur when blood vessels in the brain overreact, contracting and expanding abnormally.

This doesn't mean, though, that you can reach for feverfew to relieve a migraine.

"Feverfew has no beneficial effect on migraine attacks once they're in gear," says Varro E. Tyler, Ph.D., professor of pharmacognosy at Purdue University School of Pharmacy in West Lafayette, Indiana, and author of *The Honest Herbal.* "It works as a *preventive,* and that means taking it regularly over a long period."

Researchers suspect that feverfew may also help combat menstrual cramps and arthritic inflammation, although these uses are not as well substantiated.

Using Feverfew

Prescription medications are available for migraines, but they don't work for everybody. According to Daniel B. Mowrey, Ph.D., director of the American Phytotherapy Research Laboratory in Salt Lake City, Utah, and author of *The Scientific Validation of Herbal Medicine,* "The people feverfew works best for are usually those who don't respond to any other form of medication."

To duplicate the doses used in the migraine research, says Dr. Mowrey, "most people must eat a leaf or two or take a capsule or two each day." That's assuming you're getting perfectly potent feverfew, and that could prove difficult.

"The problem with feverfew in the United States," says Dr. Tyler, "is that you're very unlikely to get a quality product." Several investigators, he points out, have tested commercial feverfew preparations, such as tablets or extracts, and found that they contain little or no active ingredient.

For this reason, Dr. Tyler suggests taking more than the recommended dosage of any store-bought feverfew preparation to increase the odds of getting an adequate dose of the active ingredient, parthenolide. He recommends taking up to six 300- to 400-milligram tablets of the herb daily. Taking this much feverfew in tablet form is perfectly safe, he says.

You can also grow your own supply of fresh feverfew, says Dr. Mowrey. In fact, he suspects that whole feverfew leaves may work better than taking the active ingredient in concentrated form. "The research suggests strongly that the whole leaf has to be used," he says. "In some studies, people who just chewed on the leaf had better results than those who used pills filled with ground, dried plant material or an extract."

There is one potential drawback to eating feverfew leaves: They may cause irritation or ulcers of the lips, tongue and lining of the mouth. Otherwise, feverfew is generally considered safe. (If chewing feverfew leaves irritates your mouth, discontinue use immediately.)

It's also a good idea to steer clear of feverfew altogether if you are allergic to chamomile, chrysanthemum and other members of the daisy family. And since feverfew may also affect the clotting components of blood, people with a clotting disorder or those who take anti-clotting drugs probably shouldn't take it. And, just to be on the safe side, pregnant women should also avoid it.

Ginger

Spicy Weapon against Nausea

POTENTIAL HEALING POWER

May help:
- Prevent motion sickness
- Fight nausea and diarrhea from stomach flu
- Relieve gas and indigestion

A beloved spice in kitchens around the world, ginger can do more than perk up food and beverages. It has proven merit for fighting nausea and may hold promise for the treatment of other conditions as well.

Ginger looks like a root, but botanically it is a rhizome, or underground stem. Cooks use it as a seasoning in various forms—sliced fresh, candied or powdered. But when it's used as a medicine, its pungency limits how much can be taken in one dose. Thanks to the invention of the gelatin capsule, more potent and convenient formulations of powdered ginger can now be used medicinally.

Spin Control

It's rare for an herbal remedy to be taken seriously in the pages of a major medical journal, but in 1982 ginger got the nod as an effective preventive for motion sickness from the prestigious British medical journal *Lancet.*

Daniel B. Mowrey, Ph.D., director of the American Phytotherapy Research Laboratory in Salt Lake City, Utah, and author of *The Scientific Validation of Herbal Medicine,* and a colleague compared the effects of powdered ginger to a standard dose of the over-the-counter antihistamine dimenhydrinate (Dramamine) in 36 college students who had a strong tendency to get motion sickness. After being spun in a tilted rotating chair, the ginger-treated students experienced less nausea and vertigo than the Dramamine-treated group. As a bonus, ginger causes none of the sleepy side effects associated with Dramamine and other antihistamines.

Nausea is a complex reaction involving various areas of the brain as well as the digestive tract, says Dr. Mowrey. Ginger appears to work directly on the stomach as well as on the brain to calm the heaves, he says.

In addition to its usefulness in battling motion sickness, ginger can also help reduce the nausea and diarrhea that often accompany stomach flu, says Dr. Mowrey.

All of these research findings bear out traditional uses of ginger in Chinese medicine to relieve indigestion and gas.

A Warming Trend

Other uses for ginger, although less firmly proven, have been suggested by various researchers. Scattered reports have linked ginger with relief of headaches, lowering of high blood cholesterol, reduction of rheumatoid arthritis symptoms and prevention of stomach ulcers.

A significant—and therapeutic—amount of ginger may be ingested by eating ginger-spiced food or drinking ginger ale (at least the kind flavored with real ginger, not a synthetic flavoring). Ditto for a cup of ginger tea made with a teaspoon of grated fresh root or dried powder. But to take ginger for motion sickness as needed at sea or on the road, capsules containing powdered ginger are quicker and easier.

In Dr. Mowrey's experiment, the dose (taken before motion began) was 940 milligrams, or about two standard ginger capsules. But he has a simpler guideline for knowing how much ginger to take to obtain results: "If you don't taste a little ginger on your breath or in your throat about five minutes after swallowing the capsule, you haven't taken enough."

There have been several scientific reports that ginger can help relieve morning sickness, including cases so severe that the women required hospital care. So far, there is no evidence that ginger has any adverse effects on an unborn child, but the risk has never been subjected to rigorous study. Herbal authorities say that a few ginger pills in the morning to quell nausea are probably safe, but just a few may not be effective—and higher doses increase the small but unknown risk. Play it safe. If you're pregnant, don't take any medicine or supplement—including ginger—without the consent of your obstetrician.

Ginkgo

Asian Guard against Aging

Talk about late bloomers! Ginkgo, the oldest living tree species on earth, has been used medicinally by the Chinese for some 4,000 years. Yet only in the last two decades have Western medical researchers found evidence that ginkgo may offer hope for a host of age-related problems.

Ginkgo trees, also known as maidenhair trees, are often planted on city streets. The tree's fruit

POTENTIAL HEALING POWER

May help:

- Improve tinnitus (ringing in the ears)
- Relieve symptoms of Alzheimer's disease, including short-term memory loss and depression
- Reduce inflammation due to asthma and allergies
- Fight damage from stroke
- Ease outbreaks of multiple sclerosis
- Lessen symptoms of peripheral vascular disease and Raynaud's disease

smells awful when decomposed and can cause skin irritation, but the almondlike seed within is prized as a commodity in Asian markets.

It is the ginkgo's pretty, fan-shaped leaf, not its foul fruit, that excites scientists these days. Although little known in this country outside of health food stores, a concentrated extract of the plant has been the number-one prescription drug in Germany, where it is used to help asthma and circulation problems. And unlike many plant-based therapeutic agents, "ginkgo preparations have been extensively tested in people, not just in animals and test tubes," says Norman R. Farnsworth, Ph.D., director of the Program for Collaborative Research in the Pharmaceutical Sciences at the University of Illinois at Chicago.

Powerful Medicine

What's in ginkgo extract, and what can it do? The active constituents include unique compounds called ginkgolides. One of these compounds, ginkgolide B, has been shown to suppress a clot-promoting substance in the human body called platelet activating factor, or PAF. Since PAF is a key player in body processes such as allergic inflammation and asthma, the disease-fighting potential of ginkgo is intriguing.

This and other substances in ginkgo extract have shown various benefits for the ills of old age, especially those resulting from decreased blood supply to the brain and other parts of the body. These effects are believed to stem from ginkgo's ability to dilate arteries and capillaries, the tiny blood vessels that nourish the body's tissues.

Perhaps most exciting is ginkgo's potential for improving short-term memory loss and depression in elderly people. "The research on ginkgo and Alzheimer's disease is producing extremely good results in France and Germany," says Daniel B. Mowrey, Ph.D., director of the American Phytotherapy Research Laboratory in Salt Lake City, Utah, and author of *The Scientific Validation of Herbal Medicine.* "It seems that the earlier you catch the disease, the greater the chances that you can reverse it by taking ginkgo extract."

The extract has also reduced symptoms of peripheral vascular disease and Raynaud's disease, two painful conditions involving impaired circulation in the feet and hands. And "there are many clinical studies showing it can reduce tinnitus, or ringing in the ears, which affects many older people," according to Dr. Farnsworth.

German research performed on laboratory rats confirmed previous evidence that ginkgolide B may minimize the devastation of stroke. And a French study on humans showed that it may even allay bouts of multiple sclerosis.

Rx: Going Ginkgo

Remember, though, the only well-demonstrated benefits of ginkgo have been from a concentrated extract, not from the leaves themselves. Such extracts are available in the United States, and they are labeled as food supplements, not drugs, in accordance with U.S. regulations. Regular use of such products is widespread in Europe, according to Varro E. Tyler, Ph.D., professor of pharmacognosy at Purdue University School of Pharmacy in West Lafayette, Indiana, and author of *The Honest Herbal*.

Ginkgo extract is generally considered safe, says Dr. Tyler, although it has been noted to cause some generally mild side effects, including restlessness and digestive upset. If you experience such symptoms, he advises, discontinue use. And since ginkgo also affects the body's clotting mechanism, Dr. Tyler warns, use it cautiously if you take anti-clotting medications, including aspirin, or have a clotting disorder.

Dr. Tyler also warns against ginkgo hype aimed at older folks. "While ginkgo has apparently been effective in treating ailments associated with decreased cerebral blood flow in old age," he says, "claims that ginkgo extract will 'reverse the aging process' and increase longevity are, of course, unproven."

Ginseng

The Inscrutable Root

In 1711, a Jesuit missionary stationed in China gave the West its first glimpse of ginseng. "Nobody can imagine that the Chinese and Tartars would set so high a value on this root, if it did not constantly produce a good effect," he wrote. Surely it was only a matter of time, he said, before European pharmacists figured out how to use this age-old remedy.

POTENTIAL HEALING POWER

May help:
- Relieve stress
- Improve stamina
- Regulate blood pressure
- Enhance immunity

Almost 300 years later, ginseng, perhaps the most researched herb on earth, remains a mystery. Some claim it's a panacea, others insist it's worthless—and medical researchers suggest that the power of ginseng, if any, may lie in its complexity.

Name That Herb

Ginseng refers to at least three different plants. The mother of all ginseng is the Asian variety, *Panax ginseng*, prescribed in 2,000-year-old Chinese texts to "quiet the spirit and increase wisdom." A close cousin is American ginseng (*P. quinquefolius*). Just to confuse matters, a distantly related plant called Eleuthero, or Siberian ginseng, has recently become popular as a cheap substitute for "real" ginseng.

All three types of ginseng are traditionally used as tonics—to strengthen and regulate body functions and thus treat a host of ailments. Some of the fleshy roots look vaguely like a human figure, which possibly explains their reputation as a body-wide cure-all.

Is there anything to this tradition? Many scientists have tried to test the powers of ginseng, with results as frustrating as a Chinese puzzle. "I'm sure ginseng does *something*, but there's so much conflicting information that it's impossible to say just what this herb does in human beings," says Norman R. Farnsworth, Ph.D., director of the Program for Collaborative Research in the Pharmaceutical Sciences at the University of Illinois at Chicago.

Experts agree that ginseng contains a variety of compounds called ginsenosides. And various ginsenosides have been shown in test-tube and animal studies to have contradictory effects. Some of these chemicals appear to raise blood pressure; others seem to lower it. Some act as sedatives, others as stimulants.

Some herbalists argue that the complex nature of ginseng is exactly what makes it a good tonic—that is, a remedy that helps the body achieve balance, warding off damage from disease and other stresses. A more scientific term for a tonic is *adaptogen*—something that helps the body adapt (for example, by regulating temperature or blood pressure up or down toward normal).

Studies have shown that substances found in Asian and American ginseng may indeed bolster the immune system and have a positive effect on conditions ranging from diabetes to high blood pressure.

As for Siberian ginseng, it is widely used by Russians, including cosmonauts and athletes, to improve stamina and resist stress. And Russian research offers evidence that some of these effects may be real.

Despite all the research that's been done on ginseng, it will still take some large, well-done studies on humans to confirm its benefits, says Dr. Farnsworth.

Using the Mystery Herb

Many American products are simply labeled "ginseng," but Chinese medicine differentiates among the three types. For example, Asian ginseng has "warming" properties, and should be used "to reinvigorate the body, as after a long illness," says Albert Leung, Ph.D., a pharmacognosist and author of *Chinese Healing Foods and Herbs*. But American ginseng is "cooling," he says, and should be used by people who are "overheated and excited."

Unfortunately, debating such fine points may sometimes be moot—because there's no guarantee that a ginseng product contains any ginseng at all! Since ginseng is so costly, packagers are tempted to dilute or substitute cheaper ingredients. One 1978 study analyzed 54 ginseng products and found that 25 percent contained no ginseng

whatsoever. Your best bet is to buy ginseng products only from a reputable source.

Ginseng consumption seems to have few reported side effects. As with any herb, however, possible risk increases with higher intake over longer periods. If you decide to take any ginseng product, start low and go slow.

Dried ginseng root may be powdered and taken in capsule form or brewed as a tea. Extracts are also available in various formulations for use internally and externally, and these should include instructions for proper dosage. As with any herb, experts advise against taking ginseng if you are pregnant or nursing, unless you're under the care of a medical specialist.

Goldenseal

Yellow Cure for Sore Throats

POTENTIAL HEALING POWER

May help:
- Soothe sore throat
- Relieve indigestion
- Kill germs internally and externally
- Ease red, tired eyes
- Prevent and treat diarrhea caused by microorganisms

Cherokee warriors once ground goldenseal's roots as a source of bright yellow face paint. And Cherokee medicine men used the herb medicinally, applying it to arrow wounds and inflamed eyes. Early American colonists also learned to appreciate goldenseal—as a digestive tonic, as an astringent rinse for sore throats and canker sores and to stop bleeding after childbirth.

A wildflower of North American forests, goldenseal soon leaped the Atlantic and became popular in Europe as well. To this day, it remains a favorite among herbalists throughout the Western world, who still use it to treat eye irritations, minor skin wounds and indigestion. They also swear by goldenseal as an infection fighter and immune system booster.

But does science bear out folklore as to the herb's medicinal powers?

The effects of goldenseal on human beings have not been extensively studied. But chemical analysis has turned up two main active chemicals in the roots. These alkaloid compounds— berberine and hydrastine—have a wide array of effects on the human body.

Berberine reduces hemorrhaging and is a powerful antiseptic, medical experts say. In the gastrointestinal tract, it has been shown to fight diarrhea-causing microorganisms, including *Giardia*—a parasite common in water supplies around the world—and even cholera. Berberine also acts as a mild local anesthetic on mucous membranes. This lends scientific confirmation to the use of goldenseal tea as a gargle to treat sore throat.

Hydrastine has long been used as an ingredient in commercial eyewashes. This compound constricts tiny blood vessels—an action that may "get the red out" of tired eyes but may also cause a rise in blood pressure throughout the body when the compound is taken internally.

Unproven Remedy with a Potent Reputation

Overall, this herb's safety and effectiveness for various health problems remain unclear—at least until further study is done. Although goldenseal would make any herbalist's list of "greatest hits," there is still controversy and disagreement as to what it's good for and in what forms and dosages.

"Goldenseal tea may be a modestly effective astringent for sore mouth and lips," says Varro E. Tyler, Ph.D., professor of pharmacognosy at Purdue University School of Pharmacy in West Lafayette, Indiana, and author of *The Honest Herbal*. But as for taking it internally, he warns: "Unless you take doses large enough to be nearly toxic, the effects are too uncertain to be useful."

Although there is little evidence of harm caused by taking goldenseal, if you're going to use goldenseal internally, it's a good idea to take it under the supervision of a doctor who knows about herbs. And don't take goldenseal, or an herbal blend containing it, if you are pregnant or have high blood pressure. (In addition to its potential for raising blood pressure, the herb contains compounds that can stimulate contractions of the uterus.)

To make a tea that you can use for sore throats, pour a cup of boiling water over one teaspoon of the dried herb. Allow the tea to cool until lukewarm and use it as a gargle.

Gotu Kola

Far Eastern Wound Healer

POTENTIAL HEALING POWER

May help:
- Heal wounds
- Improve circulation in the legs
- Relieve anxiety
- Promote sleep

T his creeping, marsh-loving plant isn't well known outside its native range of China, India and the South Pacific. In those regions, however, gotu kola has quite a reputation. In China, it's considered the herb of choice to promote longevity, in part because it was used regularly by the Chinese herbalist Li Ching Yun, who, legend says, lived to celebrate his 256th birthday.

In India, gotu kola is known as the herb of enlightenment. "This plant is called *bramhi*, or 'greatest of the great,' " says Jay L. Glaser, M.D., medical director of the Maharishi Ayurvedic Health Center in Lancaster, Massachusetts. (Ayurvedic medicine is the traditional medicine of India.) "Gotu kola's most important use is to bring the nervous system to such an extreme degree of refinement that the individual can see his or her nature as unbounded and infinite—in other words, to become enlightened," says Dr. Glaser.

Gotu kola is also used in Ayurvedic medicine as a cure for agitation, memory loss, anxiety, insomnia, epilepsy and hyperactivity, Dr. Glaser says.

As intriguing as these claims and uses may sound, gotu kola has yet to be checked out in any organized way or with modern scientific techniques. But the two most common forms of the herb, *Centella asiatica* and *Hydrocotyle asiatica,* are known to contain several active ingredients that apparently do offer anti-inflammatory, antibacterial and sedative effects. "This herb has been described as representing an entire apothecary shop, and indeed it has many, many uses," says Daniel B. Mowrey, Ph.D., director of the American Phytotherapy Research Laboratory in Salt Lake City, Utah, and author of *The Scientific Validation of Herbal Medicine*.

In India, Indonesia and Europe, gotu kola has traditionally been used (and is still employed) to promote healing of tissue, including surgical wounds, burns, tears that occur during childbirth, anal fissures and skin ulcers, Dr. Mowrey says. "Clinical studies done overseas indicate that standardized extracts of gotu kola can greatly aid wound repair," he says. And, he says, it works equally well when taken orally or put on the skin. The herb apparently enhances cells' ability to manufacture protein and thus stimulates the growth of new tissue, he says.

Gotu kola also seems to help improve blood flow through the veins in the legs. In one study, it improved such symptoms as heaviness in the lower legs, numbness, nighttime cramps, swelling and distended veins. "It's thought to help keep veins strong and resistant to bulging by promoting the growth of connective tissues, which helps keep vein walls strong," Dr. Mowrey says.

Gotu kola contains compounds that researchers are very interested in right now—flavonoids, or terpenes. Some of this group of biochemicals are known to have anti-cancer activity. "Whether gotu kola contains those particular flavonoids that offer protection from cancer remains to be seen," Dr. Mowrey says.

Exotic but Available

You can find gotu kola at many health food stores. Capsules containing powdered *H. asiatica*, the weaker variety of gotu kola, are most commonly available. "People using this herb for health maintenance usually take two to four 400-milligram capsules a day of *H. asiatica*, which is the cheaper variety," Dr. Mowrey explains. The stronger kind, *C. asiatica*, is available as capsules or extract. "The extract is more expensive and is usually reserved for treating serious illness such as epilepsy," Dr. Mowrey says. People using the extract for a medical condition generally take one to two ounces a day, Dr. Glaser says.

The Food and Drug Administration considers gotu kola an herb of "undefined safety." Two side effects are possible—sedation and skin rash. If you are thinking about taking gotu kola for a medical condition, it's best to talk with a health professional who's familiar with herbs to determine whether it is a wise choice for you, Dr. Glaser says.

Guarana

A Potent Source of Energy

With a healthy population of poisonous spiders, plants and snakes as neighbors, the folks who live in the Amazon Basin need all the help they can get to stay alert and on their toes. And they get a major assist from guarana, a woody vine native to that region of the world.

"A cup of the beverage made from guarana has three times more caffeine than a cup of coffee," says William J. Keller, Ph.D., professor and head of the Division of Medicinal Chemistry and Pharmaceutics at the Northeast Louisiana University School of Pharmacy in Monroe. "People in South America either chew a spoonful of the seeds or crush the seeds with a mortar and pestle, add a sprinkle of water and mix up a paste. The dried paste is then used to make a hot beverage like coffee.

"Back in the 1970s, the dried paste was made into tablet form and sold under the name 'Zoom!'" he adds. "One tablet had the caffeine equivalent of four or five tablets of Nō-Dōz."

Other than keeping you moving in a dangerous environment, guarana may also have the ability to keep your red blood cells moving when they have a tendency to clump together and trigger a heart attack.

In a laboratory study conducted at the University of Sao Paulo in Brazil, researchers found that guarana extract reduces the clumping of red blood cells in rabbits anywhere from 27 to 37 percent.

Does it do the same in humans? Nobody knows for sure, the researchers report. They're still trying to figure out exactly what it is that keeps the blood cells from clumping together. While guarana may hold potential as a heart protector, it's still too soon to recommend it.

What about using guarana to stay awake? While you can still purchase the herb at health food stores, you might want to reach for a cup of coffee instead. Guarana packs a mighty potent dose of caffeine—enough to give many people the jitters.

Hawthorn

Hope for Heart Health

POTENTIAL HEALING POWER

May help:
- Regulate blood pressure
- Reduce angina pain

The hawthorn, a small thorny tree belonging to the rose family, has long been a symbol of hope—ancient Greek brides carried it on their wedding day. Herbalists have kept it in their repertoire for thousands of years, but only since the turn of this century has it been explored for a truly hopeful purpose: to heal the human heart.

The small reddish fruits of the hawthorn are used as food in many countries. In the 19th century, an Irish doctor included them in a "secret remedy" for heart disease. His discovery was popularized in the 1890s by a group of American physicians known as the Eclectics. These doctors used hawthorn preparations to treat cardiac troubles such as weak heartbeat and angina. It seems they may have been onto something.

Over the past 80 years, research on both animals and people has confirmed that hawthorn has positive effects on the cardiovascular (heart and blood vessel) system, probably through the action of plant pigments called flavonoids.

Hawthorn seems to work in two main ways, according to Varro E. Tyler, Ph.D., professor of pharmacognosy at Purdue University School of Pharmacy in West Lafayette, Indiana, and author of *The Honest Herbal.* "First, it dilates the blood vessels, especially the coronary arteries that nourish the heart muscle. This may help lower blood pressure and reduce angina," he explains. When the arteries dilate, or open wider, pressure throughout the blood vessel system is lowered—just like opening the nozzle wider on a garden hose. "Second," says Dr. Tyler, "hawthorn seems to have a direct positive action on the heart itself when taken over the long term. Apparently, it's a mild and harmless heart tonic."

So why aren't more people using hawthorn? In Germany they are. German pharmacies carry three dozen hawthorn preparations, both prescription and nonprescription, to treat heart-related ailments, says Dr. Tyler. There, hawthorn is recommended to treat very mild cases of circulatory disorders or in addition to therapy with stronger heart drugs such as digitalis.

Don't Doctor Your Own Heart

Given these observations—plus the fact that hawthorn has no record of dangerous side effects—why shouldn't the millions of Americans with heart and blood vessel problems take hawthorn pills and extracts, which are available in health food stores?

Because with cardiovascular problems, there's no good reason for self-doctoring, say herbal experts. "People who dose themselves usually do so because they've diagnosed themselves—and with a vital system like the heart and blood vessels, that can be a very dangerous thing to do," warns Dr. Tyler. "For this reason, I don't recommend self-treatment with hawthorn."

"Don't fiddle around with the heart," warns Norman Farnsworth, Ph.D., director of the Program for Collaborative Research in the Pharmaceutical Sciences at the University of Illinois at Chicago and a heart attack survivor. "There are well-established synthetic drugs available for cardiac trouble, and some herbal products could possibly interact with them. Taking them along with prescription medications wouldn't be wise—I wouldn't do it myself."

If you're already under a doctor's care for heart or blood vessel problems, you might ask about adding a hawthorn preparation to other forms of therapy—but don't be surprised if your doctor is unfamiliar with the herb. Most American doctors don't know hawthorn.

And if you take any prescription heart medications or blood pressure drugs, play it safe and avoid adding any herbal remedies to the mix, advises Dr. Farnsworth.

Horehound

A Traditional Cough Remedy

POTENTIAL HEALING POWER
May help: • Relieve coughs

Once upon a time, Europeans believed horehound would help ward off witches' spells. But whatever the herb's anti-ghoul properties, they apparently weren't powerful enough to prevent the Food and Drug Administration (FDA) from casting a spell over horehound in 1989. Over the protests of herbalists that year, the

FDA ruled horehound ineffective against coughs and banned it from over-the-counter cough remedies.

That was news to traditional herbalists. They've been recommending horehound to treat coughs for literally thousands of years. You might think the FDA ruling was the end of the story, but it's not. You can still buy the herb, you can still buy horehound candies, and some herbal experts say the final word has not yet been said on this topic.

David P. Carew, Ph.D., professor emeritus of medicinal and natural products chemistry at the University of Iowa in Iowa City, for example, actually whips up his own tasty, old-fashioned horehound candy at home. "I like the flavor of horehound myself," says Dr. Carew. "I also think there's some mucus-ejecting action in horehound, but I'm sure it all depends on how strong the extract is that you put in."

Horehound's phlegm-evicting component is thought to be released when the herb is cooked. Called marrubiin, this chemical apparently irritates the lining of the throat, causing horehound's expectorant action, according to Varro E. Tyler, Ph.D., professor of pharmacognosy at Purdue University School of Pharmacy in West Lafayette, Indiana, and author of *The Honest Herbal*.

During one study, marrubiin was found to increase the production of bile in laboratory animals, says John Michael Edwards, Ph.D., associate dean of the School of Pharmacy at the University of Connecticut at Storrs. "Presumably this means it would stimulate all sorts of secretions," says Dr. Edwards. "Think of it this way: Something that increases one secretion is likely to stimulate others."

Horehound has never been just a cough remedy. It has had other uses over the years as well, from luring bees to gardens and adding a flavorful punch to English ales to featured status as a bitter herb during Jewish Passover. One group of physicians in 19th-century America also prescribed it for colds, asthma, intestinal worms and menstrual complaints. None of these uses has been scientifically investigated, however.

Old-Fashioned Relief?

If you'd like to try horehound tea, pour a cup of boiling water over one teaspoon of dried horehound leaves and steep for ten minutes. Sweeten to taste. The candies are hard to find, and if you do find them, you'll see that they no longer come with a medicinal label.

You can judge for yourself whether the ancients were right about horehound's ability to relieve a cough. You can also enjoy the candies just as a treat, although the sweet/bitter taste is unusual, to say the least.

Hyssop

Potential Anti-AIDS Weapon

Hyssop has a history of medicinal use as old as the Bible. But at least one study shows the herb could serve as a potent weapon in the very modern fight against AIDS.

The investigation into hyssop's anti-AIDS properties began after a 29-year-old female heroin addict suffering from the virus arrived for treatment at North Shore University Hospital in Manhassett, New York. Among other ailments at the time, the woman had contracted Kaposi's sarcoma—a deadly cancer characterized by bluish-red lesions that frequently develops in people who have AIDS.

A year later, a checkup revealed that the woman's skin lesions had improved "significantly" and she was feeling "much better," says Willi Kreis, M.D., Ph.D., an oncologist at North Shore University Hospital and research professor at Cornell Medical College in New York City.

The source of her improvement was a mystery—until the woman's mother told researchers her daughter had been drinking an old Jamaican tea remedy made from hyssop and a few other herbs. What were the doctors to think?

They weren't used to seeing Kaposi's sarcoma get better. In fact, until the time of her death from AIDS-related pneumonia, the woman continued to drink her tea, and her Kaposi's sarcoma continued to regress, says Dr. Kreis. "After we heard that, we decided we had to study hyssop," he says.

The team's lab work, chronicled in a leading medical journal, seems to confirm hyssop's preliminary promise, says Dr. Kreis. "Our study was done just with tissue cultures in the laboratory, but hyssop was very effective as an antiviral, anti-HIV treatment in the test systems that we used," he says. (Doctors say that the human immunodeficiency virus—HIV—causes AIDS.)

It Fights Colds, Too

Of course, ancient herbalists weren't using hyssop against AIDS, but they were enthusiastic about its healing properties. A member of the mint family, hyssop has had advocates since antiquity. Among them were two of the biggest names in ancient medicine, Hippocrates and Galen. Both suggested hyssop for bronchitis. Other folk uses of hyssop include treating coughs, colds, hoarseness, fevers, sore throats and herpes.

An ingredient in some liqueurs, hyssop's leaves and flowers contain a volatile oil that gives it a bitter taste and strong odor, says William J. Keller, Ph.D., professor and head of the Division of Medicinal Chemistry and Pharmaceutics at North-east Louisiana University School of Pharmacy in Monroe. "That's one thing generally common to mint plants: They produce a lot of volatile oil, the thing that gives spearmint and peppermint their characteristic flavor," he says. "As it turns out, a chemical in the volatile oil is good for treating irritations of the respiratory tract and congestion due to colds. It also acts as an expectorant."

To make hyssop tea, steep two teaspoons of the fresh or dried herb in a cup of boiling water. Add sugar, honey or lemon to taste.

Juniper

Nature's Ultimate Water Pill

POTENTIAL HEALING POWER

May help:
• Reduce water retention

If you occasionally enjoy a dry martini, you can thank juniper berries. Actually, you can thank a 17th-century Dutch physician named Franciscus de la Boe, otherwise known as Dr. Sylvius. Dr. Sylvius was well aware that juniper berries are a powerful diuretic that helps the body flush away excess water. And it was while trying to distill the essence of juniper berries into alcohol that he inadvertently created gin.

His herbal concoction proved ex-tremely popular, especially with the English, who didn't give two hoots that it was *supposed* to be medicinal.

The use of the oil from juniper berries as medicine goes way back. Egyptian doctors used it as a laxative as early as 1550 B.C. Since then, in various times and places, the oil has been used to treat an incredible variety of human ailments, everything from cancer and arthritis to gas and warts. Also appearing on this unlikely list:

swelling, bronchitis, tuberculosis, gallstones, colic, heart failure, intestinal diseases, gonorrhea, gout, hysteria and back pain.

Over time, herbalists finally focused on the kidneys as the favored organ for treatment with juniper. They recommended the herb for kidney disease, kidney stones and inflamed kidneys.

Little Berries with a Powerful Punch

It wasn't until the current century that doctors discovered that juniper actually *irritates* the kidneys, says William J. Keller, Ph.D., professor and head of the Division of Medicinal Chemistry and Pharmaceutics at Northeast Louisiana University School of Pharmacy in Monroe. While juniper is a potent diuretic, it's actually harmful to any-

one with a kidney problem. What's more, as little as six drops of the oil can have a toxic effect whether or not you have kidney disease.

That's why you should never just pick a handful of berries and munch, says Dr. Keller. "The safest way to use juniper oil is to buy it in health food stores as an ingredient in over-the-counter 'water pills.' And as long as you're not pregnant, just follow the dosage instructions on the label.

"Under no circumstances should a pregnant woman use juniper in any form," adds Dr. Keller. It's known to cause miscarriage.

The best use of juniper? Probably as the flavoring agent in gin-and-tonic, chuckles Dr. Keller. These days, there's just enough juniper oil to give the drink its characteristic flavor and smell, but not enough to have a pharmacological effect.

Kola

It's a Real Herb

Colas account for more than half of the enormous U.S. soft drink market. Yet few Americans know that the tropical nut that flavors cola has several medicinal benefits.

> **POTENTIAL HEALING POWER**
>
> May help:
> - Relieve drowsiness
> - Temporarily increase stamina
> - Enhance the pain-relieving effects of aspirin

West Africans have used kola since prehistoric times for its stimulant effect, and no wonder—kola contains caffeine. In one 12-ounce can of cola, you'll find about 40 milligrams. For comparison, a 6-ounce cup of brewed coffee contains about 100 milligrams of caffeine, and a cup of instant coffee contains about 60.

When slaves brought kola to the New World, its stimulant action was adopted medicinally as an antidepressant pick-me-up. Pharmacists stocked it, including John Pemberton of Atlanta, who aspired to developing a kola-based "nerve tonic." Legend has it that in 1886, Pemberton mixed some sugar with extracts of kola and coca (the source of cocaine) in a three-legged brass pot in his backyard. He added carbonated water to his sweet syrup and created a refreshing drink that his bookkeeper dubbed Coca-Cola. Today, Coca-Cola is one of the best-known brand names in the world. Its formula has always been a closely guarded secret, but regardless of whether Coke ever contained cocaine, you can be sure that today its kick comes entirely from caffeine.

Soda with a Gentle Kick

As with coffee, kola's caffeine content accounts for both its medicinal benefits and its potential problems. On the plus side, caffeine increases the pain-relieving action of aspirin. It is also a stimulant that may open (dilate) the bronchial passages and temporarily increase athletic stamina. On the minus side, large amounts of caffeine can cause insomnia, jitters, irritability and upset stomach and, some experts say, may increase risk of heart attack. It's also addictive. Once you are accustomed to caffeine, sudden elimination often causes a headache that can last for several days.

"In moderate amounts—no more than 250 milligrams a day—caffeine is reasonably safe," says Varro E. Tyler, Ph.D., professor of pharmacognosy at Purdue University School of Pharmacy in West Lafayette, Indiana, and author of *The Honest Herbal*. "Most healthy people can consume up to that much before they need to get too concerned."

Cola beverages, although they tend to be loaded with sugar, are the most convenient way to consume this herb. But for a medicinal tea, add one to two teaspoons of powdered kola nut to a cup of water. Bring to a boil and simmer ten minutes. Drink up to three cups a day.

Kola nut may be difficult to find in your neighborhood grocery store. Two suppliers that do stock it are Herb and Spice Collection, 3021 78th Street, P.O. Box 118, Norway, IA 52318-0118 and Nature's Herb Company, 1010 46th Street, Emeryville, CA 94608.

Licorice

Sweet-Tasting Ulcer Therapy

POTENTIAL HEALING POWER

May help:
- Soothe sore throat
- Relieve coughs
- Heal peptic ulcers

Say "licorice," and most people think of candy. But licorice is actually a potent and controversial herb. Just to confuse matters, not all licorice-flavored candy contains real licorice—some is artificially flavored.

Traditionally used to soothe sore throat and cough, real licorice comes from the roots of a tall plant that has been cultivated in both China and Europe since ancient times. Ancient herbalists, both Western and Chinese, used the sweet-tasting root to treat ulcers, respiratory problems and many other ailments. In fact, licorice is still found in about one-third of all Chinese herbal prescriptions.

Today, licorice is most widely used as flavoring in tobacco products. It may also be found in some throat lozenges, in European licorice candies and in some American candies.

Licorice owes its sweetness to glycyrrhizin, a compound 50 times sweeter than sugar. Every so often, a medical journal will report serious illness from an "overdose" of real licorice. The overdose isn't from taking the herb, however.

Usually it's from eating literally pounds of the candy or from swallowing saliva from licorice-laced chewing tobacco. Overdose symptoms include high blood pressure, weakness and water retention. The substance responsible for the herb's sweetness is also the culprit in overdose symptoms. Medical experts report that glycyrrhizin mimics a naturally occurring hormone that affects the body's metabolism and water content.

Powerful Ingredients

What about the positive side of the herb? Few people, after all, consume licorice candy by the pound.

During World War II, a Dutch doctor observed that licorice extract helped heal peptic ulcers but also caused swelling of the face and limbs. This discovery led to the widespread use of a licorice-based compound—carbenoxolone—to treat ulcers. In the 1970s, the discovery of safer and more effective anti-ulcer drugs knocked carbenoxolone, with its potentially dangerous side effects, out of the running.

Licorice as an ulcer remedy has refused to stay in the dustbin of medical history, however. When researchers removed glycyrrhizin from licorice root and then tested it again, they found that the root *still* healed ulcers. Clearly, there was healing power in some other component of licorice.

Today, some herbal practitioners remain enthusiastic about the anti-ulcer powers of this "safe," or *deglycyrrhizinated*, licorice, called DGL. "This product is wonderful for healing peptic ulcers," says Alan R. Gaby, M.D., a Baltimore physician who practices nutritional and natural medicine and is president of the American Holistic Medical Association. "In some studies it has worked about as well as standard anti-ulcer therapies like Tagamet and Zantac, for a lower cost and with virtually no risk."

Use with Caution

Because licorice—the real stuff, with glycyrrhizin—can cause such serious side effects in high doses, consume only modest amounts of any product labeled "real licorice." Limit your enjoyment to a few pieces. And, to be on the safe side, avoid all licorice products if you have high blood pressure, heart disease or glaucoma.

Ulcer treatment is not something you should undertake on your own. If you have ulcer symptoms, you should see your doctor, says Dr. Gaby, "but DGL is worth a try." If you'd like to use DGL, discuss it with your doctor.

And if you'd like to give the herb's traditional ability to soothe a sore throat a try, simply sprinkle a pinch of the powdered herb into hot water or tea.

Marshmallow

A Gooey Throat Soother

POTENTIAL HEALING POWER
May help: • Soothe sore throat • Relieve coughs

Floating in a steaming cup of cocoa or skewered on a sharp stick, marshmallows may seem like little more than glorified cream puffs—and rubbery ones at that. It's hard to believe that the sugary confections have a medicinal history.

Actually, our modern marshmallows—the buoyant white candy that made S'Mores famous—no longer contain the herb for which they were named.

Marshmallow, the herb, comes from a tall plant with a long root that grows (no surprise) in marshes. Nineteeth-century doctors cooked juice from the marshmallow plant's roots with egg whites and sugar and whipped them into a foamy meringue that later hardened, creating a medicinal candy used to soothe children's sore throats. This medicine proved popular with adults as well as children, mostly as a candy. Eventually, advanced manufacturing processes and improved texturing agents eliminated the need for the gooey root juice altogether.

The Power's in the Slide

Centuries before marshmallow was ever used to make candy, physicians were prescribing preparations made from marshmallow roots, flowers and leaves for coughs and sore throats. In fact, the scientific name for marshmallow is *Althaea officinalis,* from the Greek word *althaea,* meaning "to heal."

As it turns out, the leaves, light pink flowers and roots of the marshmallow plant all contain a thick, gooey substance called mucilage.

"The mucilage can soothe irritation in your throat and help you stop coughing," says Heinz Rosler, Ph.D., associate professor of medicinal chemistry at the University of Maryland School of Pharmacy in Baltimore. In fact, when pitted against two other remedies in an Eastern European study of cough suppressants, marshmallow outperformed both. Teas containing marshmallow are commonly sold in Germany for this purpose, says Dr. Rosler.

Although the herb is not as widely available here, you can sometimes purchase marshmallow teas at health food stores. You can also make a tea by boiling ½ to 1 teaspoon of crushed root per cup of water for 10 to 15 minutes.

Meadowsweet

Aspirin from the Fields

POTENTIAL HEALING POWER

May help:
- Banish headache pain
- Relieve the aches of flu
- Ease arthritis pain
- Reduce fever

Imagine your doctor dispensing a bouquet of small, creamy white flowers instead of aspirin every time your arthritis acts up.

It's actually not that farfetched. If 19th-century scientists had failed to unlock the secret of salicylic acid, you might well be picking up flowers from your doctor for things like arthritis, headaches and the flu.

That's because the bud of the meadowsweet plant naturally contains salicin, one form of the key ingredient in an aspirin tablet, says William J. Keller, Ph.D., professor and head of the Division of Medicinal Chemistry and Pharmaceutics at Northeast Louisiana University School of Pharmacy in Monroe. "Once the salicin from meadowsweet is in the stomach, it breaks down to create salicylic acid, and basically that's what happens when you take an aspirin," he explains.

For that reason, centuries-old uses for meadowsweet—for headaches, arthritis and the flu—seem justifiable, says Dr. Keller. "It definitely has an analgesic effect, and it lowers body temperature, so it's even good for fever."

Herbalists also give meadowsweet high marks as a remedy for heartburn, gastritis, peptic ulcers and urinary tract infections. There is as yet no scientific research to support these traditional uses, but research continues. Over the past few years, for example, Russian medical researchers have begun studying meadowsweet's suspected ability to inhibit blood clotting.

Have a Spot of Comfort

You can test meadowsweet's painkilling powers for yourself in the form of a tea. Add one to two teaspoons of the dried herb to a cup of boiling water and let it steep for ten minutes before drinking.

There's one traditional use of the herb that requires no scientific study to confirm. During the Middle Ages, the plant's almond-scented flowers were often strewn to improve the smell of rooms. (Back when farm animals shared living space with people, and people didn't bathe regularly, room-freshening herbs were far more important than they are today.) Meadowsweet smells just as good as it ever did—and, if you're lucky enough to have some growing in your area, the fresh wildflowers can *still* make a room smell absolutely wonderful.

Milk Thistle

Protection for the Liver

The milk thistle, a tall, spiny plant native to the Mediterranean, got its name from its milky sap—and from a legend that the plant's white-veined leaves resulted from a sprinkling of mother's milk from the Virgin Mary. (The legend accounts for its other name, Mary thistle, and its botanical name, *Silybum marianum.*)

This tale gave rise to a folk belief that the plant was good for nursing mothers. There is no proof that milk thistle helps breast-feeding. But it has shown dramatic results in healing liver problems.

Milk thistle has been used to treat the liver for some 2,000 years. In the first century A.D., the Roman naturalist Pliny wrote that the seedlike fruits of the milk thistle were "excellent for carrying off bile." Later herbalists also esteemed the herb as a liver healer. In the past two decades, research, conducted mainly in Europe, has proven them right.

The active substance in milk thistle seeds is called silymarin—a complex of various compounds that, according to medical researchers, not only protects the liver from damage due to toxins or disease but can actually regenerate liver tissue that's already in trouble.

"Silymarin is a powerful antioxidant," says Alan R. Gaby, M.D., a Baltimore physician who practices nutritional and natural medicine and is president of the American Holistic Medical Association. (Antioxidants counter the effects of naturally occurring toxins called free radicals.) "In animal studies, it has prevented liver damage, and in human studies, it has sped recovery from hepatitis," says Dr. Gaby.

Studies in Hungary, Germany and elsewhere demonstrate that silymarin holds promise for treating various liver disorders, including damage from exposure to chemical toxins and cirrhosis caused by alcohol abuse.

Don't Go It Alone

Who should reap the benefits of milk thistle, and how? First, don't fool around with liver problems. If you have hepatitis, cirrhosis or any other liver-related condition, see your doctor.

There have never been any reports of problems associated with milk thistle consumption, and some European physicians prescribe a standardized extract for liver disease. In the United States, this product, sometimes marketed under the name Thisilyn, is available as a food supplement.

A few American doctors also use milk thistle. Dr. Gaby, for example, recommends silymarin extract to some patients with chronic liver disease. He says he gets good results. "One man had elevated liver enzymes for six years—a sign of liver damage, in this case of unknown origin. Various liver specialists offered no help," he says. "But one month after he began taking silymarin regularly, the enzymes came down to normal levels and stayed there."

Traditionally, almost every part of the milk thistle has been used for food—even the leaves, with the spines removed. But the therapeutic substances in milk thistle are not water-soluble, so a tea would be ineffective, points out Varro E. Tyler, Ph.D., professor of pharmacognosy at Purdue University School of Pharmacy in West Lafayette, Indiana, and author of *The Honest Herbal*. And since silymarin is poorly absorbed by the human digestive system, he adds, capsules of concentrate are the only source of the compound that's effective.

If you want to take milk thistle products, it might be a good idea to discuss it with your doctor.

Mullein

The Velvety Respiratory Soother

POTENTIAL HEALING POWER

May help:
- Relieve coughs
- Reduce congestion
- Ease indigestion
- Soothe stings and scrapes

Mullein (rhymes with sullen) is generally considered a minor medicinal herb. But James A. Duke, Ph.D., a botanist retired from the U.S. Department of Agriculture and author of *The CRC Handbook of Medicinal Herbs,* laments this status: "I'm a real believer in mullein," he explains. "Once my wife and I returned from a trip to China, and we both had bronchitis. She went to the doctor and did what he said. I took mullein tea. My bronchitis cleared up before hers did."

Mullein grows almost everywhere, and its velvety leaves, rod-like stem and striking yellow flowers are hard to miss. Mullein has a long history in herbal medicine. Its botanical family name—Scrophulariaceae—is derived from *scrofula,* an old term for chronically swollen lymph glands, later identified as a form of tuberculosis. Early on, this herb gained a reputation as a respiratory remedy. And physicians from India to England touted it as a remedy for coughs and chest congestion.

In a 1986 survey of folk medicine in Indiana, Varro E. Tyler, Ph.D., professor of pharmacognosy at Purdue University School of Pharmacy in West Lafayette, Indiana, and author of *The Honest Herbal,* discovered that the herb remains "very popular" for respiratory complaints.

Dr. Duke is not the only herb expert to value mullein. Daniel B. Mowrey, Ph.D., director of the American Phytotherapy Research Laboratory in Salt Lake City, Utah, and author of *The Scientific Validation of Herbal Medicine,* says it soothes not only the respiratory tract but also the digestive system: "It's a shame there's been so little research on mullein. I think it's very valuable. For stings and scrapes while hiking, for example, crush a few leaves in your hand and apply it on the wound as a poultice. It's very soothing." However, like any hairy plant, mullein has the potential for being irritating. It is not likely that irritation will occur, but discontinue use if it does.

To brew a medicinal tea, use 1 to 2 teaspoons of dried leaves per cup of boiling water. Steep for ten minutes. Drink up to three cups per day. Mullein tastes bitter, so you might want to add sugar or honey and lemon, or mix it into an herbal beverage blend. In a tincture, take ½ to 1 teaspoon up to three times a day. There have been no reports of mullein causing adverse effects.

Oregano

It's Not Just for Pizza

POTENTIAL HEALING POWER
May help:
• Soothe coughs
• Aid digestion

Rumor has it that oregano didn't become a popular seasoning in the United States until after World War II, when soldiers who'd been stationed in the Mediterranean returned home with a penchant for pizza.

Whether that's true or not, this pungent herb has been around for centuries, and many of its early uses were medicinal rather than culinary. The ancient Greeks made poultices from the leaves and used them to treat sores and aching muscles. Traditional Chinese doctors have used oregano for centuries to relieve fever, vomiting, diarrhea, jaundice and itchy skin. In Europe, the herb is still used to improve digestion and soothe coughs.

Little contemporary research has been done on the medical uses of oregano. The work that has been done shows that this herb contains two essential components, thymol and carvacol, which are also found in another herb, thyme.

Thymol can be used to help loosen phlegm in the lungs, according to Norman R. Farnsworth, Ph.D., director of the Program for Collaborative Research in the Pharmaceutical Sciences at the University of Illinois at Chicago.

In Germany, where herbal medicine is popular, syrups containing thymol are frequently prescribed for even the most serious kinds of coughs. In the United States, you're most likely to find thymol in cough remedies such as Vicks Menthol Cough Drops and in topical cough and cold products such as Vicks VapoRub.

The ingredients in oregano that soothe coughs also help unknot muscles in the digestive tract. So there's some scientific basis for using this herb as a digestive aid, Dr. Farnsworth says. Oregano also has a reputation as a menstruation promoter. "Pregnant women may safely use this herb as a seasoning, but they should avoid taking large amounts," Dr. Farnsworth warns.

For a warm, spicy tea that can settle the stomach or soothe a cough, use one to two teaspoons of dried herb per cup of boiling water. Let it steep for ten minutes.

Peppermint

After-Dinner Digestive Aid

The fragrance and flavor of mint put a refreshing zing into thousands of products, from candy and chewing gum to cosmetics and medicines. But mint—in particular, peppermint—is more than just another pleasant taste. It lives up to its centuries-old reputation for easing indigestion and other ailments.

Today's custom of taking a mint after dinner is nothing new. The ancient Romans used mint after meals to aid digestion. Peppermint, a hybrid of other mint species, is a relative newcomer, first identified in England around 1700. (Spearmint, a related plant, is also used for flavoring but is not considered medicinally potent like peppermint.) As early as 1801, American herbalists recommended peppermint preparations for gas, colic,

---

POTENTIAL HEALING POWER

May help:

- Ease intestinal gas
- Relieve indigestion and diarrhea
- Reduce congestion
- Soothe muscle soreness
- Treat irritable bowel syndrome
- Calm menstrual cramps

---

hiccups and nausea.

"Peppermint is probably our best-known remedy for stomach problems," says Daniel B. Mowrey, Ph.D., director of the American Phytotherapy Research Laboratory in Salt Lake City, Utah, and author of *The Scientific Validation of Herbal Medicine*. The herb tames tummy trouble through several actions, he says: Its essential oils stimulate the gallbladder and encourage bile secretion while helping the muscles that line the stomach and intestines to function smoothly. Peppermint oil in extremely high concentrations may also inhibit and kill many microorganisms associated with digestive and other problems.

Peppermint can produce a relieving burp after a big, heavy meal or calm the crampiness of indigestion or diarrhea. In recent years, medical researchers have found peppermint helpful for irritable bowel syndrome, a common and hard-to-treat ailment with no known cause. The anti-spasmodic action of peppermint has also given the plant a possibly undeserved reputation for soothing menstrual cramps. Its effectiveness has not been proven.

The active ingredient that gives peppermint its kick is menthol—a potent aromatic chemical in the plant's volatile oil. Menthol (usually a synthetic version) is one of the pungent key ingredients in many popular products, from Vicks VapoRub to Noxzema. Mentholated remedies help clear congestion in the head and upper respiratory passages and, applied externally, help ease sore muscles and cool inflammation.

Tapping In to Menthol Power

Few herbal remedies are more innocuous than peppermint tea, which is widely available loose or in tea bags. It's a refreshing remedy enjoyed by thousands to relieve digestive upset. Peppermint candies are also a popular option, but these may not contain sufficient oil to actually be therapeutic. Peppermint oil is highly concentrated and should be used only in small, recommended amounts. (Pure menthol is poisonous, and should never be taken internally.)

Although peppermint is a time-honored remedy for colicky babies, some authorities discourage its use. "Don't give the tea to infants or very young children," counsels Varro E. Tyler, Ph.D., professor of pharmacognosy at Purdue University School of Pharmacy in West Lafayette, Indiana, and author of *The Honest Herbal*. "The menthol may give them a choking sensation." If you do give peppermint tea to older youngsters, make sure it's a very weak dilution.

Rosemary

Fragrant Cancer Fighter

In ancient Greece, students tucked sprigs of this spicy, pine-scented herb in their hair, supposedly to improve their ability to study. That's how rosemary came by its reputation as a memory sharpener.

That particular ability has yet to be proven, but other traditional uses for rosemary are holding up under scrutiny in the laboratory, and some additional benefits are being discovered as well.

Rosemary works so well at preventing fats from becoming rancid that the food industry sometimes uses extracts of rosemary oil as a food preservative. Rosemary oil is a strong antioxidant—which means it protects fats from being attacked by oxygen. Because oxygen damage is also known to be a factor in the development of cancer, researchers have been looking at its potential in this area as well.

Several studies done in the last several years show that oil from the leaves of the very plant sold as a spice for flavoring can help prevent the development of cancerous tumors in laboratory animals.

In one study, led by Chi-Tang Ho, Ph.D., professor in the Department of Food Science at Rutgers University in New Brunswick, New Jersey, applying rosemary oil to the skin of experimental animals reduced their risk of cancer to half that found in animals that did not receive the application of oil.

In other studies by the same research team, animals whose diets contained some rosemary oil had about half the incidence of colon cancer or lung cancer compared with animals not eating rosemary. And researchers at the University of Illinois in Urbana found that rosemary cut by half the incidence of breast cancer in animals at high risk for developing the disease.

"In the few studies done so far, rosemary has proven to be a strong inhibitor of the development and growth of cancerous tumors," says Dr. Ho. "Given orally or used topically, it has consistently reduced the incidence of cancer by about half." Further studies will demonstrate whether rosemary offers cancer protection to humans as well, he adds.

Like many culinary herbs, rosemary also helps to relax muscles, including the smooth muscles of the digestive tract and uterus. So it's sometimes used to soothe digestive upsets and relieve menstrual cramps. In large amounts, however, it appears to have the opposite effect—causing intestinal irritation and cramping. (In fact, larger doses of rosemary oil and other rosemary preparations can be a risk to pregnancy.)

Enjoying Rosemary

Rosemary makes a wonderful addition to meats such as pork, lamb, beef and chicken and can turn an ordinary pizza into a culinary masterpiece, especially when it's paired with a healthy dose of garlic. One holiday Italian bread combines rosemary and raisins in a braided eggbread that makes fragrant, delicious toast.

But is the small amount of rosemary you would typically use to season a dish enough to give you a therapeutic effect? Surprisingly, the answer may be yes.

"We've done studies that looked at both large amounts and smaller amounts in the diet and found benefits even with small amounts," Dr. Ho says. "When animals were fed a diet that contained 2 percent (by weight) of rosemary, we saw significant cancer protection. But when we cut that amount way back, to 1/100th of that amount, rosemary still had a very strong effect. Even just using a fraction of a teaspoon a day could have potential health benefits."

If you prefer a tea, you can make a pleasant-tasting brew with one teaspoon of crushed dried leaves in a cup of boiling water. Let steep for ten minutes.

Avoid using rosemary oil in any amount, though. Even small doses can cause stomach, kidney and intestinal problems, and large amounts may be poisonous.

Pregnant women should not use the herb medicinally, although it's okay to use it as a seasoning.

Sage

A Potential Diabetes Fighter

You may recall the scene in *Zorba the Greek* where Anthony Quinn refuses an offer of sage tea and calls instead for rum. But other Greeks in Zorba's fictional world drank sage tea. And real-world Greeks do as well.

For centuries in Greece sage was believed to have medicinal value. As a tea it was thought to slow menstrual bleeding, while mixed with wine it was thought to stimulate menstruation. Throughout history sage has also been used as a muscle relaxant, an antiperspirant and a treatment for sore throats, diarrhea, venereal disease and a host of other conditions. It was also applied to wounds and insect bites.

The use of sage over time has been so extensive, in fact, that one text lists some 60-plus medical uses for it. Its Latin name—*Salvia officinalis*—seems appropriate, as it is derived from *salvere*, meaning to heal or be healthy.

Sweet Relief

Does sage live up to its sterling reputation when medical science takes a look at it? In some ways, yes.

Because of its antiseptic qualities, sage does have merit as a gargle for sore throat, says Varro E. Tyler, Ph.D., professor of pharmacognosy at Purdue University School of Pharmacy in West Lafayette, Indiana, and author of *The Honest Herbal*. In fact, it's used extensively for that purpose in Germany.

There's also compelling new research indicating that sage may be of value to people with diabetes. In Type II (non-insulin-dependent) diabetes, the hormone insulin does not work as efficiently as it should. Insulin has the job of helping the body's cells use glucose—the simple sugar your body uses as fuel. Laboratory studies indicate that sage may boost insulin's action, says Richard Anderson, Ph.D., lead scientist in vitamin and mineral nutrition at the U.S. Department of Agriculture's Human Nutrition Research Center in Beltsville, Maryland. Sage was among 24 herbs tested that were found to boost insulin activity two- to fivefold or more, says Dr. Anderson.

For people who have diabetes, this means that drinking sage tea in conjunction with their insulin treatments is worth a try, says Dr.

Anderson. "It may be that they will need less insulin," he says.

The exact mechanism by which sage improves the activity of insulin is not yet known, and that's the next phase of research to be undertaken, says Dr. Anderson.

Putting Sage to Work

A person with diabetes can use sage any way that's convenient, says Dr. Anderson. You can use the herb as a spice or drink it as a tea, as long as you ingest it, he says.

To make a tea, pour a cup of boiling water over one to two teaspoons of dried leaves and steep for ten minutes. If you have diabetes, it would be a good idea to discuss using sage with your doctor.

For sore throat, allow the tea to cool till warm, then gargle as needed.

St.-John's-Wort

A Natural Antidepressant

St.-John's-wort has been used in herbal healing for more than 2,000 years. Herbal healers thought they had a pretty good handle on what it can do, but its most exciting potential medical use was discovered in 1988. That's when researchers at New York University found that St.-John's-wort has dramatic action against the type of virus that causes acquired immune deficiency syndrome (AIDS). Since then, some AIDS patients have reported positive results using the herb, and a study sanctioned by the Food and Drug Administration is under way, testing the effects of

POTENTIAL HEALING POWER
May help:
• Fight AIDS
• Heal burns
• Relieve depression
• Treat minor wounds

some of the herb's constituents in people who have AIDS.

Initial studies of St.-John's-wort have caused tremendous excitement among people with AIDS. Since early 1989, according to *AIDS Treatment News*, "almost all the reports we have heard from users have been good." And medical researchers are hopeful that within the next few years, a chemical component of St.-John's-wort (hypericin) will be used to treat AIDS.

"I'm very intrigued by hypericin," says Varro E. Tyler, Ph.D., professor of pharmacognosy at Purdue University School of Pharmacy in West Lafayette, Indiana, and author of *The Honest Herbal*. "Many AIDS drugs have not panned out, but everything I've heard about hypericin looks positive. I'm eager to see the results of the trial."

Wound Healer of Old

The leaves and flowers of St.-John's-wort contain special glands that release a red oil when pinched. Early Christians named the plant in honor of John the Baptist, because they believed it released its blood-red oil on August 29, the anniversary of the saint's beheading. (*Wort* is Old English for "plant.")

Perhaps because of its oil's blood-red color, St.-John's-wort has a long history of use as a wound treatment. Several scientific studies have confirmed this use. Medical researchers have found that St.-John's-wort does, in fact, contain antiviral, antibacterial and anti-inflammatory chemicals. One German study showed that, compared with conventional treatment, a St.-John's-wort ointment substantially cut the healing time of burns and caused less scarring. (This ointment is not available as an approved drug in the United States.)

That's not all the herb does, however. There's more.

"Initially, hypericin, one compound in St.-John's-wort, was considered the strong inhibitor of monoamine oxidase (MAO)," says Bernie Olin, Pharm.D., editor of *The Lawrence Review of Natural Products*, a St. Louis–based newsletter that summarizes scientific research on medicinal herbs. New studies suggest that two other constituents of St.-John's-wort, xanthones and flavonoids, are the active MAO inhibitors, which are an important class of antidepressant medication. (Prescription MAO inhibitors include Nardil and Parnate.) In a small German study, six depressed women were given a St.-John's-wort preparation. "After six weeks," Dr. Olin explains, "they all showed improvement."

Tapping This Herb's Many Uses

To make an antidepressant tea, use one to two teaspoons of dried herb per cup of boiling water. Steep 10 to 15 minutes. Drink up to three cups a day. St.-John's-wort tastes initially sweet, then bitter and astringent.

After eating large quantities of St.-John's-wort, cattle often develop severe sunburn with blistering (photosensitization). Several sources say the same is true for humans, especially those with fair skin. If you have fair skin, use St.-John's-wort cautiously, and wear protective clothing when you're out in the sun.

For AIDS, St.-John's-wort should only be taken under the guidance of a physician. The preparation used is not the bulk herb but rather a standardized hypericin extract. People with AIDS say the herb is relatively nontoxic, but some have reported sun sensitivity, drowsiness, nausea and diarrhea.

For wound treatment, apply crushed leaves and flowers to the affected area.

Saw Palmetto

Promise for Prostate Problems

POTENTIAL HEALING POWER
May help: • Improve symptoms of enlarged prostate

Young men don't want to think about it. Older men don't want to talk about it. But the reality is that more than half of all men over age 50 will experience the discomfort of an enlarged prostate gland.

In the not-too-distant past men sometimes relied on remedies made from saw palmetto berries for relief. These days there are more treatment options available—usually prescription drugs or surgery—but a man can *still* seek relief from saw palmetto. The only difference these days is that the herb increasingly has the blessing of modern medical science.

What exactly is this prostate unpleasantness that so many men have to deal with? The prostate is a tiny gland located at the base of a man's bladder. It completely encircles the urethra—the narrow tube through which urine exits the body. When the gland enlarges as a man ages, it sometimes blocks the urethra, creating a frequent, urgent need to urinate, a weak or interrupted flow and difficulty emptying the bladder.

Berries versus Blockage

Saw palmetto is a palm that grows throughout the southeastern United States, and its therapeutic value lies in its dark red berries.

The herb's active ingredient is unknown. But studies done in Europe show that an extract from the berries appears to counteract the effects of androgens, male sex hormones that may cause prostate enlargement, says Varro E. Tyler,

Ph.D., professor of pharmacognosy at Purdue University School of Pharmacy in West Lafayette, Indiana, and author of *The Honest Herbal*. In Europe, Dr. Tyler notes, medications based on saw palmetto are routinely prescribed for enlarged prostate.

Saw palmetto products are available in this country, although they are not labeled for use in treating an enlarged prostate. That's because the Food and Drug Administration (FDA) has banned marketing saw palmetto medications for this problem, claiming there is too little proof that they work. The FDA evidently "overlooked" the European research when it made that ruling, notes Dr. Tyler.

But the FDA did not ban saw palmetto here; it simply restricted marketing claims. In fact, some American health practitioners and herbalists recommend the herb highly.

"I recommend saw palmetto berry extract for men with enlarged prostate glands," says Alan R. Gaby, M.D., a Baltimore physician who practices nutritional and natural medicine and is president of the American Holistic Medical Association. "Studies have shown that it can improve urinary flow rates and reduce symptoms like urinary hesitancy and weak flow. In many cases, it works as well or better than the prescription drug—and it's cheaper and safer."

No Substitute for the Doctor

Just because some herbalists believe saw palmetto works doesn't mean you should use it on your own. Dr. Gaby and other herb experts caution against self-medicating for an enlarged prostate.

Seeking medical care for prostate symptoms can be a lifesaver, points out Dr. Gaby. "Taking this or any herb does not eliminate the need for older men to get a routine checkup for prostate cancer," he says. Alert your doctor if you take any saw palmetto product, he warns, because the herb may change the results of blood tests that are used to detect prostate cancer. It's also inadvisable to take saw palmetto products plus prescription medication for an enlarged prostate, he adds. They could interact.

Finally, the form in which you take the herb is important, says Dr. Tyler. An oil-based extract was used in the scientific studies. "A water-based saw palmetto preparation, such as a tea, would give little or no benefit," says Dr. Tyler.

If you want to take saw palmetto, use an extract prepared by a reputable herbal medicine company and follow dosage directions on the package. The commonly recommended dose is 320 milligrams of oil-based extract daily. And make sure you discuss it with your doctor.

Senna

A Powerful Laxative

> **POTENTIAL HEALING POWER**
>
> May help:
> • Relieve constipation

During the ninth century, legend has it, the great caliph of Baghdad became dissatisfied with the medicines available in his court, particularly the laxatives. It seems they did more harm than good, causing severe abdominal distress. The caliph sent for a famous physician, Mesue the Elder, who brought new medicines to the court, including a "gentler" laxative, senna.

If senna was the gentler alternative, the caliph's old laxatives must have been real gut-wrenchers. Senna is such a powerful laxative that it can cause cramping and abdominal distress if not used with caution.

"Like aloe, buckthorn and cascara sagrada, senna contains anthraquinone glycosides, chemicals that stimulate the colon," says James A. Duke, Ph.D., a botanist retired from the U.S. Department of Agriculture and author of *The CRC Handbook of Medicinal Herbs*.

It's quite possible that you've taken small doses of senna without being aware of it. The herb is an ingredient in many over-the-counter laxatives, including Fletcher's Castoria, Senokot, Perdiem and Innerclean Herbal Laxative.

Anthraquinone laxatives should be considered as treatment for constipation only as a last resort, says Anne Simons, M.D., assistant clinical professor of family and community medicine at the University of California's San Francisco Medical Center. "First, eat a diet that's higher in fiber, drink more fluids and get more exercise," she recommends. "If that doesn't provide relief, try a bulk-forming laxative." One such laxative is psyllium (Metamucil). "If that doesn't help," advises Dr. Simons, "try ingesting the lubricant laxative mineral oil. And if that doesn't provide relief, try an anthraquinone laxative in consultation with your physician."

Senna is certainly effective, but most authorities consider two other anthraquinone laxatives to be gentler—buckthorn and cascara sagrada.

A Moving Experience

Senna tastes awful. Herbalists generally discourage using the plant material and instead recommend over-the-counter products containing it. However, if you're interested in trying the unprocessed herb, you can brew a medicinal tea from one to two teaspoons of dried leaves per cup of boiling water. Let steep for ten minutes. Add sugar, honey and lemon to taste. You can also mix it with pleasant-tasting herbs, such as anise, fennel, peppermint, chamomile, ginger, coriander or licorice. Drink up to one cup a day in the morning or before bed for no more than a few days. To take senna in capsule form, simply follow the package directions.

Senna should not be given to children under 2. For older children and people over 65, start with a low-strength preparation and in-crease strength if necessary.

Don't, under any circumstances, be tempted to use more than these small amounts of senna. Larger doses can cause diarrhea, nausea and severe abdominal cramping, with possible dehydration. Senna's powerful action means it should not be used by those with chronic gastrointestinal conditions, such as ulcers, colitis or hemorrhoids. Pregnant and nursing women should not take senna. And senna should never be used for more than two weeks, because over time, it can cause what's known as lazy bowel syndrome—the inability to move stool without chemical stimulation.

Slippery Elm

Early American Throat Soother

> **POTENTIAL HEALING POWER**
>
> May help:
> - Relieve sore throat
> - Soothe burns and skin irritation
> - Treat minor wounds
> - Ease indigestion

When alumni come to visit the University of Connecticut School of Pharmacy in Storrs, John Michael Edwards, Ph.D., is more than happy to show them around the old alma mater. But all the while he's got at least one eye on the department's jar of slippery elm.

It seems that the graduates developed a taste for the stuff when they were students—and they aren't afraid to raid the jar when they're back in town, says Dr. Edwards, associate dean of the school of pharmacy.

"In the old days, the pharmacy students had to be able not only to identify powdered drugs but to identify them in chunks—and slippery elm was one of them," says Dr. Edwards. "And if you suck on a piece of slippery elm, you get this mucilage out of it that's sort of sweet. Every so often, we have an alumnus who comes back and pounces on the jar of slippery elm bark."

Former pharmacy students aren't the first to covet slippery elm bark. Before Dutch elm disease decimated the great slippery elm forests of the northeastern United States, this plant was perhaps the country's favorite home remedy—used in sore throat lozenges and as a hot cereal like oatmeal for ulcers, heartburn and common digestive complaints.

That sweet mucilage apparently coats and soothes mucous membranes. "There's a polysaccharide in the bark that's very soothing, there's no question about that," says Christopher W. W. Beecher, Ph.D., associate professor of pharmacognosy in the Department of Medicinal Chemistry and Pharmacognosy at the University of Illinois at Chicago. A polysaccharide is a kind of carbohydrate.

Soothing Relief

You don't have to scout the forests for slippery elm trees to take advantage of this old-fashioned herb. You can still buy slippery elm throat lozenges in health food stores and some drugstores.

If you prefer a pleasant-tasting tea, add a cup of boiling water to a teaspoon of slippery elm powder or to slippery elm tea that you can buy at a health food store. Add sugar or honey to taste.

For a poultice to pack on burns, boils, minor wounds and inflamed skin, simply add enough water to slippery elm powder to create a paste. Some people are allergic to slippery elm. If you find that the paste irritates your skin, discontinue use.

Tarragon

Anti-cancer Activist

Although tarragon has a long and venerable history as a healing plant, you probably know it as a kitchen herb—the

POTENTIAL HEALING POWER
May help: • Prevent certain cancers • Heal herpes outbreaks • Fight flu

pretty, green, spiky-looking plant that's used in expensive bottles of tarragon vinegar. You can still enjoy it just for its flavor, of course, but there's plenty of reason to think of it as a therapeutic agent as well.

Tarragon contains 72 potential cancer preventives, according to James A. Duke, Ph.D., a botanist retired from the U.S. Department of Agriculture and author of *The CRC Handbook of Medicinal Herbs*. The herb's main cancer-blocking punch comes from a chemical called caffeic acid, which has the ability to cleanse the body of naturally occurring harmful substances known as free radicals. Caffeic acid also has some ability to kill viruses. "Caffeic acid is one ingredient in tarragon I would seek if I were looking to prevent cancer, flu or herpes," says Dr. Duke.

Help for Herpes

If I had herpes I would be drinking lemon balm tea with tarragon in it, and I would be applying the tea bag to the blisters," says Dr. Duke. "Both have antiviral activity, and I'm a great believer in synergy." Besides, tarragon will add a pleasant flavor to the tea, he says.

For relief from either oral or genital herpes, you can try a cup of tea with a lemon balm tea bag and one teaspoon of dried tarragon. (You can purchase lemon balm tea in many health food stores.) Let the brew steep for 10 to 15 minutes before drinking. Drink up to three cups a day.

Tea

A Cup of Comfort

It's the world's most popular herbal remedy and the second most popular beverage, after water. Technically, any concoction of plants steeped in water is a tea. But when most people say "tea," they mean the bracing brew beloved by everyone from Chinese peasants to the English aristocracy: the fragrant leaves of an Asian evergreen shrub called *Camellia*

POTENTIAL HEALING POWER

May help:
- Stimulate the nervous system
- Clear congestion
- Prevent certain cancers
- Ward off heart disease

---

sinensis. Several related species are also known simply as tea.

As it happens, a nice cup of tea may give you more than just a morning lift. Research suggests that tea, especially the green tea popular in the Orient, may have beneficial actions against heart disease and cancer.

Caffeine Plus

Tea contains several stimulant compounds, including caffeine and theophylline. An average cup of tea contains between 10 and 50 milligrams of caffeine, depending on the type of tea and the preparation method. (By comparison, a cup of brewed coffee has about 100 milligrams.) Both caffeine and theophylline act as bronchodilators, agents that can help open clogged respiratory passages. So your grandmother was right if she gave you hot tea to ease the misery of colds, flu or bronchitis.

There's no firm evidence that caffeine in moderation poses any risk to most people, although in excess, it can cause jitters and insomnia.

The Green Scene

Recently, scientists have been finding that tea may offer broader health benefits. Mostly, their research has been on green tea, a type more popular in the Orient than in the United States, where black tea is the leading seller. Green tea supplies generous amounts of substances called polyphenols, including one called catechin. Black tea leaves, which undergo an added process of fermentation, contain less catechin.

There's a small but growing body of evidence that the catechin and some related substances in green tea may have cancer-fighting properties.

For example, one research team found that catechin derived from a traditional Himalayan tea helped prevent skin tumors in laboratory animals. Other studies using laboratory animals have shown that green tea has a protective effect against tumors of the lung, stomach and liver. Can humans reap the same benefits? Only more research will tell, say the experts.

Tea for the Heart

It's well established that moderate tea drinking does no harm to the heart, and it may do some good.

An Israeli study of more than 5,000 tea drinkers found a link between tea consumption and lower blood cholesterol, although the cause-and-effect relationship wasn't clear. Japanese researchers, however, found that green tea polyphenols seemed to lower blood cholesterol and blood pressure in laboratory animals.

Researchers have also found that tea is a mild diuretic, helping to rid the body of excess fluid.

To enjoy the multiple benefits of tea—including its wonderful taste—simply buy a commercial product and follow the directions on the package.

Thyme

Ace Antiseptic

Thyme has a centuries-long history of use, in both the pharmacy and kitchen. This fragrant, ground-hugging shrub was grown in monastery gardens in southern France and in Spain and Italy during the Middle Ages for use as a cough remedy, digestive aid and treatment for intestinal parasites.

These days sprigs of its pungent, minty leaves are mandatory in a *bouquet garni*—the mixture of seasonings used to spice up just about every French food from soup to salad.

And it's still being used medicinally. A solution of thyme's most active ingredient, thymol, is used in such over-the-counter products as Listerine mouthwash and Vicks VapoRub. "Thymol is added to these products because of its well-known antibacterial and antifungal properties," explains Brian M. Lawrence, Ph.D., a research scientist and editor of the *Journal of Essential Oil Research.*

Thymol apparently also has a therapeutic effect on the lungs. "The oil from the leaves of this plant, when ingested or inhaled, helps to loosen phlegm and relax the muscles in the respiratory tract," explains Norman R. Farnsworth, Ph.D., director of the Program for Collaborative Research in the Pharmaceutical Sciences at the University of Illinois at Chicago.

In Germany, where herbal medicine is considerably more mainstream than it is in the United States, concoctions of thyme are frequently prescribed for coughs, including those resulting from whooping cough, bronchitis and emphysema. In the United States, thyme extract was included in a popular cough syrup, Pertussin, that is no longer on the market. "These days, you are most likely to find thyme in 'cold formula' herbal teas or remedies for coughs that are distributed by small companies and sold at health food stores," Dr. Farnsworth says.

Taking Thyme

To use thyme safely and effectively, brew a tea or infusion, Dr. Farnsworth suggests. Use two teaspoons of dried herb per cup of boiling water and steep for ten minutes.

The Food and Drug Administration includes thyme on its list of herbs generally regarded as safe. "As with many herbs, though, too large a dose may produce intestinal problems," Dr. Farnsworth warns. If you experience diarrhea or bloating, cut back on the amount you're using or discontinue use altogether. And make sure you take thyme as tea, not as oil. Undiluted thyme oil can be toxic, causing headache, nausea, vomiting and weakness, as well as thyroid, heart and lung problems.

Turmeric

India's Amazing Medicinal Plant

POTENTIAL HEALING POWER

May help:
- Aid digestion
- Relieve arthritis
- Treat dysentery
- Protect the liver
- Combat heart disease
- Ward off ulcers
- Prevent certain cancers

Most Americans are only vaguely aware of turmeric as an ingredient in Indian curry. We certainly don't think of it as a healing herb. Indians do, however.

A great deal of scientific research—almost all of it Indian—shows that turmeric aids digestion, prevents ulcers, protects the liver, helps prevent heart disease and may one day be used to treat cancer.

A relative of ginger, turmeric has held a place of honor in India's traditional Ayurvedic medicine for thousands of years. It was used as a digestive aid and treatment for fever, wounds, infections, dysentery, arthritis, jaundice and other liver problems. The Chinese adopted turmeric and used it similarly.

"Turmeric stimulates the flow of bile," says Pi-Kwang Tsung, Ph.D., former assistant professor of pathology at the University of Connecticut Medical School in Farmington and currently editor of *The East-West Medical Digest*. "This means it helps digest fats, confirming its traditional use as a digestive herb."

"Turmeric has strong liver-protective properties," agrees Bernie Olin, Pharm.D., editor of *The Lawrence Review of Natural Products*, a St. Louis–based newsletter that summarizes scientific research on medicinal herbs. If you drink alcohol regularly and/or take high doses of many pharmaceutical drugs—including the common pain reliever acetaminophen (Tylenol)—medical researchers say you may be at risk for liver damage. Using turmeric may offer a degree of protection.

The latest studies show that turmeric also protects the stomach lining and helps prevent ulcers, says Alan R. Gaby, M.D., a Baltimore physician who practices nutritional and natural medicine and is president of the American Holistic Medical Association. "Turmeric's anti-ulcer effect should be cause for celebration among curry lovers with Type-A personalities, like myself." And several studies show that curcumin, an active chemical in turmeric, has anti-inflammatory action, lending credence to the herb's traditional use in treating arthritis.

Like most culinary herbs, turmeric helps retard food spoilage because it has antibacterial action. In laboratory tests, turmeric also fights protozoa—microbes that cause a multitude of human ills. These tests lend credence to the herb's traditional use in treating dysentery, which is caused by this type of microorganism.

Powerful Protection

Several medical studies now suggest that turmeric may also help prevent heart disease by lowering cholesterol and preventing the formation of the internal blood clots that trigger heart attack (and many strokes). These findings come from studies done with laboratory animals and cannot necessarily be applied to people. But turmeric is a tasty spice that does no harm, and these studies suggest it might do some real good.

After a while, you begin to wonder if there's anything turmeric *can't* do. Sure enough, it even has potential as a cancer fighter. Several studies on laboratory animals show that curcumin has anti-cancer activity, probably because it is a powerful antioxidant. (Antioxidants are substances that counteract naturally occurring toxic substances called free radicals.)

Evidence from a recent study, a human trial in smokers, makes this herb look even more beneficial. Smokers' urine contains substances (mutagens) that cause genetic mutation. Mutagens are often carcinogens, or cancer causers. Indian researchers added 1.5 grams of turmeric a day (about a teaspoon) to the diet of 16 smokers for a month. The result was a significant reduction in urinary mutagens.

Giving Turmeric a Try

Since Indian research shows that even a teaspoon of turmeric has medicinal value, it makes a lot of sense to enjoy turmeric as the Indians do—as a seasoning in foods. Turmeric tastes pleasant, but in large amounts it becomes somewhat bitter.

If you'd prefer to make a medicinal drink to aid digestion and possibly help prevent heart disease, use one teaspoon of turmeric powder per cup of warm milk. Drink up to three cups a day. Unusually large amounts of turmeric may cause stomach upset. If you find the drink doesn't agree with you, discontinue use.

Ulcers, arthritis, liver disease, heart disease and cancer all require professional treatment. If you'd like to use turmeric in addition to standard therapies, discuss it with your doctor.

Medicinal turmeric preparations should not be given to children under 2. For older children and people over 65, start with low-strength preparations and increase strength if necessary.

Valerian

A Safe Aid to Slumber

Valerian smells funky—sort of like a forgotten washrag left in a basement corner. And it tastes funny . . . as you might imagine sucking on that washrag *would* taste. (Cats don't share this view. They think valerian is the hottest thing since catnip.) Taste notwithstanding, herbalists for hundreds of years have relied on the woody roots of valerian to calm the anxious and relax the sleepless. But does it really work?

Numerous studies have shown that valerian does indeed help people with insomnia get to sleep faster and sleep better—without the groggy "morning-after" effects of standard prescription sedatives.

> ## POTENTIAL HEALING POWER
>
> May help:
> - Ease insomnia
> - Calm nerves
> - Relieve menstrual cramps and muscle spasms

No one is quite certain how valerian performs this magic.

"According to the latest information available, we simply don't know what the active ingredients are," says Varro E. Tyler, Ph.D., professor of pharmacognosy at Purdue University School of Pharmacy in West Lafayette, Indiana, and author of *The Honest Herbal*.

Chemicals in valerian called valepotriates act as muscle relaxants, making the herb potentially useful against menstrual cramps and other types of spasms. But even valerian preparations *without* valepotriates help slumbertime come faster—raising the possibility that some still-unidentified chemical, or a synergistic reaction among various compounds in the root, may confer its calming action.

Smart Use

In Europe, where herbal preparations are part of mainstream medicine, there are dozens of valerian preparations available to treat nervousness and insomnia. In this country, the root is available in the form of teas, tinctures, capsules and extracts.

Since the herb has a good record of safety, with few reported side effects, many herbalists—and a few doctors—suggest trying it if you toss and turn at night.

"I recommend it to my patients, and they say it helps," says Alan R. Gaby, M.D., a Baltimore physician who practices nutritional and natural medicine and is president of the American Holistic Medical As-

sociation. "For some people, only the big guns—the prescription tranquilizers—will offer relief," he adds. "But for those with mild insomnia, it's the first thing I try, usually in capsule form." Simply follow the directions on the package. When using a tincture or extract, one teaspoon daily is the usual recommended dose. If taken as a tea, one cup should be sufficient.

As with any herbal remedy, be cautious about using large amounts over a long period, especially if you're using concentrated extracts; valerian in high doses has been reported to cause headaches and grogginess.

An important note: Don't be confused by the similarity of the herb's name to Valium. Valium is one of those "big gun" prescription sedatives. This powerful drug has no relation to valerian and should be used only under the strict supervision of a physician.

Vervain

A Neglected Tonic

During the Middle Ages, healing herbs were often called simples, and herbalists were known as simplers. Ver-

POTENTIAL HEALING POWER

May help:
- Aid digestion
- Relieve depression
- Thwart headache
- Ease minor aches and pains

vain was prescribed so frequently for so many conditions, it became known as simpler's joy. The name has some basis in fact. It turns out that vervain acts like mild aspirin, relieving minor pains and inflammation. It also has mild antidepressant effects.

In Egyptian mythology, vervain grew from the tears of Isis, goddess of fertility, as she grieved for her murdered brother/husband, Osiris. A thousand years later, vervain entered Christian mythology as the herb pressed into Christ's wounds to stanch his bleeding, hence one of its names, herb-of-the-cross.

Vervain has been used medicinally for thousands of years. Hippocrates recommended it for fever and plague. The 12th-century German abbess and herbalist Hildegard of Bingen prescribed a medicinal tea of vervain and vermouth for "toxic blood" (infections), toothache and "discharges from the brain to the teeth." Our word *vervain* comes from the Celtic *ferfaen*, from *fer-*, "to drive away," and *-faen*, "stone"—a reference to its traditional use in treating kidney stones.

The Rodney Dangerfield of Herbs

In modern times, vervain has fallen by the medicinal wayside because its actions are mild. "But that's no reason to neglect this herb," says Daniel B. Mowrey, Ph.D., director of the American Phytotherapy Research Laboratory in Salt Lake City, Utah, and author of *The Scientific Validation of Herbal Medicine*. "It's a valuable tonic. Unfortunately, tonics don't get much respect in American pharmacology."

A tonic is a substance that doesn't have a dramatic action, but over time, its subtle effects strengthen the body and contribute to vitality. Vervain, Dr. Mowrey says, is slightly astringent, which helps digestion. It's mildly pain-relieving and anti-inflammatory, so it helps control minor aches and pains. Vervain has mild laxative action to help keep the digestive tract running smoothly. And it's a mild antidepressant, so it may improve mood, says Dr. Mowrey. No wonder medieval herbalists called vervain simpler's joy.

To make an infusion to treat headache, mild arthritis and other minor pains, use 2 teaspoons of dried herb per cup of boiling water. Steep for 10 to 15 minutes. Drink up to three cups a day. You can mask vervain's bitter taste with sugar, honey and lemon, or mix it with some other herbal beverage tea. If you buy a tincture, use ½ to 1 teaspoon up to three times a day.

White Willow

Herbal Aspirin

POTENTIAL HEALING POWER

May help:

- Reduce fever
- Relieve pain and inflammation
- Ward off heart attack and stroke
- Combat certain cancers
- Prevent migraine headache

Mention "willow," and most people say "weeping." But the graceful tree should actually be seen as a source of joy. White willow is Nature's aspirin. In fact, pharmaceutical aspirin was originally created from a chemical very similar to one found in white willow bark.

Today there are more reasons than ever to use this herb. Medical research shows that this chemical in white willow (called salicin) not only reduces fever and relieves pain and inflammation but also may help prevent heart attack, stroke, digestive tract cancers and migraine headaches.

Chinese physicians have used willow to relieve pain since ancient times, but it took 2,000 years for this use to catch on in the West—an event that occurred almost by accident.

During the mid-1700s, British minister/physician Edmund Stone was trying to find a cheap substitute for cinchona bark, the rare, costly South American herb used to treat malaria (and later shown to contain the antimalarial drug, quinine). Cinchona was a bitter-tasting bark, and near Stone's Oxfordshire home, he found another bark that looked and tasted similar—white willow. As an experiment, he gave willow bark tea to people with fevers. Their fevers and pain subsided.

Never mind that by today's scientific standards, Stone's experiment left a great deal to be desired. The thermometers of his day were so crude that he couldn't be sure if his subjects really had fevers to begin with. Nonetheless, the herb quickly became the treatment of choice for fever and subsequently for pain and inflammation as well.

During the early 19th century, European chemists created aspirin from white willow bark's active chemical—salicin. Aspirin hit the market for the first time in 1899, and within a few years, it was one of the most popular drugs on earth.

Bark Still Packs a Punch

Herbal experts say that white willow bark will work on almost anything you take aspirin for—most likely, fever, pain and inflammation. It will stand in for aspirin, but perhaps not quite as well.

"The salicylate content of willow bark varies considerably," says Varro E. Tyler, Ph.D., professor of pharmacognosy at Purdue University School of Pharmacy in West Lafayette, Indiana, and author of *The Honest Herbal*. "You may need several cups of white willow bark tea to approach the effectiveness of two standard aspirin tablets."

Recent studies show that taking about half an aspirin a day can significantly reduce risk of heart attack and stroke by reducing the likelihood of the internal blood clots that trigger these medical emergencies. Studies of aspirin's effectiveness have not been duplicated for willow bark, but Dr. Tyler says that in the body, "they become the same thing, salicylic acid."

The problem with using willow bark to prevent heart attack and stroke is uncertainty about the herb's salicin content. "But the preventive dose is quite low," Dr. Tyler says. "Many willow bark samples should contain enough. If you have a willow bark sample that helps reduce pain, it probably contains enough salicin to produce aspirin's preventive benefits."

James A. Duke, Ph.D., a botanist retired from the U.S. Department of Agriculture and author of *The CRC Handbook of Medicinal Herbs*, agrees: "I have used willow bark for toothache pain, and if I were at risk, I would drink willow bark tea for heart attack prevention." How much is enough? Given adequate salicin content, a cup or two a day should be enough, says Dr. Duke.

According to American Cancer Society researchers, the same low aspirin dose that helps prevent heart attack and stroke also significantly reduces deaths from four digestive tract cancers: tumors of the esophagus, stomach, colon and rectum. According to Dr. Tyler, if willow bark contains enough salicin, it should produce the same effects.

The herb may also help people who suffer from migraine headaches, since use of low-dose aspirin has been shown to significantly reduce attacks.

Brewing Up Some Bark

To take advantage of the healing powers of white willow bark, soak one teaspoon of powdered bark per cup of cold water for eight hours. Strain it and drink up to three cups a day. White willow tastes bitter and astringent. To improve the taste, you can add sugar or honey and lemon. You can also mix it into an herbal beverage tea.

Aspirin upsets some people's stomachs, but most herbalists say white willow bark rarely causes this problem. If stomach upset, nausea or ringing in the ears develops, reduce your dose or discontinue use. Pregnant women and those with chronic gastrointestinal conditions such as ulcers, colitis or Crohn's disease should not use this herb.

When children under 18 who have colds, flu or chicken pox take aspirin, they are at risk for Reye's syndrome, a potentially fatal condition. White willow has never been linked to Reye's syndrome, but because of its aspirin-like action, do not give it to children with fevers from those conditions. For complaints not involving fever, start children over 2 on low-strength preparations and increase strength if necessary. People over 65 should also begin with low-strength preparations.

Heart attack, stroke, cancer and migraines are serious conditions requiring professional care. If you'd like to use white willow bark in addition to standard therapies, discuss it with your doctor.

Wild Cherry

An Airway Cleaner

POTENTIAL HEALING POWER
May help:
• Loosen phlegm

Early colonial settlers didn't have the option of running down to the corner drugstore for cough syrup or an expectorant when their kids had a cold. Instead, they stripped bark from a wild cherry tree, steeped it in hot water and offered it to their children as a hot, soothing beverage.

Today, not much has changed. Parents can run down to the corner drugstore for a bottle of cough syrup, all right. But chances are that the bottle is still going to contain wild cherry.

"Wild cherry is a flavoring agent that has a slight expectorant activity," says James E. Robbers, Ph.D., professor of pharmacognosy in the Department of Medicinal Chemistry and Pharmacognosy at Purdue University in West Lafayette, Indiana, and editor of the *Journal of Natural Products*. It contains benzaldehyde, a substance that loosens phlegm.

Generally, other ingredients with a more intense chemical activity are included in wild cherry cough syrups to boost the cherry's natural abilities and to provide the actual cough suppressant, says Dr. Robbers.

Loosening Things Up

Although the bottled variety of wild cherry cough syrup is more effective than wild cherry tea, the tea can be soothing to someone who's not feeling well.

If you'd like to make some tea, place one teaspoonful of wild cherry bark or leaves in a cup of boiling water. Steep for ten minutes and strain. Add honey, sugar or lemon to taste and enjoy. When using a tincture, follow the package directions.

Just two caveats: Do not give wild cherry tea to children under age two, and do not drink more than three cups a day. Wild cherry leaves, bark and fruit pits all contain hydrocyanic acid, which can be toxic in large amounts.

Witch Hazel

The Herb Even Doctors Recommend

POTENTIAL HEALING POWER

May help:
- Soothe skin irritation
- Heal minor wounds
- Treat hemorrhoids

Witch hazel is a popular home remedy for cuts, bruises, hemorrhoids and sore muscles. More than a million gallons of witch hazel water are sold each year in the United States, making it one of the nation's most widely used healing herbs. But ironically, commercial witch hazel water would be just as effective without its witch hazel.

Despite this herb's name, witch hazel has nothing to do with witchcraft. In medieval English, *witch* was spelled *wych*, and it meant flexible. Witch hazel is a tree with branches that are indeed flexible—so springy, in fact, that American Indians used them to make bows. The Indians also rubbed witch hazel tea on cuts, bruises, insect bites and aching muscles and joints, and they drank it for a variety of ailments, including colds and menstrual problems.

During the 1840s, an Indian medicine man introduced the herb's astringent properties to Theron T. Pond of Utica, New York, who began marketing it. Witch hazel water has been with us ever since.

The Astringent That Isn't

Early witch hazel water was simply tea on a large scale. This herb is high in astringent tannins, which dissolved in water-based witch hazel preparations, thus making them effective astringents. But about a century ago, manufacturers switched to steam distillation, a simpler process but one that eliminated the tannins— and all herbal astringent benefits. Nonetheless, Americans kept on using witch hazel water and swearing by it as a treatment for cuts, rashes and hemorrhoids.

Today it can be found in any pharmacy. "It's the active ingredient in Tucks hemorrhoid pads," says James A. Duke, Ph.D., a botanist retired from the U.S. Department of Agriculture and author of *The CRC Handbook of Medicinal Herbs*.

How can tannin-free witch hazel water have astringent benefits? "Witch hazel water isn't water anymore. It's 14 percent alcohol, which is also astringent," says Varro E. Tyler, Ph.D., professor of pharmacognosy at Purdue University School of Pharmacy in West Lafayette, Indiana, and author of *The Honest Herbal*.

If you want to get the astringent benefits of natural witch hazel, you'll have to brew up a batch yourself. Boil one teaspoon of powdered leaves or twigs per cup of water for ten minutes. Strain and cool. Apply the solution directly or mix it into an ointment.

The medical literature contains no reports of harm from external use of witch hazel. But if witch hazel causes minor discomforts, such as skin irritation, dilute it or discontinue use.

IV

MEDICATIONS

Medications

Therapeutic Wonders of Science

Of all the advances in modern science, drugs are arguably the most impressive. In fact, there are few conditions that can't at least be treated—if not always cured—with one or more of the thousands of medications on the market today.

This was not always the case. In fact, only 50 years ago, physicians had but a handful of scientifically proven drugs in their black bags. More often, they relied on folk remedies and sympathy, says E. Don Nelson, Pharm.D., professor of clinical pharmacology at the University of Cincinnati College of Medicine. Administered by a trusted physician, these early treatments may have made some people feel better. Real cures, however, were rare.

Then, in the early 1940s, researchers began testing a revolutionary new drug called penicillin. "There was a profound change in the way medicine was practiced," explains Dr. Nelson. Diseases that had plagued mankind for millennia could now be effectively treated—and cured. Thus began the "golden age" of antibiotics and other modern drugs. Good physicians, of course, continued to dispense comfort along with the new tablets.

Help for Every Condition

Today, doctors and consumers can choose from well over 300,000 over-the-counter (OTC) and prescription products. Acetaminophen alone, one of our most popular pain relievers, is found in over 100 different capsules, tablets, powders, liquids and even suppositories.

With so many drugs to choose from, and so many forms, strengths and brand names, it's not surprising that consumers—and even physicians—can be hard-pressed to keep up! Don't let the numbers throw you. Although there are thousands of medications, they all work in just a few basic ways:

By replacing something that should have been there in the first place. Your body requires a number of chemicals—such as insulin, endorphins, thyroid hormone and more—to work efficiently. If one or more of these substances is in short supply, your doctor may give you drugs to replace them.

By changing how your body works. Many drugs act directly on individual cells to change the ways in which they function. Taking aspirin, for example, blocks the production of specialized chemicals (prostaglandins) that cause pain.

By attacking invaders or abnormal cells. Drugs such as penicillin (an antibiotic) and amantadine (an antiviral drug) help control the tiny creatures that cause infection. Cancer drugs, on the other hand, are designed to target malfunctioning cells while leaving healthy tissue alone.

By making you think you're better. There's no question that the mind is powerful medicine. Studies have shown that when people with a variety of symptoms are given inactive tablets, or placebos, as many as 40 percent will improve, at least for a while, says Joe DiPiro, Pharm.D., professor of pharmacy and clinical professor of surgery at the University of Georgia College of Pharmacy in Augusta. To some extent, most medications have this effect.

Strict Safety Standards

A new drug doesn't just miraculously appear, however. Long before it reaches pharmacy shelves, the manufacturer will have spent millions of dollars and years of research ensuring that it not only works but is safe. Only after numerous studies are done—both in the laboratory and in hospitals—will the Food and Drug Administration decide whether to allow it to be sold.

"The number of drugs that make it all the way to market is a very small fraction of those that are evaluated," says Hartmut Derendorf, Ph.D., chairman of the Department of Pharmaceutics at the University of Florida College of Pharmacy in Gainesville. "The more we know about drugs and their negative effects, the more we want to be sure that new drugs are safe and effective."

Despite these safeguards, few medications are entirely problem-free, says Dr. DiPiro. Virtually all drugs can cause side effects, ranging from mildly uncomfortable to downright dangerous. In addition, even the safest drug can be harmful if it's taken inappropriately. "A lot of people think if they can get it over the counter, then there's no risk associated with it," he says. "That's just not true."

Using Them Safely

We're so accustomed to taking drugs—everything from aspirin for a headache to decongestants for a stuffy nose—that we forget how powerful they can be. Here's how to get the most from your medications with a minimum of problems.

Get to know your pharmacist. With money being tighter than ever, it's tempting to shop around for the lowest prices. But what you save in dollars, you may lose in personal service, says Peter P. Lamy, Ph.D., professor and chairman of geriatric pharmacotherapy at the University of Maryland School of Pharmacy in Baltimore. "It's very important to use a pharmacist who knows you, what your problems are and what other drugs you're taking," he says.

Store them correctly. Although the car glove compartment is a handy place to store medications, summer's broiling temperatures

---

QUESTIONS YOU SHOULD ASK ABOUT YOUR MEDICATION

The best drugs are only as reliable as the people taking them—and that's not always good enough.

"A third of patients will take their medicines correctly sometimes, a third will never take them and only a third will take them correctly all the time," says Paul Doering, professor of pharmacy practice at the University of Florida College of Pharmacy in Gainesville. "That's a little scary."

Before leaving your doctor's office or the drugstore, Doering says, you should always ask the following questions:

What's the name of the drug? It's not enough to know your medication by its color ("the green one") or flavor ("it tastes like bubble gum"), Doering says. You should always know both the name (such as penicillin) and why you're taking it (to treat an infection).

How do I take it? Some drugs are taken at bedtime, while others should be taken in the morning. Ask your doctor or pharmacist: Do I take it with meals or on an empty stomach? Is it safe with other drugs? Can I take it with aspirin? With antacids? What if I miss a dose? What if I accidentally take too many? Don't stop asking questions until you know exactly how to use the medication, Doering says.

Are there side effects? Most medications do cause some unintended effects, such as headache or fatigue. But even minor discomfort can be frightening if you don't know what's causing it or how serious it may be. You should always know what to expect—both the best and the worst, Doering says.

How long should I take it? Some drugs are meant to be taken only as needed—like aspirin for a headache—while others must be taken every day, even when you're feeling fine.

PRESCRIPTION DESCRIPTIONS

When your doctor fills out a prescription form—which he then signs with an illegible scrawl—he's giving the pharmacist crucial information about you and your medication. You should always double-check the information—on the prescription and the bottle—to ensure it's accurate. Here are some things to look for.

Your name. If you should ever get a prescription that doesn't have your name exactly right, *don't* use it. It may be nothing more than a spelling error, but there's also the chance that you've been given the wrong medicine by mistake.

Drug name and dose. This tells what the drug is and in what strength. It also tells how much medication is contained in the bottle.

Generic substitute instructions. Your doctor may check a box allowing the pharmacist to give you a generic medication. In most cases these no-name drugs work just as well as their name-brand counterparts, at considerably less cost.

How to take it. These instructions—usually written in medical shorthand—tell you exactly how to use the medication. Here are some common abbreviations taken from the Latin:

ac (*ante cibos*): before meals

bid (*bis in die*): twice a day

pc (*post cibum*): after meals

po (*per os*): by mouth

qid (*quater in die*): four times a day

tid (*ter in die*): three times a day

can quickly render them ineffective. The medicine chest isn't much better, says Paul Doering, professor of pharmacy practice at the University of Florida College of Pharmacy. "The bathroom is subjected to huge changes in humidity and temperature, which are not good storage conditions for medicines."

Some drugs require refrigeration, but most will stay fresh if stored in a cool, dry place, such as the top shelf of a closet, says Dr. DiPiro. In time, however, even properly stored medications tend to lose their potency. Most drugs have marked expiration dates. It's a good idea to sift through them at least twice a year and discard the old ones as well as those you're no longer using.

Take the right dose. "There's a commonplace belief that if one is good, then two is twice as good," Doering says. Unfortunately, the opposite is likely to be true. Taking too much of a drug can cause serious problems. If you accidentally take too much medication and begin having problems, call your doctor, pharmacist or poison control center immediately.

Know exactly what you're taking. People who wake up at midnight and fumble for the right bottle are looking for trouble. "A person should never take a medication in the dark," Doering says.

"It's essential that you verify the medication to be sure it's the one you *think* you're taking."

Stick to a schedule. Taking one drug a day is easy. Remembering to take two, three or more—each of which may be taken at different times—can get confusing. To help yourself remember, try taking them at the same times every day—after brushing your teeth, for example, or at bedtime. Keeping a medication diary can also be a big help, Doering says.

Ask if you still need them. Many people continue taking drugs long after the original problem has

---

PROTECTING THE UNBORN

Drugs are complicated enough when there's just one person taking them. But when a pregnant woman uses medications, her fetus may be affected as well. That's why doctors are extremely cautious about giving drugs to women during pregnancy.

"For the vast majority of drugs," says E. Don Nelson, Pharm.D., professor of clinical pharmacology at the University of Cincinnati College of Medicine, "the specific risk in pregnancy is unknown."

Researchers very rarely test drugs in pregnant women, explains Dr. Nelson. As a result, it can be difficult to say for sure which drugs are safe during pregnancy. To complicate things still further, the risk of taking drugs varies with the stage of pregnancy. The danger may be highest during the first six weeks—a time when many women may be taking medications without knowing that they're pregnant.

It's not always possible, of course, for pregnant women to do without medications, says Hartmut Derendorf, Ph.D., chairman of the Department of Pharmaceutics at the University of Florida College of Pharmacy in Gainesville. "The advice, obviously, is to be very, very careful," he says. "Women should use as little medication as possible during pregnancy and consult a doctor or pharmacist before taking *any* drug—even if it's for a cold or headache."

gone away. "Every three to six months, you should ask your doctor or pharmacist, 'Do I still need these drugs?'" says Dr. Lamy. "You want to reduce the number of drugs that you're taking to the absolute minimum."

Using This Section

To help you find the medications you're interested in, we've arranged this section in 60 easy-to-remember categories: arthritis drugs, gout drugs, painkillers and so on. We've also included a comprehensive "Cure Finder" chart at the beginning of the book. By referring to any condition, you will see at a glance most of the drugs that may be used to treat it and where in this section to find them.

Each chapter gives a brief explanation of conditions the drugs are commonly used for. This is followed by a discussion of the medications themselves. You'll also find hundreds of easy-to-read "At a Glance" charts, boxed charts that show each drug's effects, side effects and more.

Finally, you'll find a special feature throughout called "Natural Alternatives," in which we describe some powerful, doctor-tested home remedies that may reduce or eliminate your need for medications.

It's nearly impossible to overestimate the effects drugs have had on our daily lives. By learning how they work and how to use them wisely, you can play a more active role in all your health needs. This section will help you to do just that. But, remember to check with your doctor or pharmacist if you have any questions regarding any medication.

Acne Medications

Skin Savers

Sure, you had them when you were a teenager, but that was *decades* ago. So why are pimples once again spotting your smooth skin?

Because acne, which plagues eight out of ten teenagers, sometimes wreaks its wrath on adults as well. Caused by a combination of bacteria, oil glands and blocked

---

NATURAL ALTERNATIVES

From the time you got your first pimple to the time you get your last, you'll have heard the following gems a hundred times.

"You need to wash your face more often."

"Lay off the chocolate."

"Don't pick, you'll make scars."

Sure, they *sound* good, but are they true? Let's start with face-washing. No one would say hygiene isn't important. But it has little or nothing to do with acne. In fact, "vigorous face-washing is probably detrimental. You don't want to overscrub and irritate the cells," says Barbara D. Reed, M.D., associate professor of family practice at the University of Michigan in Ann Arbor.

Another enduring myth is that chocolate, potato chips or french fries are pimple-making bombs. In fact, there's little scientific evidence that diet—good or bad—affects acne, doctors say. On the other hand, a few people *know* that certain foods make them break out. If you feel this is true with you, then avoiding those foods is worth a try, says Dr. Reed.

The third caveat—to keep your fingernails off your face—is good advice, says Dr. Reed. Picking at pimples can cause them to rupture beneath the skin, spreading germs. This can cause a secondary infection that looks worse—and can cause worse scarring—than the original eruption.

hair follicles, acne typically waxes and wanes. If you're interested in seeing it wane more than wax, certain drugs can be of great help, says Paul Zanowiak, Ph.D., R.Ph., professor of pharmaceutics and director of continuing pharmaceutical education at Temple University in Philadelphia.

Applied Relief

Many acne outbreaks can be tamed with topical medications alone. For example, soaps, creams and pads containing sulfur or salicylic acid (Clearasil, Oxy Medicated Cleanser, Stri-Dex) can unblock clogged hair follicles. This often helps cool acne hot spots, says Dr. Zanowiak.

The most popular acne medication is benzoyl peroxide (Benzac W, Desquam-X 5, Oxy-10). Available over the counter and by prescription, it kills bacteria and slows the activity of pore-clogging glands. "For mild to moderate cases of acne, you usually can see quite a change within a month of treatment," says Barbara D. Reed, M.D., associate professor of family practice at the University of Michigan in Ann Arbor.

In one study, people were treated with benzoyl peroxide or an antibiotic cream. After ten weeks, 63 percent of those in the benzoyl peroxide group had "good to excellent results"—nearly twice the success rate of those in the antibiotic group.

AT A GLANCE

SALICYLIC ACID

Brand names: Clearasil, Oxy Medicated Cleanser, Stri-Dex

How taken: Cream, gel, lotion, pads, shampoo, soap

Prescription: Sometimes, depending on strength

	YES	NO
Generic substitutes	✓	
Potentially addicting		✓
May cause drowsiness		✓
Alcohol discouraged		✓

Possible drug interactions include: Using this drug may increase the effects of other topical medications.

Possible side effects include: Skin irritation and stinging.

BENZOYL PEROXIDE

Brand names: Benzac W, Desquam-X 5, Oxy-10

How taken: Cream, gel, lotion, soap

Prescription: Sometimes, depending on strength

	YES	NO
Generic substitutes	✓	
Potentially addicting		✓
May cause drowsiness		✓
Alcohol discouraged		✓

Possible drug interactions include: Interactions are unlikely (unless using other topical skin medications).

Possible side effects include: Stinging, burning and peeling of the skin.

357

Unfortunately, benzoyl peroxide often causes dry skin, peeling and irritation, although these side effects usually subside after a few weeks. "For most people, benzoyl peroxide is tolerated pretty well," says Dr. Reed.

Still more potent is a prescription drug called tretinoin (Retin-A). Derived from vitamin A, it helps dry up existing pimples and prevents new ones from forming. Like benzoyl peroxide, however, tretinoin can irritate the skin. It also works slowly: Improvements may not be visible for several weeks, Dr. Zanowiak says.

For acne that is infected and inflamed, your doctor may recommend antibiotics. Creams containing erythromycin (Erygel, Staticin, T-Stat) or clindamycin (Cleocin T Lotion) often are used in conjunction with benzoyl peroxide or tretinoin. In one study, German doctors treated more than 1,000 blemished faces with a tretinoin-erythromycin cream. After 14 weeks, 47 percent were pimple-free; an additional 41 percent were at least somewhat smoother.

AT A GLANCE

TRETINOIN

Brand name: Retin-A

How taken: Gel, cream, lotion

Prescription: Yes

	YES	NO
Generic substitutes		✓
Potentially addicting		✓
May cause drowsiness		✓
Alcohol discouraged		✓

Possible drug interactions include: Using this drug may increase the effects of other topical medications containing sulfur, resorcinol or salicylic acid.

Possible side effects include: Burning, redness, swelling, irritation, blistering and lightening or darkening of the skin.

CAUTION: Do not use this drug if you spend a lot of time in the sun.

ERYTHROMYCIN

Brand names: Erygel, Staticin, T-Stat

How taken: Gel, ointment, lotion

Prescription: Yes

	YES	NO
Generic substitutes	✓	
Potentially addicting		✓
May cause drowsiness		✓
Alcohol discouraged		✓

Possible drug interactions include: Interactions are unlikely (unless using other topical skin medications).

Possible side effects include: Stinging, burning, itching, scaling or dryness of the skin

AT A GLANCE

ISOTRETINOIN

Brand name: Accutane

How taken: Capsule

Prescription: Yes

	YES	NO
Generic substitutes		✓
Potentially addicting		✓
May cause drowsiness		✓
Alcohol discouraged		✓

Possible drug interactions include: Taking this drug may increase the side effects of vitamin A supplements.

Possible side effects include: Nausea, dry skin, dryness of the nose or mouth and inflamed lips.

CAUTION: This drug can cause birth defects and should not be taken if you are pregnant or planning a pregnancy.

TRIAMCINOLONE

Brand names: Aristocort, Kenacort, Trilone

How taken: Tablet, liquid, injection

Prescription: Yes

	YES	NO
Generic substitutes	✓	
Potentially addicting		✓
May cause drowsiness		✓
Alcohol discouraged	✓	

Possible drug interactions include: Taking this drug may decrease the effects of anti-clotting drugs.

Possible side effects include: Increased appetite, indigestion, weight gain, fluid retention, nervousness, insomnia and mood changes.

Internal Affairs

Severe acne can't always be controlled with lotions and creams. Your doctor may prescribe isotretinoin (Accutane)—the biggest gun in the acne war.

Like tretinoin, isotretinoin is derived from vitamin A. Unlike tretinoin, it's taken orally, sometimes for up to five months. For many people, it will virtually eliminate acne, sometimes for as long as six years.

A wonder drug? Not quite. For one thing, it works slowly. Months may pass before your skin improves. More serious is its tendency to cause uncomfortable, sometimes dangerous, side effects. These include itching, headache, muscle pain, hair loss, vomiting, high cholesterol levels and, if taken by pregnant women, birth defects.

Women of child-bearing age *must* have pregnancy tests before taking the drug and be prepared to practice strict contraception as long as treatment lasts, says James J. Leyden, M.D., professor of dermatology at the University of Pennsylvania in Philadelphia.

Less dangerous than isotretinoin—but still needing careful supervision—are steroids. Drugs such as cortisone (Cortone) or triamcinolone (Aristocort, Kenacort, Trilone) can be injected directly into the pimples or taken orally, says Dr. Leyden. "For very severe, generalized acne, a short course of systemic steroids may be used to calm down the destructive inflammation," he says. "They work very fast."

Women with severe acne sometimes are treated with estrogen, which suppresses the production of skin oils. (Because estrogen is a female sex hormone, it can't be given to men.) This therapy, however, increases the risk for clots in the bloodstream. It may be used only when safer treatments don't work.

AIDS Drugs

Allies in a Terrible War

There's no doubting the destructive power of the AIDS virus. It has infected more than 14 million people worldwide, and the number is rising. Once a person is infected, the long-term prognosis is anything but good. The virus essentially destroys the major portion of the body's immune system.

Treating AIDS has proved to be extremely difficult. And finding a cure for this deadly disease could be years away. In the meantime, doctors may choose from a number of powerful drugs that can help people with AIDS live longer lives.

A Strong Weapon

The number-one drug on the AIDS front is called AZT, or zidovudine (Retrovir). Usually taken orally, this prescription medication attacks the virus during its replication cycle, the stage at which it begins to multiply. Zidovudine can't destroy the virus, but it can slow the rate at which it multiplies. Researchers at Johns Hopkins University School of Medicine found that people treated with zidovudine lived about four times longer once they started the drug than those who didn't take the drug (approxi-

AT A GLANCE

ZIDOVUDINE (AZT)

Brand name: Retrovir

How taken: Capsule, injection, liquid

Prescription: Yes

	YES	NO
Generic substitutes		✓
Potentially addicting		✓
May cause drowsiness		✓
Alcohol discouraged		✓

Possible drug interactions include: The effects of this drug may decrease if taken with clarithromycin (an antibiotic). This drug taken in combination with drugs for cancer, gout, thyroid problems or fungal infections may result in blood problems.

Possible side effects include: Anemia, fever, headache, nausea, fatigue, sore throat and muscle soreness.

DIDANOSINE (ddI)

Brand name: Videx

How taken: Powder, tablet

Prescription: Yes

	YES	NO
Generic substitutes		✓
Potentially addicting		✓
May cause drowsiness		✓
Alcohol discouraged	✓	

Possible drug interactions include: This drug taken in combination with estrogen, diuretics (water pills), immune system suppressants or some antibiotics may result in pancreatitis (inflammation of the pancreas); taking it with cancer drugs or medications for mood disorders may result in tingling, numbness, burning or pain in the hands or feet.

Possible side effects include: Cramps, diarrhea, nausea or vomiting and tingling, numbness, burning or pain in the hands or feet.

mately 770 days compared to 190).

In the past, people usually were given zidovudine only when AIDS-related symptoms—a type of pneumonia, for example—began to appear. Today, the drug may be given as soon as the immune system begins to decline, even if symptoms haven't occurred, says Joseph R. Thurn, M.D., assistant professor of medicine at the University of Minnesota Medical School and a staff physician in the infectious disease section of the Veterans Administration Medical Center in Minneapolis.

Although zidovudine is one of the strongest weapons in the AIDS war, it is far from ideal. It frequently causes side effects, including anemia (a blood condition that can bring on extreme fatigue). In addition, the virus usually becomes resistant to the

AT A GLANCE

ZALCITABINE (ddC)

Brand name: Hivid

How taken: Tablet

Prescription: Yes

	YES	NO
Generic substitutes		✓
Potentially addicting		✓
May cause drowsiness		✓
Alcohol discouraged	✓	

Possible drug interactions include: This drug taken in combination with some cancer, blood pressure or anti-seizure medications may result in tingling, numbness, burning or pain in the hands or feet.

Possible side effects include: Diarrhea, mouth sores and tingling, numbness, burning or pain in the hands or feet.

medication within one to two years, says Dr. Thurn. When that happens, it may be time to try other drugs instead.

New Treatments, New Hopes

Researchers are excited about a relatively new prescription drug called didanosine, or ddI (Videx). Taken orally, this medication acts in a manner similar to zidovudine. At the same time, it causes different side effects. This means it can be taken when zidovudine is no longer effective or when side effects are too severe, says Dr. Thurn.

Until recently, didanosine was used only when zidovudine was no longer effective. There is some research, however, that suggests it may work as well as the older drug. In a study conducted by the AIDS Clinical Trial Group sponsored by the National Institutes of Health, people who had been taking zidovudine for at least 16 weeks either stayed on the drug or switched to didanosine. After an average of 12 months, those treated with didanosine had fewer AIDS-related infections than those in the zidovudine group.

"The study suggests that after 16 weeks you're better off switching to didanosine," says James O. Kahn, M.D., associate director of the AIDS program at San Francisco General Hospital and assistant clinical professor of medicine at the University of California, San Francisco, School of Medicine.

Unfortunately, just as is the case with zidovudine, didanosine eventually loses its effectiveness. It's also rife with side effects, including diarrhea, nerve problems and a dangerous inflammation of the pancreas called pancreatitis. "In some cases, didanosine may be a front-line drug, but in general, I think people tolerate zidovudine better than didanosine," says Dr. Thurn.

Combination Power

Many researchers believe that the future of AIDS therapy lies not in any one drug but in using different drugs together, a technique they call convergent combination therapy.

The principle is simple: By using two or more drugs to attack the virus, it may be possible to destroy it before it has time to spread or develop resistance. In laboratory studies, Dr. Thurn explains, a three-drug combination has been shown to temporarily stop the virus without destroying healthy cells in the process.

In studying people, researchers have tried several drug combinations. For example, when zidovudine is combined with didanosine—either at the same time or given in alternating cycles—the results may be superior to when either drug is used alone. Zidovudine also has been combined with oral antiviral prescription drugs such as zalcitabine, or ddC (Hivid).

Thus far, the treatments for AIDS haven't been ideal, says Dr. Kahn. "Better drugs or combinations of drugs need to be developed to help our patients."

Anal and Rectal Drugs

Help for Sitting Easy

Sometimes it seems that the anus is the body's equivalent of Rodney Dangerfield: It gets no respect, even when afflicted with itches, hemorrhoids and fissures. "You'll get to the bottom of this," chuckle your well-meaning but irreverent friends, "with no ifs, ands or butts!"

Easy for them to laugh. But when it's your end that's aching, you don't need comic relief. You just need relief—and the quicker the better.

Help for Hemorrhoids

Perhaps the most common affliction of the nether region is hemorrhoids. Informally known as piles, these distended anal veins can be aggravated by pregnancy or straining during bowel movements. Hemorrhoids inside the rectum are painless and usually require no medical treatment. But those that occur outside can be excruciating, says Lee E. Smith, M.D., director of the Division of

NATURAL ALTERNATIVES

The best way to treat anal and rectal problems, doctors say, is to prevent them from getting started. Try these proven prevention strategies.

Fill up on fiber. The average American eats only about half the amount of fiber doctors recommend. By eating plenty of fiber—available in whole grains, fruits and vegetables—your stools will be softer and easier to pass and less likely to cause problems.

Try wet wipes. When your bottom is throbbing, even soft paper can feel like sandpaper. To reduce the rasp, moisten the paper before using it. Then *pat* yourself clean.

Be patient. Anal problems are often caused by trying to force a bowel movement when you're not ready. Don't push it, doctors say. If nothing happens after five to ten minutes, try again later.

Colon and Rectal Surgery at George Washington University in Washington, D.C.

To ease the ache of external hemorrhoids, your doctor may recommend anesthetic creams or ointments. Over-the-counter creams containing dibucaine (Nupercainal), benzocaine (Americaine Hemorrhoidal) or pramoxine (Fleet Relief, ProctoFoam/non-steroidal, Tronolane) can provide quick relief, says Edmund Leff, M.D., a colon and rectal specialist with practices in Phoenix and Scottsdale, Arizona.

But, he adds, some people become sensitive to the "caine" anesthetics and may develop irritation. That's why these medications are best used only when absolutely necessary.

For reducing swelling, over-the-counter creams containing 1 percent (or less) hydrocortisone (Anusol-HC, Cort-Dome, Proctocort) can be very helpful, says Dr. Leff. The overuse of hydrocortisone creams, however, can cause a permanent thinning of the skin. To be safe, don't use them for more than a week without checking with your doctor.

To protect sensitive hemorrhoids from being scraped by passing stool, lubricating creams, ointments or suppositories can be a help, says Dr. Smith. There are dozens of over-the-counter lubricants, also called protectants. These include glycerin (Fleet Babylax, Sani-Supp), zinc oxide or even plain petroleum jelly.

Perhaps the best-known hemorrhoid preparation of all contains a live yeast cell derivative and shark liver oil (Preparation H). According to the manufacturer, it helps relieve pain, itching and

AT A GLANCE

BENZOCAINE

Brand name: Americaine Hemorrhoidal

How taken: Ointment

Prescription: No

	YES	NO
Generic substitutes	✓	
Potentially addicting		✓
May cause drowsiness	✓	
Alcohol discouraged		✓

Possible drug interactions include: Interactions are unlikely.

Possible side effects include: Redness, swelling and burning of the anal area.

PRAMOXINE

Brand names: Fleet Relief, Procto-Foam/non-steroidal, Tronolane

How taken: Cream, foam, suppository, ointment

Prescription: No

	YES	NO
Generic substitutes	✓	
Potentially addicting		✓
May cause drowsiness	✓	
Alcohol discouraged		✓

Possible drug interactions include: Interactions are unlikely.

Possible side effects include: Rash, irritation, burning and itching of the anal area.

HYDROCORTISONE

Brand names: Anusol-HC, Bactine Hydrocortisone Anti-Itch Cream, Cort-Dome, Proctocort, Cortaid, CaldeCORT Anti-Itch

How taken: Cream, suppository

Prescription: Sometimes, depending on strength

	YES	NO
Generic substitutes	✓	
Potentially addicting		✓
May cause drowsiness		✓
Alcohol discouraged		✓

Possible drug interactions include: Interactions are unlikely.

Possible side effects include: Long-term regular use may cause thinning of the skin.

ZINC OXIDE

Brand name: Generic only

How taken: Ointment, suppository

Prescription: No

	YES	NO
Generic substitutes	✓	
Potentially addicting		✓
May cause drowsiness		✓
Alcohol discouraged		✓

Possible drug interactions include: Interactions are unlikely.

Possible side effects include: Nervousness, sleeplessness and nausea.

swelling. Experts say it can be a useful but expensive way to lubricate the anus and protect painful hemorrhoids against passing stools. On the other hand, petroleum jelly probably would do just as well, says Dr. Smith.

Fighting Fissures

Although the anus is one of the most elastic parts of your body, there are limits to what it can accommodate. Passing an unusually large, hard stool can cause it to tear. The resulting split, or fissure, says Dr. Smith, can be terribly painful—so much so that some people won't see a doctor because

---

AT A GLANCE

GLYCERIN

Brand names: Fleet Babylax, Sani-Supp

How taken: Suppository, enema

Prescription: Sometimes, depending on strength

	YES	NO
Generic substitutes	✓	
Potentially addicting		✓
May cause drowsiness		✓
Alcohol discouraged		✓

Possible drug interactions include: Interactions are unlikely.

Possible side effects include: Irritation of the anal area.

---

they don't want their bottom touched!

As with hemorrhoids, one good way to deal with fissures is with lubricants such as glycerin and petroleum jelly. "A glycerin suppository may lubricate a stool so it slips out easier," says Dr. Smith.

For short-term use, over-the-counter anesthetics such as benzocaine can help numb the pain. But again, there's always the possibility of having allergic-type reactions. As a result, they shouldn't be used too often, says Dr. Smith.

The best "treatment" for fissures is to use over-the-counter stool softeners and bulking agents, says Dr. Smith. Preparations containing methylcellulose (Citrucel, Cologel), psyllium (Effer-syllium, Fiberall, Metamucil) or docusate sodium (Colace, Pro-Sof, Surfak) don't actually heal fissures, but they do make stools softer and easier to pass, reducing the chance of splitting the anal skin again.

Easing Itches

Doctors call it *pruritus ani.* You know it as "itchy anus," and it can occur whenever the skin's normally protective barriers break down. Scratching only makes it worse, says Dr. Smith, and it may take several weeks before improving.

To speed things along, doctors often recommend hydrocortisone (Bactine Hydrocortisone Anti-Itch Cream, CaldeCORT Anti-Itch, Cortaid). Available over the counter and applied directly to the anus several times a day, it reduces inflammation and provides fast relief from itching.

When used regularly for long periods of time, however, hydrocorti-sone may cause anal tissues to become more delicate. If itching persists for more than a couple of weeks, says Dr. Smith, see your doctor.

Angina Medications

Aids to Circulation

We cross it for promises, cover it for pledges and draw an arrow through it on Valentine's Day. We even, at certain special times, give it away!

Yet the heart, for all its special purposes, is extremely vulnerable: It cannot thrive, or even survive, without oxygen. Reduce the supply of oxygen and the heart complains—loudly!—with tightness and sharp pains behind the breastbone. Doctors call this pain angina pectoris, or angina for short.

Approximately three million Americans experience angina pain. The cause, in most cases, is the accumulation of fatty deposits in the arteries, a condition called atherosclerosis. Blood and oxygen still travel through the arteries, but in reduced amounts. During times of exertion—exercise, for example—the heart notices the difference. And doesn't like it.

"Angina is a supply-and-demand issue," says Alan D. Forker, M.D., professor of medicine at the University of Missouri–Kansas City School of Medicine and chief of cardiology at Truman Medical Center in Kansas City. "When you decrease the supply of blood or increase the demand, you may have angina pain."

Reducing Demand, Boosting Supply

Angina isn't always recognized for what it is. Some people expect severe, unbearable pain and overlook milder forms of discomfort. "It can be mild enough that some people mistake it for indigestion," says Robert DiBianco, M.D., director of cardiology re-

NATURAL ALTERNATIVES

Angina pectoris—chest pain caused by a shortage of oxygen to the heart—often can be relieved just by making some simple lifestyle changes. For example:

Give up cigarettes. This is perhaps the most important thing you can do to safeguard your health. Not only does smoking promote the accumulation of blood-blocking deposits in the arteries, it also robs the heart of needed oxygen.

Lay off the high-fat foods. A steady diet of hot dogs, doughnuts and other foods high in saturated fats does more than fill you up (and out). It also can lead to artery-blocking deposits that contribute to angina pain.

Lose those extra pounds. The more weight you're carrying around, the harder your heart has to work.

Give yourself a workout. If you're out of shape, a vigorous exercise session may initiate angina pain. Those who keep themselves fit, however, are less likely to have problems. Check with your doctor, of course, before beginning any exercise program.

---

search and the Heart Failure Clinic and Risk Factor Reduction Center at Washington Adventist Hospital in Takoma Park, Maryland. In more serious cases, however, it can be excruciatingly painful.

To stop angina pain, your doctor may recommend prescription medications called fast-acting nitrates. Drugs such as nitroglycerin (Nitrostat), placed under the tongue at the first sign of angina, reduce the heart's demand for oxygen, says Dr. DiBianco. At the same time, they cause arteries to expand, boosting the flow of oxygen-rich blood within minutes.

"A tiny little tablet of nitro under your tongue is the number-one defense against angina," says Dr. Forker. The drugs are quite safe, although headache, flushing and dizziness may sometimes occur, he adds. An alternative to the tablet that is just as effective is a nitroglycerin oral spray (Nitrolingual).

Fast-acting nitrates work well in a pinch, but people who have frequent attacks may require a longer-lasting preparation. Popular options include isosorbide dinitrate (Isonate, Isordil, Sorbitrate) and the new isosorbide mononitrate (Ismol), both of which are usually taken orally. Nitroglycerin may be taken orally (Nitrocap, Nitroglyn, Nitrong) or applied to the skin as a cream (Nitro-Bid Ointment, Nitrol) or patch (Deponit, Nitrodisc, Nitro-Dur). This allows the medication to slowly enter the bloodstream. Rather than stopping attacks, slow-acting nitrates help prevent them from occurring.

Unlike the fast-acting drugs, however, the slower preparations often become less effective as your body builds up a tolerance. They're also more likely to cause side effects, including headache and dizziness. To prevent these problems, your doctor will prescribe the medication in the lowest possible dose, says Dr. Forker.

Because angina reflects a probable narrowing in the arteries that supply the heart with blood, it is potentially very dangerous. You must tell your doctor if you notice any changes in pain or the frequency of attacks, warns Dr. DiBianco. It's also important to keep your medicine fresh. Nitrates lose their effectiveness very quickly. To

---

AT A GLANCE

NITROGLYCERIN

Brand names: Deponit, Nitro-Bid Ointment, Nitrocap, Nitrodisc, Nitro-Dur, Nitroglyn, Nitrol, Nitrolingual spray, Nitrong, Nitrostat

How taken: Capsule, ointment, patch, tablet, spray

Prescription: Yes

	YES	NO
Generic substitutes	✓	
Potentially addicting		✓
May cause drowsiness		✓
Alcohol discouraged	✓	

Possible drug interactions include: This drug taken in combination with beta-blockers, calcium channel blockers and other heart and blood pressure medicines may result in very low blood pressure.

Possible side effects include: Headache, nausea, flushing, restlessness, dizziness and a fast heart rate.

ISOSORBIDE DINITRATE

Brand names: Isonate, Isordil, Sorbitrate

How taken: Capsule, tablet

Prescription: Yes

	YES	NO
Generic substitutes	✓	
Potentially addicting		✓
May cause drowsiness		✓
Alcohol discouraged	✓	

Possible drug interactions include: This drug taken in combination with beta-blockers, calcium channel blockers and other heart and blood pressure medicines may result in very low blood pressure.

Possible side effects include: Headache, nausea, flushing, restlessness, dizziness and a fast heart rate.

AT A GLANCE

PROPRANOLOL

Brand name: Inderal

How taken: Capsule, liquid, tablet, injection

Prescription: Yes

	YES	NO
Generic substitutes	✓	
Potentially addicting		✓
May cause drowsiness	✓	
Alcohol discouraged	✓	

Possible drug interactions include: Taking this drug may decrease the effects of theophylline and other asthma drugs and may blunt the effects of insulin or oral diabetes medications. This drug taken in combination with other heart and blood pressure medications may result in low blood pressure; taking it with monoamine oxidase (MAO) inhibitors (used for depression) may result in increased blood pressure.

Possible side effects include: Fatigue, insomnia, dizziness, weakness and decreased sex drive.

ACEBUTOLOL

Brand name: Sectral

How taken: Capsule

Prescription: Yes

	Yes	No
Generic substitutes		✓
Potentially addicting		✓
May cause drowsiness	✓	
Alcohol discouraged	✓	

Possible drug interactions include: Taking this drug may decrease the effects of theophylline and other asthma medications and may blunt the effects of insulin or oral diabetes drugs. This drug taken in combination with other heart and blood pressure medications may result in low blood pressure; taking it with monoamine oxidase (MAO) inhibitors (used for depression) and nonprescription nasal decongestant sprays may result in increased blood pressure.

Possible side effects include: Fatigue, insomnia, dizziness, weakness and decreased sex drive.

prevent this, they should be stored in a dark, tightly closed bottle, he says.

Pain Prevention

Nitrates aren't the only medications that can prevent attacks. A class of drugs called beta-adrenergic blocking agents, or beta-blockers, can be very effective as well, says Dr. DiBianco.

Prescription drugs such as metoprolol (Lopressor) and propranolol (Inderal), usually taken orally, work by inhibiting the transmission of nerve signals to the heart. This slows the heart, which in turn causes it to use less oxygen, Dr. Forker explains.

Although beta-blockers can help prevent attacks, they have a slow onset of action. For added protection, people taking beta-blockers should always carry fast-acting nitroglycerin for use under the tongue as well.

Beta-blockers have been extensively tested and are considered quite safe. However, they may cause insomnia, nightmares, fatigue and other uncomfortable side effects. They also can cause a slight rise in cholesterol levels, possibly leading to *more* angina pain. But a new generation of beta-blockers—for example, acebutolol (Sectral)—can help stop angina pain without causing dangerous rises in cholesterol, says Dr. Forker.

On balance, beta-blockers are hard to beat. "Beta-blockers are the only group of angina drugs shown to prolong survival rates for coronary artery disease or heart attack victims," says Dr. Forker.

AT A GLANCE

DILTIAZEM

Brand name: Cardizem

How taken: Capsule, tablet, injection

Prescription: Yes

	YES	NO
Generic substitutes		✓
Potentially addicting		✓
May cause drowsiness	✓	
Alcohol discouraged	✓	

Possible drug interactions include: Taking this drug may increase the effects of other heart medications and certain anti-seizure drugs. This drug taken in combination with glaucoma medications such as betaxolol and timolol may result in low blood pressure or slowed heart rate.

Possible side effects include: Dizziness, fatigue, headache, flushing and constipation.

VERAPAMIL

Brand names: Calan, Isoptin, Verelan

How taken: Capsule, injection, tablet

Prescription: Yes

	YES	NO
Generic substitutes	✓	
Potentially addicting		✓
May cause drowsiness		✓
Alcohol discouraged	✓	

Possible drug interactions include: Taking this drug may increase the effects of other heart drugs and certain anti-seizure medications. This drug taken in combination with glaucoma medications such as betaxolol and timolol may result in low blood pressure or slowed heart rate.

Possible side effects include: Headache, dizziness, fatigue, flushing and constipation.

Pipe Expanders

A third class of angina drugs your doctor may recommend is called calcium channel blockers.

Prescription medications such as diltiazem (Cardizem), nifedipine (Adalat, Procardia) and verapamil (Calan, Isoptin, Verelan), taken orally, work by relaxing muscles that surround the blood vessels. This causes the vessels to widen, which allows more blood—and oxygen—to reach the heart.

As with beta-blockers, these drugs should be augmented with fast-acting nitroglycerin to stop unexpected attacks, says Dr. DiBianco.

Although calcium blockers rarely cause serious side effects, they can reduce blood pressure and, at times, make you feel dizzy and light-headed. They also may cause ankle swelling.

Antacids

Stomach Settlers

With so much holiday food on the table—smoked turkey, stewed onions and scalloped potatoes—who could resist having seconds? What a wonderful meal! What a terrible case of heartburn!

You may know heartburn as dyspepsia, sour stomach or acid indigestion. The term your doctor uses is *esophageal reflux*. This simply means that stomach acid, rather than staying where it belongs, is splashing upward into the esophagus, the pipe between your stomach and your mouth, explains Richard McCallum, M.D., professor of medicine and chief of the Division of Gastroenterology, Hepatology and Nutrition at the University of Virginia Health Sciences Center in Charlottesville.

If you frequently have heartburn with abdominal discomfort, he adds, you should see a doctor, because it may indicate a serious problem such as ulcers. But in most cases, heartburn is easily treated at home with safe, inex-

NATURAL ALTERNATIVES

There are many things you can do to quell the flames of heartburn fires. Here are a few tips from the experts.

Don't overeat! A stomach that's bursting at the seams is likely to erupt burning acid.

Avoid fatty, greasy foods. These are champion acid makers.

Avoid coffee, chocolate and mints. At the bottom of the esophagus is a valve that helps keep stomach acid where it belongs. But these three foods tend to relax the valve, possibly allowing acid to surge upward.

Stay away from cigarettes. People who smoke are far more likely to have heartburn than those who don't.

Tip your bed upward. When you tilt the head of the bed up to eight inches, gravity becomes a nighttime ally and helps keep stomach acid down. Solid wooden blocks under the two headboard posts should do the trick.

Don't eat before bedtime. Where there's food, there's acid. At night when you're lying down, it's easy for that acid to creep upward and cause heartburn.

pensive, over-the-counter medications called antacids.

The Acid Test

Antacids are among the most commonly used drugs in the United States. Here's why. Your stomach's fluids are highly corrosive. On the acid scale, they lie somewhere between pure lemon juice and battery acid. This makes them very efficient at digesting tough food fibers.

Your stomach has a very efficient lining that protects it from the corrosiveness of these acids, but the stomach's upstairs neighbor has no such protection.

So after big meals, when food and acid rise to the top of the stomach and splash into the esophagus, the result is mild to moderate burning pain—heartburn, in other words.

Antacids, by neutralizing stomach acid, can help bank heartburn's fires.

There are dozens of antacids to choose from, but most contain aluminum, calcium, magnesium, sodium, magaldrate or a combination of these ingredients. All are effective but may cause mild side effects, Dr. McCallum says. You might need to try several brands to find the one that works best for you.

AT A GLANCE

SODIUM BICARBONATE

Brand names: Alka-Seltzer, Arm & Hammer Pure Baking Soda

How taken: Tablet, powder

Prescription: No

	Yes	No
Generic substitutes	✓	
Potentially addicting		✓
May cause drowsiness		✓
Alcohol discouraged	✓	

Possible drug interactions include: Taking this drug may decrease the effects of some antibiotics, anti-infectives and antifungal drugs; it may increase the effects of mecamylamine (a blood pressure drug).

Possible side effects include: Side effects are unlikely.

CALCIUM CARBONATE

Brand names: Alka-Mints, Calcium Rich/Sodium Free Rolaids, Tums

How taken: Chewing gum, liquid, tablet

Prescription: No

	YES	NO
Generic substitutes	✓	
Potentially addicting		✓
May cause drowsiness		✓
Alcohol discouraged	✓	

Possible drug interactions include: Taking this drug may decrease the effects of cellulose sodium phosphate (used to prevent kidney stones) and some antibiotics, anti-infectives and antifungal drugs; it may increase the effects of mecamylamine (a blood pressure drug).

Possible side effects include: Side effects are unlikely.

An Old-Time Favorite

Perhaps the oldest antacid—and for some people the most effective—is sodium bicarbonate, or baking soda (Alka-Seltzer, Arm & Hammer Pure Baking Soda). Available over the counter and taken orally, either as a tablet or as a powder mixed into water, this potent antacid can quickly relieve heartburn. A related product that contains sodium citrate and sodium bicarbonate (Citrocarbonate Ant-

acid) also can be very effective.

Unfortunately, many people dislike the salty taste of the sodium-based antacids. They're also short-acting and may need to be taken many times a day. They may also cause a condition known as acid rebound, in which more acid is present after taking the drug than there was before. But this usually is a problem only when large doses are taken.

Perhaps the biggest drawback to sodium-based antacids is that they can raise blood pressure and increase water retention. People who have heart, kidney or blood pressure problems should avoid sodium-based antacids and try other medications instead.

Aluminum Alternatives

Many antacids contain calcium carbonate (Alka-Mints, Calcium Rich/Sodium Free Rolaids, Tums). Sold over the counter and taken orally, calcium carbonate may neutralize twice as much stomach acid as sodium bicar-bonate, without the associated danger of high blood pressure.

As with sodium bicarbonate, however, calcium carbonate occasionally may cause acid rebound. It also may cause constipation, belching and flatulence.

Yet there's a bonus: Doctors say the calcium in calcium carbonate can double as a dietary supplement. For example, taking three antacids a day not only can help relieve heartburn but also can help you meet your daily need for calcium. This may help prevent the bone-thinning disease called osteoporosis.

AT A GLANCE

ALUMINUM HYDROXIDE

Brand names: Gaviscon, Mylanta

How taken: Liquid, tablet, gel, capsule

Prescription: No

	YES	NO
Generic substitutes	✓	
Potentially addicting		✓
May cause drowsiness		✓
Alcohol discouraged	✓	

Possible drug interactions include: Taking this drug may decrease the effects of some antibiotics, antifungal drugs and isoniazid (a tuberculosis drug); it may increase the effects of mecamylamine (a blood pressure medication).

Possible side effects include: Side effects are unlikely.

ALUMINUM and MAGNESIUM

Brand names: Alamag, Maalox

How taken: Liquid, tablet

Prescription: No

	YES	NO
Generic substitutes	✓	
Potentially addicting		✓
May cause drowsiness		✓
Alcohol discouraged	✓	

Possible drug interactions include: Taking this drug may decrease the effects of some antibiotics, anti-infectives, antifungal drugs and isoniazid (a tuberculosis drug); it may increase the effects of mecamylamine (a blood pressure medication).

Possible side effects include: Side effects are unlikely.

Aid from Aluminum

Many of today's antacids are made with aluminum hydroxide (Gaviscon, Mylanta). The main advantage of these medications, available over the counter and taken orally, is that they're sodium-free. They're often mixed with other active ingredients such as magnesium hydroxide.

One problem with aluminum antacids is that they may cause constipation. They also may block the absorption of other drugs and vitamins, including iron, tetracycline antibiotics and some sedatives. So don't take other medications at the same time as aluminum antacids. Instead, space them at least two hours apart, doctors say.

More from Magnesium

One antacid that's pure magnesium is milk of magnesia (Phillips' Milk of Magnesia). In fact, most magnesium antacids also contain aluminum, says Dr. McCallum.

This is because magnesium mixed with aluminum (Alamag, Maalox) is more potent and long lasting than either drug used alone and can neutralize stomach acid in just a few

---

AT A GLANCE

MAGNESIUM HYDROXIDE

Brand name: Phillips' Milk of Magnesia

How taken: Liquid, tablet

Prescription: No

	YES	NO
Generic substitutes	✓	
Potentially addicting		✓
May cause drowsiness		✓
Alcohol discouraged	✓	

Possible drug interactions include: Taking this drug may decrease the effects of some antibiotics and anti-fungal drugs; it may increase the effects of mecamylamine (a blood pressure medication).

Possible side effects include: Side effects are unlikely.

MAGALDRATE

Brand name: Riopan

How taken: Liquid, tablet

Prescription: No

	YES	NO
Generic substitutes	✓	
Potentially addicting		✓
May cause drowsiness		✓
Alcohol discouraged	✓	

Possible drug interactions include: Taking this drug may decrease the effects of some antibiotics and anti-fungal drugs; it may increase the effects of mecamylamine (a blood pressure medication).

Possible side effects include: Side effects are unlikely.

minutes. Another reason for mixing the two is that magnesium, taken alone, often acts as a laxative. Aluminum, on the other hand, tends to be constipating. When both are taken together in small and infrequent doses, the side effects often cancel each other out, says Dr. McCallum. In large quantities, however, diarrhea may result.

With so many choices, chances are that most people will be able to find a suitable antacid, be it a liquid or a tablet.

Antibiotics

Arsenal against Infection

In the bad old days before antibiotics, even minor conditions—a bout with bronchitis or even an earache—could have major consequences.

"The mortality rate was very high for many diseases," says Mitchell L. Cohen, M.D., director of the Division of Bacterial and Mycotic (fungal) Diseases at the Centers for Disease Control and Prevention in Atlanta. "People tended to accept the fact that they would lose some of their children in the first five or ten years of life to infectious diseases."

This began to change in the early 1940s when penicillin became widely available. For the first time ever, killer diseases like pneumonia could be cured, often within days.

Since then, dozens of antibiotics have joined penicillin in the war on germs. Why so many drugs? Because there are hundreds of strains of bacteria, and nearly as many places in the body that they can infect you. Your doctor or pharmacist will consider both factors—what you probably have and where—before deciding which antibiotic is right for you.

Germ-Killing Basics

Before discussing individual antibiotics, it might be helpful to consider how these drugs actually work.

All antibiotics, whether taken by tablet, liquid, injection or cream, are either bacter*icidal* or bacteri*static*. Bactericidal drugs destroy bacteria outright. Bacteristatic drugs, on the other hand, prevent them from multiplying. With fewer bugs to contend with, your body's immune system then can finish the job.

Which drug you take depends on which bacterium is trouble. "There could be ten different organisms that could cause pneumonia," explains Dr. Cohen. "One particular antibiotic, erythromycin, is able to kill many of those organisms." By contrast, a person with a strep throat infection will harbor a different strain of bacteria. This person might be treated with penicillin instead.

One problem with antibiotics is that they kill not only harmful bacteria but also beneficial ones. When your normal internal balance of microorganisms is disturbed, diarrhea or yeast infections may result. Normally, these side effects are mild and will go away on their own. If they don't, tell your doctor. Lowering the dose or, in some cases, changing the drug may clear things up.

Internal Infections

Few conditions are as annoying—or occur as often—as urinary tract infections, or UTIs. Often caused by bacteria that migrate from the anus to the urethra (the urinary tract canal), UTIs can cause fever, pelvic pain and other uncomfortable symptoms.

Most UTIs are easily knocked out with antibiotics, says Joshua Hoffman, M.D., an internist and assistant clinical professor of medicine at the University of California, Davis, Medical Center in Sacramento. Prescription antibiotics such as ampicillin (Omnipen, Principen), taken orally, concentrate in the urine. This means even low doses can eliminate most UTIs within a week to ten days, says Dr. Hoffman.

In fact, some doctors treat UTIs in just one day, using prescription drugs such as trimethoprim (Proloprim, Trimpex) or trimethoprim plus sulfamethoxazole (Bactrim, Septra). "The effectiveness rates are slightly less than seven- to ten-day therapy, but studies show they're very close," says Dr. Hoffman.

Yet another common condition is pneumonia. Fifty years ago, this

---

AT A GLANCE

AMPICILLIN

Brand names: Omnipen, Principen

How taken: Capsule, injection, liquid

Prescription: Yes

	YES	NO
Generic substitutes	✓	
Potentially addicting		✓
May cause drowsiness		✓
Alcohol discouraged		✓

Possible drug interactions include: Taking this drug may decrease the effects of some oral contraceptives.

Possible side effects include: Nausea, mild diarrhea and mouth irritation.

CAUTION: May cause serious allergic reactions in some people.

TRIMETHOPRIM

Brand names: Proloprim, Trimpex

How taken: Tablet

Prescription: Yes

	YES	NO
Generic substitutes	✓	
Potentially addicting		✓
May cause drowsiness		✓
Alcohol discouraged		✓

Possible drug interactions include: The effects of this drug may decrease if taken with other antibiotics. Taking this drug may increase the effects of phenytoin (an anti-seizure drug).

Possible side effects include: Headache, nausea, loss of appetite and diarrhea or stomach cramps.

AT A GLANCE

NEOMYCIN–POLYMYXIN B–BACITRACIN

Brand names: Maximum Strength Mycitracin Triple Antibiotic First Aid Ointment, Neosporin Ointment

How taken: Ointment

Prescription: Sometimes, depending on strength

	YES	No
Generic substitutes	✓	
Potentially addicting		✓
May cause drowsiness		✓
Alcohol discouraged		✓

Possible drug interactions include: Interactions are unlikely.

Possible side effects include: Rash, itching and other skin irritations.

CEFACLOR

Brand name: Ceclor

How taken: Capsule, liquid

Prescription: Yes

	Yes	No
Generic substitutes		✓
Potentially addicting		✓
May cause drowsiness		✓
Alcohol discouraged		✓

Possible drug interactions include: This drug may stay in the body longer when taken with probenecid (used to treat gout).

Possible side effects include: Mild stomach cramps, nausea and a sore mouth or tongue.

lung infection could be, and often was, fatal, says Dr. Cohen. Today, however, when diagnosed early, it's often readily treated with penicillin V (Beepen VK, Pen Vee K, Robicillin VK) or newer oral antibiotics, such as vancomycin (Vancocin), cefaclor (Ceclor) or ciprofloxacin (Cipro).

Of course, not all bacterial infections are easy to treat. For example, meningitis, an infection that causes inflammation of the membrane surrounding the brain, may require injections containing more than 20 million international units of penicillin—200 times the dose needed to treat pneumonia.

On the Surface

Not all bacterial infections are treated with liquids, tablets and injections. Many common infections can be eliminated—or prevented—with antibiotic ointments and creams.

For example, acne that has become inflamed can be treated with prescription creams containing erythromycin (E-Mycin, Robimycin) or clindamycin (Cleocin T Lotion).

For minor cuts and scrapes, doctors often recommend *triple* antibiotics—over-the-counter ointments and creams containing three active ingredients, such as neomycin, polymyxin B and bacitracin (Maximum Strength Mycitracin Triple Antibiotic First Aid Ointment, Neosporin Ointment).

These ointments may do more than treat infection, doctors say. In one study, researchers at the University of Pennsylvania in Philadelphia treated blister wounds either with antiseptics such as iodine or with a triple antibiotic containing neomycin, polymyxin B and bacitracin. They found that blisters treated with the antibiotic ointment healed about four days sooner than those treated with the other drugs. The antibiotics also don't sting like iodine!

Smart Advice

In the approximately 50 years since antibiotics have been on the market, bacteria have become increasingly difficult to kill. This is starkly illustrated by the re-emergence of tuberculosis. After a century in decline, this dangerous,

---

AT A GLANCE

PENICILLIN V

Brand names: Beepen VK, Pen Vee K, Robicillin VK

How taken: Injection, liquid, tablet

Prescription: Yes

	YES	NO
Generic substitutes	✓	
Potentially addicting		✓
May cause drowsiness		✓
Alcohol discouraged		✓

Possible drug interactions include: The effects of this drug may decrease if taken with antacids or other antibiotics. Taking this drug may decrease the effects of some oral contraceptives.

Possible side effects include: May encourage yeast infections by killing off "friendly" bacteria in the body.

ERYTHROMYCIN

Brand names: E-Mycin, Robimycin, T-Stat

How taken: Capsule, injection, liquid, ointment, tablet

Prescription: Yes

	YES	NO
Generic substitutes	✓	
Potentially addicting		✓
May cause drowsiness		✓
Alcohol discouraged		✓

Possible drug interactions include: Taking this drug may increase the side effects of carbamazepine (an anti-seizure drug), digoxin (used for heart problems), ergotamine (used for migraines), methylprednisolone (an anti-inflammatory drug), theophylline (used for asthma) and warfarin (an anti-clotting drug); taking it may decrease the effects of other antibiotics.

Possible side effects include: Nausea, mild diarrhea, abdominal cramps and skin irritation.

sometimes-deadly disease is making a comeback. Worse, some of the bacteria now can resist many of the drugs in use today.

Paradoxically, this problem has occurred, at least in part, because antibiotics work so well. Suppose, for example, that someone has been sick for days. Then he takes an antibiotic. Within 24 hours, he feels dramatically better. Believing himself cured, he throws the remaining tablets in the trash.

But he wasn't really cured. Al-though the antibiotic quickly eliminated some of the bacteria, "there will be some organisms that are slightly resistant," explains Dr. Hoffman. By stopping treatment early, he gave the survivors a chance to rally. This means he might get sick again. He also helped create a drug-resistant strain of bacteria.

That's why it's so important to finish *all* of your prescription, Dr. Hoffman says, even when you're feeling better.

Antidepressants

The Blues Bashers

There's nothing unusual about feeling sad, gloomy or dejected. We all have these feelings occasionally. In most cases we begin to feel better once a little time passes.

For people who are seriously depressed, however, feeling better can be a long time coming. Many will need a doctor—and, perhaps, antidepressant drugs.

Experts estimate that as many as one in five people will, at some point in their lives, have a bout with serious depression, says Michael Feinberg, M.D., Ph.D., professor of psychiatry at Hahnemann University School of Medicine in Philadelphia. For many of these people, antidepressants such as amitriptyline, imipramine and fluoxetine (Prozac) can help restore the confidence and energy they need to feel themselves again.

But antidepressants do more than fight depression, Dr. Feinberg

ARE YOU DEPRESSED?

Doctors estimate that as many as 20 million Americans may suffer from major depression, and millions more are afflicted with lesser degrees of lethargy, loss of appetite and other mood changes. According to the American Psychiatric Association, if you have five or more of the following symptoms, you may have a major depression and should see your doctor.

- Depression of mood

- Loss of interest or pleasure in normal activity

- Significant weight change or change in appetite

- Changes in sleep patterns

- Changes in activity—you slow down or become nervous and anxious

- Loss of energy

- Feelings of worthlessness or excessive guilt

- Inability to think, concentrate or make decisions

- Recurrent thoughts of death or suicide

adds. They are also used to treat sleep disorders, tension and migraine headaches, irritable bowel syndrome and long-term pain. It's not surprising, then, that some of these drugs are among the most widely used medications in America.

Restoring Balance

There are many types of antidepressants. Doctors usually divide them into three broad categories: tricyclic antidepressants, monoamine oxidase (MAO) inhibitors and new-generation antidepressants. Each works in slightly different ways, but all have one thing in common: They boost the activity of various chemicals, called neurotransmitters, in the brain.

Cells in our brain normally release neurotransmitters, which help us maintain our good moods and energy levels. Sometimes, however, the movement of these neurotransmitters from cell to cell isn't as efficient as it's supposed to be. This can cause anxiety, moodiness, loss of appetite and other symptoms of depression, says Dr. Feinberg.

Essentially, antidepressant drugs help neurotransmitters do their job. This, in turn, can help relieve depression—and a host of other problems in some people—in as little as three to six weeks, says Raymond Pary, M.D., associate professor of psychiatry at the University of Louisville School of Medicine and staff psychiatrist at the Veterans Affairs Medical Center in Louisville, Kentucky.

Antidepressants are designed to relieve you of depression—not to make you walk around all day with a silly grin on your face. "These pills don't make people 'high,'" says Dr. Pary.

Therapy in a Bottle?

Not everyone with depression needs to take antidepressants. Nor are antidepressants necessarily a substitute for psychological coun-

---

AT A GLANCE

FLUOXETINE

Brand name: Prozac

How taken: Capsule, liquid

Prescription: Yes

	YES	NO
Generic substitutes		✓
Potentially addicting		✓
May cause drowsiness	✓	
Alcohol discouraged	✓	

Possible drug interactions include: Taking this drug may increase the effects of sedatives, cold medications or antihistamines; taking it may interfere with anti-clotting drugs and some heart medications. This drug taken in combination with monoamine oxidase (MAO) inhibitors (used for depression) may cause serious side effects.

Possible side effects include: Headache, nausea, nervousness, decreased appetite, insomnia and decreased sexual ability.

AMITRIPTYLINE

Brand names: Elavil, Endep

How taken: Tablet, injection

Prescription: Yes

	YES	NO
Generic substitutes	✓	
Potentially addicting		✓
May cause drowsiness	✓	
Alcohol discouraged	✓	

Possible drug interactions include: Taking this drug may increase the effects of sedatives such as diazepam or of blood pressure medications such as clonidine; taking it may increase or decrease the effects of diabetes medications. This drug taken in combination with appetite suppressants, cold medications or antihistamines may result in heart problems; taking it with or within two weeks of taking monoamine oxidase (MAO) inhibitors (used for depression) may cause severe side effects.

Possible side effects include: Headache, nausea, dizziness, dry mouth, constipation, increased appetite and weight gain.

AT A GLANCE

IMIPRAMINE

Brand names: Janimine, Tofranil

How taken: Tablet, injection

Prescription: Yes

	YES	NO
Generic substitutes	✓	
Potentially addicting		✓
May cause drowsiness	✓	
Alcohol discouraged	✓	

Possible drug interactions include: Taking this drug may increase the effects of sedatives such as diazepam or of blood pressure medications such as clonidine; taking it may increase or decrease the effects of diabetes medications. This drug taken in combination with appetite suppressants, cold medications or antihistamines may result in heart problems; taking it with or within two weeks of taking monoamine oxidase (MAO) inhibitors (used for depression) may cause severe side effects.

Possible side effects include: Headache, nausea, dizziness, dry mouth, constipation, increased appetite and weight gain.

CLOMIPRAMINE

Brand name: Anafranil

How taken: Capsule

Prescription: Yes

	YES	NO
Generic substitutes		✓
Potentially addicting		✓
May cause drowsiness	✓	
Alcohol discouraged	✓	

Possible drug interactions include: Taking this drug may increase the effects of sedatives such as diazepam or of blood pressure medications such as clonidine; taking it may increase or decrease the effects of diabetes medications. This drug taken in combination with appetite suppressants, cold medications or antihistamines may result in heart problems; taking it with or within two weeks of taking monoamine oxidase (MAO) inhibitors (used for depression) may cause severe side effects.

Possible side effects include: Headache, nausea, dizziness, dry mouth, constipation and changes in appetite or weight.

seling. Some cases of depression may not be linked to faulty brain chemicals at all. Experts aren't sure just how big a role these chemicals play.

But one thing seems clear. In at least some cases of depression, a single prescription for an antidepressant may be more effective than *years* of couch time, says Dr. Feinberg.

"One of my patients was a woman of about 35 who came to see me feeling very depressed," he says. "She was convinced that she was in imminent danger of losing her job, even though her supervisor told her it wasn't so." The woman had seen several therapists but still felt miserable much of the time. Upon being treated with antidepressant drugs, however, her fears—and her depression—lifted.

AT A GLANCE

DOXEPIN

Brand name: Adapin, Sinequan

How taken: Capsule, liquid

Prescription: Yes

	YES	NO
Generic substitutes	✓	
Potentially addicting		✓
May cause drowsiness	✓	
Alcohol discouraged	✓	

Possible drug interactions include: Taking this drug may increase the effects of sedatives such as diazepam or of blood pressure medications such as clonidine; taking it may increase or decrease the effects of diabetes medications. This drug taken in combination with appetite suppressants, cold medications or antihistamines may result in heart problems; taking it with or within two weeks of taking monoamine oxidase (MAO) inhibitors (used for depression) may cause severe side effects.

Possible side effects include: Headache, nausea, dizziness, dry mouth, constipation, increased appetite and weight gain.

Studies have shown that at least seven out of ten people who are down in the dumps will see their spirits rise after several weeks on antidepressants.

Versatile Remedies

Antidepressants are by no means prescribed only by psychiatrists. In fact, the majority of prescriptions are written by family physicians, sometimes for conditions that affect the body more than the mind.

For example, "antidepressants are useful for chronic pain," says Dr. Pary. In one British study, people with facial pain (including temporomandibular joint disorders, or TMDs) were given a tricyclic antidepressant. After nine weeks, 71 percent were judged to be pain-free.

Doctors have also found that the drug amitriptyline (Elavil, Endep) is effective for treating tension and migraine headaches, low back pain and diabetic neuropathy—painful foot problems that sometimes strike people with diabetes.

While people with long-term pain often are depressed, "it doesn't necessarily mean that the patient has to be depressed to benefit from antidepressants," Dr. Pary says. In other words, the drugs appear to have painkilling abilities apart from their potential to relieve depression. They also have varied potential in other areas.

One drug, imipramine (Janimine, Tofranil), has been used to

reduce involuntary contractions of the bladder that cause nighttime bed-wetting. Drugs such as clomipramine (Anafranil) and doxepin (Adapin, Sinequan) have been used to treat bulimia, peptic ulcer, obsessive-compulsive behavior and many other disorders.

The Right Drug, the Right Dose

With more than a dozen equally effective antidepressants to choose from, how does your doctor decide which one is right for you?

For reasons that aren't always clear, people usually do better with one drug than with another. It may take several weeks or months before your doctor finds the drug—and dose—that's exactly right for you.

Many antidepressants are plagued by side effects, Dr. Feinberg says. These range from a dry mouth to constipation to heart palpitations.

When MAO inhibitor drugs such as phenelzine (Nardil) are combined with foods high in tyramine—a naturally occurring chemical sometimes found in wine, aged cheeses and other foods—they can cause dangerous rises in blood pressure. "One woman was doing fine for years until she got this tasty cheese," remembers Dr. Feinberg. "She said it made her feel like the top of her head was coming off."

Antidepressants often stimulate the appetite, he adds. "For a depressed patient with a depressed appetite, that's initially a plus. But

AT A GLANCE

PHENELZINE

Brand name: Nardil

How taken: Tablet

Prescription: Yes

	YES	NO
Generic substitutes		✓
Potentially addicting		✓
May cause drowsiness	✓	
Alcohol discouraged	✓	

Possible drug interactions include: Taking this drug may increase or decrease the effects of diabetes medications. This drug taken in combination with asthma medications, antihistamines or cold remedies may result in fever, high blood pressure or convulsions; taking it with or within two weeks of other types of antidepressants may cause serious side effects.

Possible side effects include: Headache, dizziness, blurred vision, insomnia, reduced levels of urine and decreased sexual ability.

CAUTION: Because of numerous possible drug interactions, take no other medications, except aspirin or acetaminophen, without talking to your doctor. Also beware of tyramine-containing foods and beverages such as aged cheeses and wines.

later on, it can be a real negative when they go up three sizes."

On the other hand, some side effects can be beneficial. For example, people who have insomnia may be given amitriptyline, which has a sedative effect. Conversely, desipramine can keep people awake.

This can be helpful for someone who often feels lethargic and fatigued.

Anti-diarrheal Drugs

Putting a Stop to Loose Bowels

Did you know that having diarrhea can be good for you? Sure, it feels terrible, but it's often your body's way of flushing out nasty substances. "It's generally best to let diarrhea run for 24 hours to clear out the system," says Edmund Leff, M.D., a colon and rectal specialist with offices in Phoenix and Scottsdale.

Still, diarrhea has a way of coming at the worst times—when you're flying at 30,000 feet, for example, and the "occupied" sign is lit. For short-term relief, anti-diarrheal medications can help stem the tide, putting you—not your bowel—in control.

Intestinal Sponges

When diarrhea is mild, over-the-counter preparations containing kaolin (Parepectolin), psyllium (Perdiem-Fiber) and methyl-cellulose (Citrucel) are often your best bet, doctors say. Taken orally, these ingredients soak up many times their weight in water. This can make the stool firmer and slower to pass.

Another absorbent-type drug is attapulgite (Donnagel, Kaopectate, Rheaban). Taken orally, this over-the-counter powder absorbs bacteria from the gut. Its job is to remove diarrhea-causing organisms before they cause further trouble.

Although the absorbent anti-diarrheal drugs are extremely safe, they aren't without problems, says Dr. Leff. One, they're not going to help you much on that airplane, since they require one to three days to be effective. Two, they sometimes work *too* well and cause constipation. To prevent this, doctors say, be sure to drink plenty of water—at least four to eight (eight-ounce) glasses every day.

NATURAL ALTERNATIVES

Approximately eight million Americans a year travel to countries where modern sanitation is lacking and exotic germs run rampant. A good third of these voyagers will experience that crampy, runny diarrhea that can turn a dream vacation into a holiday from hell.

To prevent such a fate on your next vacation abroad, doctors recommend the following:

Avoid raw foods. Diarrhea-causing organisms flourish on uncooked vegetables and fruits and undercooked meats and shellfish. The high temperatures used in cooking destroy most of these organisms.

Stay away from tap water. Don't even brush your teeth with it. Avoid ice cubes made with it. Instead, stick with bottled water. Carbonated drinks are usually safe.

Avoid street food. Those wonderfully tasty tacos and fajitas are notorious for harboring vast quantities of microscopic troublemakers. When the dinner bell rings, get off the streets and head for an established restaurant.

Turn Off the Switch

When you absolutely, positively have to stop diarrhea cold, nothing works faster than small doses of certain kinds of narcotics, says Lee E. Smith, M.D., director of the Division of Colon and Rectal Surgery at George Washington University in Washington, D.C.

Taken orally, prescription and over-the-counter narcotics such as difenoxin (Motofen), diphenoxylate (Diphenatol, Lomotil, Nor-Mil) and loperamide (Imodium, Imodium A-D) quickly interrupt nerve signals traveling through the bowel or from the brain to the bowel. This helps reduce the frequency of bowel movements as well as the "Emergency! Urgency!"

AT A GLANCE

KAOLIN

Brand name: Parepectolin

How taken: Liquid

Prescription: No

	YES	NO
Generic substitutes	✓	
Potentially addicting		✓
May cause drowsiness		✓
Alcohol discouraged	✓	

Possible drug interactions include: Taking this drug may prevent the absorption of other medications.

Possible side effects include: Constipation.

AT A GLANCE

PSYLLIUM

Brand name: Perdiem-Fiber

How taken: Powder, granules, caramels

Prescription: No

	YES	NO
Generic substitutes	✓	
Potentially addicting		✓
May cause drowsiness		✓
Alcohol discouraged		✓

Possible drug interactions include: Interactions are unlikely.

Possible side effects include: Side effects are unlikely.

DIPHENOXYLATE

Brand names: Diphenatol, Lomanate, Lomotil, Nor-Mil

How taken: Liquid, tablet

Prescription: Yes

	YES	NO
Generic substitutes	✓	
Potentially addicting		✓
May cause drowsiness	✓	
Alcohol discouraged	✓	

Possible drug interactions include: Taking this drug may increase the effects of sedatives and antidepressants. This drug taken in combination with monoamine oxidase (MAO) inhibitors (used for depression) may increase blood pressure.

Possible side effects include: Dizziness and constipation.

CAUTION: May cause dangerous side effects when taken with certain antibiotics.

feelings that precede them.

"If I were to be on a desert island and could only take one nonprescription anti-diarrheal drug with me, I would take Imodium A-D," comments Dr. Leff. But any of the narcotics can be very effective, he says.

As you might expect of narcotics, however, they may cause drowsiness and, when taken in high doses, painful cramping. And because they keep stool inside the intestine for long periods of time, there's also a chance that diarrhea-causing organisms in the gut will have more time to do their dirty work.

Narcotic anti-diarrheals, as a rule, shouldn't be taken for more than two to three days, says Dr. Smith. If the diarrhea continues or is accompanied by fever, vomiting or bloody stools, discontinue use and see your doctor.

Slow the Motion

When diarrhea is accompanied by painful cramping, your doctor may recommend medications called antispasmodics. Prescription drugs like belladonna (Bellergal-S, Donnatal) and dicyclomine (Antispas, Bentyl, Neoquess), usually taken orally, can help ease the pain. They may slow the flow as well.

Like the narcotics, antispasmodics work by interrupting nerve signals traveling through the bowel or from the brain to the bowel. Unfortunately, also like the narcotics, antispasmodics may cause side effects, including headaches, blurred vision and a dry nose, mouth or throat.

In the Pink

Perhaps the best-known anti-diarrheal among travelers is bismuth subsalicylate (Pepto-Bismol). Sold over the counter in

---

AT A GLANCE

LOPERAMIDE

Brand names: Imodium, Imodium A-D

How taken: Capsule, liquid, tablet

Prescription: Sometimes, depending on strength

	YES	NO
Generic substitutes		✓
Potentially addicting		✓
May cause drowsiness	✓	
Alcohol discouraged	✓	

Possible drug interactions include: This drug taken in combination with narcotic pain medications such as codeine may result in severe constipation; taking it with certain antibiotics may worsen diarrhea.

Possible side effects include: Constipation and loss of appetite.

BELLADONNA

Brand names: Bellergal-S, Donnatal

How taken: Liquid, tablet, suppository, capsule

Prescription: Yes

	YES	NO
Generic substitutes		✓
Potentially addicting		✓
May cause drowsiness	✓	
Alcohol discouraged	✓	

Possible drug interactions include: The effects of this drug may decrease if taken with ketaconazole (an anti-fungal drug), some other diarrhea medicines and antacids; the effects may increase if taken with other medicines used for stomach cramps or antidepressants.

Possible side effects include: Constipation, dizziness and dryness of the mouth, nose or throat.

AT A GLANCE

DICYCLOMINE

Brand names: Antispas, Bentyl, Neoquess, Spasmoject

How taken: Capsule, liquid, tablet

Prescription: Yes

	YES	NO
Generic substitutes	✓	
Potentially addicting		✓
May cause drowsiness	✓	
Alcohol discouraged	✓	

Possible drug interactions include: The effects of this drug may decrease if taken with ketoconazole (an antifungal drug), antacids and some diarrhea medicines; the effects may increase if taken with other medicines used for stomach cramps or antidepressants.

Possible side effects include: Constipation, dizziness, blurred vision and dryness of the mouth, nose or throat.

CAUTION: Because this medicine can reduce sweating, beware of exercise, hot weather and saunas. You may be a candidate for heat-stroke.

virtually every country in the world, bismuth subsalicylate works by neutralizing diarrhea-causing poisons created by bacteria in the gut, says Dr. Leff.

Indeed, research shows that travelers who take two tablets of bismuth subsalicylate four times a day often can prevent diarrhea before it occurs.

Unfortunately, bismuth subsalicylate also can turn the tongue and stool black and cause a distracting ringing in the ears called tinnitus. But when you stop taking the drug, the side effects usually subside within a few days.

Antifungal Drugs

Infection Fighters

There is fungus among us. Like bacteria, it's everywhere—in the air, on the ground and in our bodies. "We're exposed to funguses every day and our immune systems usually prevent us from acquiring any kind of significant disease," says Michael A. Amantea, Pharm.D., clinical pharmacist at Millard Fillmore Hospital in Buffalo.

But sometimes a fungus may get

NATURAL ALTERNATIVES

Does *Candida albicans* sound familiar? Even if you don't recognize the name, you may have experienced this itchy, uncomfortable fungus, best known for causing yeast infections.

"Forty percent of women will have yeast infections at some time in their lives, and 70 percent of those will have them numerous times," says Barbara D. Reed, M.D., associate professor of family practice at the University of Michigan in Ann Arbor. Women have tried many things—vinegar douches, wearing cotton underwear, even avoiding sex—to prevent yeast infections. Yet the infections often return. Here's another possibility: dieting.

In a study at the University of Utah, researchers evaluated the eating habits of 166 women who had reported frequent yeast infections. They found that women who consumed the most calories—particularly calories from carbohydrates—were the ones most likely to be afflicted.

"For some patients, diet probably does play a role," says Dr. Reed, who conducted the study. However, she adds, the results are preliminary, and more research still is needed.

AT A GLANCE

CLOTRIMAZOLE

Brand names: Gyne-Lotrimin, Lotrimin, Mycelex Troches

How taken: Cream, vaginal suppository, lozenge

Prescription: Sometimes, depending on strength

	YES	NO
Generic substitutes		✓
Potentially addicting		✓
May cause drowsiness	✓	
Alcohol discouraged	✓	

Possible drug interactions include: Interactions are unlikely.

Possible side effects include: Nausea, vomiting, diarrhea and skin irritation.

NYSTATIN

Brand names: Mycostatin, Nystex

How taken: Tablet, liquid, ointment, vaginal suppository, lozenge, powder

Prescription: Yes

	YES	NO
Generic substitutes	✓	
Potentially addicting		✓
May cause drowsiness		✓
Alcohol discouraged		✓

Possible drug interactions include: Interactions are unlikely.

Possible side effects include: Skin irritation.

the upper hand—especially when you're ill or taking antibiotics. When that happens, Dr. Amantea says, you can get a yeast infection, oral thrush or even a fungal infection of an internal organ.

"If you have a fungal disease that has been identified, it should be treated," says Charles H. Banov, M.D., clinical professor of medicine and microbiology-immunology at the Medical University of South Carolina College of Medicine in Charleston. The treatment, in most cases, is with antifungal drugs.

Common Infections, Uncommon Discomfort

The most common fungal infection is candidiasis, otherwise known as yeast (when it affects the vagina) or oral thrush. In most cases, it's easily treated with creams, lozenges or ointments, Dr. Amantea says.

For example, lozenges containing clotrimazole (Mycelex Troches) or nystatin (Mycostatin, Nystex) often are recommended for oral thrush. By sucking on a lozenge, you put the medication right where the infection is.

Yeast infections, on the other hand, usually are treated with over-the-counter creams and ointments containing miconazole (Monistat I.V., Monistat 7) or clotrimazole (Gyne-Lotrimin, Lotrimin), or with other vaginal creams available by prescription. Applied once a day, they often will eliminate yeast within a week, says Barbara D. Reed, M.D., associate professor of family practice at the University of Michigan in Ann Arbor.

Another common fungal infection is athlete's foot, which often is treated with creams, ointments, powders and sprays. Nonprescription preparations usually contain tolnaftate (Tinactin, Ting), which seems to be effective in approximately 80 percent of cases.

Other antifungal drugs available without prescription include undecylenic acid (Cruex Antifungal Spray, Powder or Cream; Desenex Antifungal Cream, Ointment or Powder) for ringworm and benzoic and salicyclic acids (Whitfield's Ointment) for athlete's foot. Your doctor or pharmacist can tell you which preparation is right for you.

In many cases, however, even mild fungal infections are tough to treat. "It can take a lot of perseverance and a lot of patience to get rid of them," Dr. Amantea says. In fact, the infections don't always go away. Or they go away, then return the minute you stop using the drugs. In either case, your doctor may recommend oral drugs, instead.

Tough Cases

A particularly troublesome infection, called onychomycosis, sometimes afflicts the fingernails and toenails. Unsightly and tough to get rid of, it rarely responds to ointments or creams, says Dr. Amantea. However, it can be treated with an

---

AT A GLANCE

MICONAZOLE

Brand names: Monistat I.V., Monistat 7

How taken: Injection, cream, liquid

Prescription: Sometimes, depending on strength

	YES	NO
Generic substitutes		✓
Potentially addicting		✓
May cause drowsiness		✓
Alcohol discouraged		✓

Possible drug interactions include: Interactions are unlikely.

Possible side effects include: Fever and chills, nausea, diarrhea and skin irritation.

GRISEOFULVIN

Brand names: Fulvicin P/G, Grisactin

How taken: Tablet, capsule, liquid

Prescription: Yes

	YES	NO
Generic substitutes		✓
Potentially addicting		✓
May cause drowsiness	✓	
Alcohol discouraged	✓	

Possible drug interactions include: Taking this drug may decrease the effects of barbiturates, anti-clotting drugs and oral contraceptives containing estrogen.

Possible side effects include: Skin irritation.

CAUTION: Exposure to sunlight while taking this drug may cause skin irritation.

AT A GLANCE

AMPHOTERICIN B
Brand names: Fungizone, Fungizone Intravenous

How taken: Injection, ointment

Prescription: Yes

	YES	NO
Generic substitutes	✓	
Potentially addicting		✓
May cause drowsiness		✓
Alcohol discouraged		✓

Possible drug interactions include: Interactions are unlikely (unless taken with steroids, cancer drugs and other medications).

Possible side effects include: Rash, diarrhea, headache and nausea.

CAUTION: May be dangerous, when taken by injection, in combination with steroids, cancer drugs and other medications.

KETOCONAZOLE
Brand name: Nizoral

How taken: Tablet, cream, liquid, shampoo

Prescription: Yes

	YES	NO
Generic substitutes		✓
Potentially addicting		✓
May cause drowsiness	✓	
Alcohol discouraged	✓	

Possible drug interactions include: The effects of this drug may decrease if taken with drugs such as antacids, antidepressants and ulcer medications. This drug taken in combination with terfenadine (an antihistamine) may result in heart problems.

Possible side effects include: Itching, stinging and skin irritation.

oral drug called griseofulvin (Fulvicin P/G, Grisactin). While effective, griseofulvin often must be given for several months. It causes headache in up to 15 percent of cases. It sometimes causes nausea and diarrhea as well.

A newer prescription drug, terbinafine, may be just as effective as griseofulvin while causing fewer side effects. In one British study, 82 percent of people with onychomycosis treated with terbinafine stayed clear of the fungus for at least nine months without recurrence.

Terbinafine works for athlete's foot as well. At Yale University School of Medicine, people were treated either with griseofulvin or terbinafine. Six to 15 months later, 94 percent of those treated with terbinafine were cured, compared with only 30 percent in the griseofulvin group.

Internal Affairs

While many fungal diseases are skin deep, they also can be systemic, meaning they affect the whole body. An example of this is a disease called histoplasmosis. It can cause fever, headache and other flulike symptoms. And, much more serious, a fungus such as Candida can travel through the body and attach itself to internal organs. The resulting infection can be deadly, Dr. Banov says.

For systemic fungal infections, the treatment of choice often is amphotericin B (Fungizone, Fungizone Intravenous). Given by injection, this drug destroys fungal invaders. At the same time, however, it also can cause fever, chills and, in rare cases, even kidney damage.

A safer drug is the tablet or liquid ketoconazole (Nizoral), which is prescribed both for internal and external infections, says Dr. Amantea. Another potent fungus fighter is fluconazole, available only through prescription.

Though very effective, these drugs are too potent for everyday use, adds Dr. Banov. "You always want to try topical drugs before using the systemic ones."

Anti-gas Drugs

Guardians against Social Embarrassment

Perhaps you glare at your neighbors or pointedly stare at the dog asleep in the corner. Or maybe you passively feign innocence while those around you clamp their noses.

There are dozens of ways of dealing with flatulence, but total prevention isn't among them. Indeed, researchers say, the average person passes gas—actually, a combination of gases, including nitrogen, hydrogen and carbon dioxide—approximately 13 times a day.

Some gas undoubtedly is caused by digestive problems. More often, it occurs as bacteria in the gut feed on the nonabsorbable portions of beans, broccoli and other

Contrary to popular belief, carbonated beverages do not play a big role in causing gas, says Michael D. Levitt, M.D., associate chief of staff for research at the Veterans Affairs Medical Center in Minneapolis. The foods you eat, however, can play a big role. To keep flatulence to a minimum:

Beware of beans. Yes, they're nutritious and filled with fiber, but beans eaten in excess can have untoward consequences. Don't give them up, just don't eat more than you can handle.

Soak them overnight. One study has found that beans soaked in water before cooking lose as much as 90 percent of their gas-producing power.

Go slow. If you're increasing your intake of high-fiber foods such as oat bran and apples, do so gradually. Give your body time to adjust.

Arrest the cow. As many as 70 percent of adults have trouble digesting the sugar, called lactose, in milk and other dairy foods. If you suspect milk and cheese are helping to fill your gas tank, try eating less—or doing without—to see if your problems go away.

AT A GLANCE

SIMETHICONE

Brand names: Gas-X, Mylanta Gas

How taken: Liquid, tablet

Prescription: Sometimes, depending on strength

	YES	NO
Generic substitutes	✓	
Potentially addicting		✓
May cause drowsiness		✓
Alcohol discouraged		✓

Possible drug interactions include: Interactions are unlikely.

Possible side effects include: Side effects are unlikely.

gas-producing foods, says Michael D. Levitt, M.D., associate chief of staff for research at the Veterans Affairs Medical Center and a professor of medicine at the University of Minnesota Medical School in Minneapolis.

Even though you can't entirely prevent flatulence, there are medications that you can take to help prevent it from becoming a serious (or seriously embarrassing) problem.

Bubble Breakers

An ingredient found in many over-the-counter anti-gas preparations is simethicone (Gas-X, Mylanta Gas, Phazyme 95). Taken orally, simethicone breaks up gas bubbles in the large intestine.

The Food and Drug Administration has recognized simethicone as being safe and effective, but many doctors aren't convinced it works. "I don't recommend it," says Dr. Levitt.

If simethicone doesn't work for you, perhaps you'll have better luck with charcoal. Not the briquettes in your outdoor grill, but activated charcoal (Actidose-Aqua, Charcocaps). Made from pure carbon, activated charcoal has been chemically treated—activated—to soak up gas. Charcoal works by trapping gases before they escape from the intestine.

Like simethicone, activated charcoal is extremely safe. It may, however, turn your stools black. And because it absorbs small particles from the intestine, it shouldn't be taken within two hours of taking other medications. Some brands of activated charcoal contain sorbitol, a sweetener. Experts say you should choose a brand *without* sorbitol, because the sweetener has been known to worsen some people's gas problems.

Digestive Aids

Intestinal gas is most often caused, remember, by bacteria feeding on particles in your large intestine. One way to interrupt this feeding process—and its odoriferous consequences—is to take special digestive enzymes that

AT A GLANCE

ACTIVATED CHARCOAL

Brand names: Actidose-Aqua, Charcocaps

How taken: Capsule, liquid

Prescription: No

	YES	NO
Generic substitutes	✓	
Potentially addicting		✓
May cause drowsiness		✓
Alcohol discouraged	✓	

Possible drug interactions include: Interactions are unlikely.

Possible side effects include: Side effects are unlikely.

ALPHA-GALACTOSIDASE

Brand name: Beano

How taken: Drops

Prescription: No

	YES	NO
Generic substitutes		✓
Potentially addicting		✓
May cause drowsiness		✓
Alcohol discouraged		✓

Possible drug interactions include: Interactions are unlikely.

Possible side effects include: Side effects are unlikely.

CAUTION: People who are galactosemic (cannot digest galactose) should not use this product.

beat bacteria to the banquet.

There are several enzymes to choose from. One over-the-counter product contains the enzyme alpha-galactosidase (Beano). Taken orally with meals, it helps break down indigestible sugars in the gut, reducing the gas caused by foods such as beans, broccoli and cauliflower.

Another digestive enzyme is lactase. Your body normally produces lactase to digest lact*ose*, a sugar found in milk and other dairy products. People who don't produce enough lactase may experience gas, cramps, diarrhea and other symptoms when they ingest lactose. Lactase supplements (Dairy Ease, Lactaid), sold over the counter and by prescription, can be a big help.

AT A GLANCE

LACTASE

Brand names: Dairy Ease, Lactaid

How taken: Liquid, capsule, tablet

Prescription: Usually nonprescription

	YES	NO
Generic substitutes	✓	
Potentially addicting		✓
May cause drowsiness		✓
Alcohol discouraged		✓

Possible drug interactions include: Interactions are unlikely.

Possible side effects include: Side effects are unlikely.

Antihistamines

Relief for Runny Noses—And More

Doctors estimate that approximately 41 million Americans wheeze, sniffle and honk their way through allergy season every year. So it's not surprising that antihistamines are among the most widely used drugs on the market.

In fact, these versatile drugs—there are more than 100 prescription and over-the-counter antihistamine products on the market today—are used not only to relieve hay fever but to ease itching, nausea and insomnia as well. What's more, they're exceptionally safe. "Most physicians tend to recommend antihistamines when there's any conceivable chance they might help," says Richard L. Mabry, M.D., a clinical professor of otolaryngology–head and neck surgery at the University of Texas Southwestern Medical Center at Dallas.

Chemical Interference

As the name suggests, antihistamines work by blocking a chemical in the body called histamine. Normally, histamine helps control a number of bodily functions, such as the contraction and expansion of muscles and blood vessels. But when histamine is released in large quantities—which may occur when you come into contact with pollen, poison ivy or other allergens—it can cause hives, itches and runny noses.

Antihistamines help control histamine's troublesome effects. At the same time, they may depress the central nervous system. This is what makes some antihistamines useful for preventing insomnia and motion sickness as well as allergic reactions.

There are a half-dozen chemical categories of antihistamines, including chlorpheniramine, dimenhydrinate (Calm X, Dimetabs, Dramamine) and dexchlorpheniramine (Dexchlor, Polaramine). In order to keep things simple, doctors typically divide them into two groups: classical and non-sedating.

NATURAL ALTERNATIVES

The best way to beat allergies, doctors agree, is to stay away from whatever it is that's causing them. Here's how.

Research your problem. If you start sneezing when the summer wind blows, your problem may be pollen. Or perhaps you're allergic to your cat or to the dust and mold in your basement. The sooner you discover what's making you sick, the sooner you can take steps to avoid it. If you need help doing the detective work, hire an allergist.

Spend the A.M. inside. Airborne pollen typically takes flight between 5:00 and 10:00 A.M. To avoid the fallout, consider staying indoors during this morning bombardment.

Plug in the dehumidifier. Dust mites, tiny relatives of ticks and a common source of allergic woes, thrive in warm, humid environments. By making the air drier, you'll force the little culprits to seek moister climes.

Keep cool. Air-conditioning helps filter pollens and other allergens from incoming air, whether at home or in the car.

DIPHENHYDRAMINE

Brand names: Aller-med, Benadryl, Nordryl

How taken: Capsule, liquid, tablet

Prescription: Sometimes, depending on strength

	YES	NO
Generic substitutes	✓	
Potentially addicting		✓
May cause drowsiness	✓	
Alcohol discouraged	✓	

Possible drug interactions include: Taking this drug may increase the effects of sedatives and some painkillers.

Possible side effects include: Dry nose, mouth and throat.

CAUTION: Do not take if you have bronchitis, pneumonia or active bronchial asthma.

HYDROXYZINE

Brand names: Atarax, Vistaril

How taken: Capsule, liquid, tablet

Prescription: Sometimes, depending on strength

	YES	NO
Generic substitutes	✓	
Potentially addicting		✓
May cause drowsiness	✓	
Alcohol discouraged	✓	

Possible drug interactions include: Taking this drug may increase the effects of sedatives and some painkillers.

Possible side effects include: Dry nose, mouth and throat.

Classical Relief

The classical antihistamines have been in use since the 1940s, and some of these old timers still are the drugs of choice for relieving hay fever, insomnia and motion sickness, says Dr. Mabry.

These drugs work in similar ways, he says, although they aren't quite interchangeable. Suppose, for example, you got into poison ivy, and your legs are so itchy that you can't stop scratching or get to sleep. Drugs such as diphenhydramine (Aller-med, Benadryl, Nordryl) or hydroxyzine (Atarax, Vistaril), usually taken orally, help in two ways: by relieving itching and making you sleepy, Dr. Mabry says.

On the other hand, the camp director with an attack of hay fever can't afford to be sleepy—not when she's responsible for hundreds of rambunctious youngsters. For her, an antihistamine like chlorpheniramine (Chlor-Trimeton Allergy Tablets, Coricidin Tablets, Triaminic Allergy Tablets) can ease the sniffles without making her groggy.

Regardless of which antihistamine you choose, they all work best when taken before you need them, adds Dr. Mabry. So if boats make you queasy, cats make you itchy and July makes you sniffly, don't wait until you're already miserable, he advises. Take your medication half an hour to an hour before you think you'll need it.

Although most people take antihistamines orally, the drugs are commonly used as ingredients in creams and sprays as well. These should be avoided, many doctors say. "Not enough is absorbed to do much good, but enough is absorbed for you to become sensitive," warns Dr. Mabry. In other words, the medicine itself may cause problems.

Though classical antihistamines are both safe and effective, they aren't without problems. For one thing, they often become less effective over time. More significant are the side effects, which include drowsiness, a dry nose and mouth and, for some older men, difficulty urinating. If side effects are a problem for you, your doctor may recommend non-sedating antihistamines instead.

Non-sedating Breakthroughs

There are three non-sedating antihistamines on the market today: astemizole (Hismanal), loratadine (Claritin) and terfenadine (Seldane, Seldane-D). Available by prescription and taken orally, these drugs help relieve most allergic symptoms while causing virtually no side effects, says Eli O. Meltzer, M.D., clinical professor of pediatrics in the Division of Allergy and Immunology at the University of California, San Diego.

"They developed larger antihistamine molecules so they are unable to get into the central nervous system and cause drowsiness," Dr.

AT A GLANCE

ASTEMIZOLE
Brand name: Hismanal
How taken: Tablet
Prescription: Yes

	Yes	No
Generic substitutes		✓
Potentially addicting		✓
May cause drowsiness	✓	
Alcohol discouraged	✓	

Possible drug interactions include: Taking this drug may increase the effects of sedatives and some painkillers, antibiotics and antifungal drugs.

Possible side effects include: Side effects are unlikely.

TERFENADINE
Brand names: Seldane, Seldane-D
How taken: Tablet
Prescription: Yes

	Yes	No
Generic substitutes		✓
Potentially addicting		✓
May cause drowsiness		✓
Alcohol discouraged		✓

Possible drug interactions include: This drug taken in combination with certain antibiotics such as erythromycin or ketoconazole (an antifungal drug) may result in heart irregularities.

Possible side effects include: Side effects are unlikely.

AT A GLANCE

DIMENHYDRINATE

Brand names: Calm X, Dimetabs, Dramamine

How taken: Capsule, injection, liquid

Prescription: Sometimes, depending on strength

	YES	NO
Generic substitutes	✓	
Potentially addicting		✓
May cause drowsiness	✓	
Alcohol discouraged	✓	

Possible drug interactions include: Taking this drug may increase the effects of sedatives and some painkillers.

Possible side effects include: Dryness of nose, mouth and throat.

DEXCHLORPHENIRAMINE

Brand names: Dexchlor, Polaramine

How taken: Liquid, tablet

Prescription: Yes

	YES	NO
Generic substitutes	✓	
Potentially addicting		✓
May cause drowsiness	✓	
Alcohol discouraged	✓	

Possible drug interactions include: Taking this drug may increase the effects of sedatives and some painkillers. This drug taken in combination with monoamine oxidase (MAO) inhibitors (used for depression) may result in low blood pressure.

Possible side effects include: Dry nose, mouth and throat.

Meltzer explains. This can be particularly important for people such as schoolteachers or police officers, who can't afford to be drowsy just because it's hay fever season.

Despite the advantages of non-sedating antihistamines, they do have limitations, says Dr. Meltzer. The onset of their action is not immediate. They require several hours in your system before they provide any benefit. In addition, because they have little effect on the brain, non-sedating antihistamines aren't helpful for conditions like insomnia and motion sickness. They also can be dangerous when taken in combination with medications such as quinidine (a heart rhythm drug), ketoconazole (an antifungal drug) or erythromycin (an antibiotic). Be sure to tell your doctor if you're taking these or other medications.

Anti-inflammatory Drugs

Aspirin and Its Many Cousins

I had a *swell* time," you exclaim to the hostess. "What a *swell* guy!" you tell your best friend. "It was a *swell* trip," you say to your sister.

"Swell" means things are wonderful, fabulous, A-okay. But when "swell" becomes "swelling"—as in painful inflammation—life doesn't seem so swell anymore. Inflammation can be more than painful. Left untreated for long periods of time, certain kinds of inflammation can cause serious problems like joint damage. That's why doctors sometimes prescribe powerful anti-inflammatory drugs. But for some people, as simple a remedy as aspirin will sometimes make swollen joints and tissues . . . er, swell once again.

An Over-the-Counter Workhorse

For hundreds of years, aspirin's active ingredient, salicin, was extracted from the bark of willow trees and used to treat pain, fever and swelling. Aspirin in its present form has been around nearly a century, and Americans today consume over 10,000 *tons* a year.

Aspirin works, at least in part, by blocking the production of chemicals in your body called prostaglandins, which are responsible for causing pain and swelling.

For minor inflammation, one to two aspirin (Alka-Seltzer Plus, Anacin, Genuine Bayer Aspirin) four times a day may work wonders. Aspirin works quickly, sometimes reducing swelling in just a few hours, says Leroy C. Knodel, Pharm.D., director of the Drug Information Service and an associate professor of pharmacology at the University of Texas Health Science Center at San Antonio. As far as aspirin's effectiveness, it doesn't matter which brand you buy, he adds. They all do the same job.

When it comes to preventing aspirin's sometimes troubling gastric side effects, however, you might wish to shop around. For example, if aspirin irritates your stomach,

NATURAL ALTERNATIVES

You twisted your ankle and now it's swelling like a water balloon. You've already taken an aspirin. What next?

For quick relief, bring on the rice. Make that RICE, which stands for rest, ice, compression and elevation. This procedure, utilized soon after injuries, can help decrease swelling, relieve pain and hasten healing, says Lourdes C. Corman, M.D., a rheumatologist and associate professor of medicine at the University of Florida College of Medicine in Gainesville.

Resting the injured part is just common sense, says Dr. Corman. Whether you've twisted an ankle or hurt your back, the best thing you can do is put it—and the rest of you—to bed for a few hours.

While you're resting, put ice on the swelling for up to 20 minutes, several times a day. (If you don't have a cold pack in the freezer, use ice cubes wrapped in a washcloth or dish towel.) "With ice, you get less blood flow to the area, which reduces swelling," says Dr. Corman. Ice also may slow the action of inflammation-causing enzymes.

Compression means wrapping the injury—gently, never too tightly—with an elastic bandage. This helps push fluids out while preventing more fluids from flooding in, says Dr. Corman.

Elevation means raising the injured area, which further helps accumulated fluids drain.

Once the swelling goes down, try to get moving again. Nothing vigorous, just some gentle stretches at first. "Once the inflammation has cooled off, what you want is *more* blood flow to help improve the chances for the tissue to recover," Dr. Corman says.

you might be better off with a buffered variety (Bufferin, Magnaprin). These are mixed with ingredients such as magnesium oxide and calcium carbonate, which help protect the stomach from aspirin's harsh effects.

Perhaps even easier on the stomach is enteric-coated, or delayed-release, aspirin (Bayer Enteric Aspirin, Norwich Enteric Safety Coated Aspirin). It dissolves in the small intestine instead of the stomach, thereby causing less irritation. Taking aspirin with meals can further reduce stomach upset, says Dr. Knodel.

Because any kind of aspirin, taken regularly, can cause ulcers, bleeding and other problems, you should check with your doctor before making aspirin a daily habit, says Lourdes C. Corman, M.D., a rheumatologist and associate professor of medicine at the University of Florida College of Medicine in Gainesville.

Also, unless recommended by a doctor, a child or teenager shouldn't take aspirin because of the risk of Reye's syndrome, a dangerous neurological condition. Instead, they can take acetaminophen (Tylenol), an aspirin substitute. It has only mild anti-inflammatory effects, but it can relieve much discomfort, says Dr. Corman.

Alternatives to Aspirin

Aspirin is the oldest member of a class of drugs called NSAIDs, or nonsteroidal anti-inflammatory drugs. When aspirin doesn't relieve inflammation (or it causes uncomfortable side

---

AT A GLANCE

ASPIRIN

Brand names: Alka-Seltzer Plus, Anacin, Genuine Bayer Aspirin, Ecotrin, Empirin

How taken: Tablet, capsule, chewing gum, suppository

Prescription: No

	YES	NO
Generic substitutes	✓	
Potentially addicting		✓
May cause drowsiness		✓
Alcohol discouraged	✓	

Possible drug interactions include: Taking this drug may increase the effects of anti-clotting drugs, methotrexate (used for psoriasis, cancer and rheumatoid arthritis), valproic acid (an anti-seizure drug) and oral diabetes drugs.

Possible side effects include: Indigestion, stomach irritation and nausea.

IBUPROFEN

Brand names: Advil, Genpril, Medipren, Motrin IB, Nuprin

How taken: Tablet, liquid

Prescription: Sometimes, depending on strength

	YES	NO
Generic substitutes	✓	
Potentially addicting		✓
May cause drowsiness	✓	
Alcohol discouraged		✓

Possible drug interactions include: Taking this drug may increase the effects of anti-clotting drugs.

Possible side effects include: Fluid retention (weight gain) and discoloration of urine.

CAUTION: Do not take if you are allergic to aspirin.

AT A GLANCE

INDOMETHACIN

Brand names: Indameth, Indocin

How taken: Capsule, liquid, suppository

Prescription: Yes

	YES	NO
Generic substitutes	✓	
Potentially addicting		✓
May cause drowsiness	✓	
Alcohol discouraged		✓

Possible drug interactions include: Taking this drug may increase the effects of anti-clotting drugs and lithium (used for manic depression).

Possible side effects include: Ringing in the ears and fluid retention.

NAPROXEN

Brand names: Anaprox, Naprosyn, Aleve

How taken: Tablet, liquid

Prescription: Sometimes, depending on strength

	YES	NO
Generic substitutes		✓
Potentially addicting		✓
May cause drowsiness		✓
Alcohol discouraged	✓	

Possible drug interactions include: Taking this drug may increase the effects of anti-clotting drugs.

Possible side effects include: Fluid retention.

fects), you might want to try another NSAID instead.

One over-the-counter NSAID is ibuprofen (Advil, Motrin IB, Nuprin). This potent inflammation fighter, usually taken as a tablet, works at least as well as aspirin, usually with fewer side effects.

A newer nonprescription NSAID is naproxen (Aleve), which also comes most often in tablet form. Its effects are longer lasting than those of aspirin or ibuprofen, so you don't have to take it as often.

When over-the-counter NSAIDs don't work, your doctor may recommend prescription drugs instead. For example, people who have spondylitis (inflammation of the back vertebrae) may be given indomethacin (Indameth, Indocin) to help quell the swelling. "Once I had a terrible back pain that lasted for several months," says a former construction worker. "Then I started taking indomethacin. A day later the pain was gone—100 percent."

Other prescription NSAIDs include naproxen (Anaprox, Naprosyn), nabumetone (Relafen), diclofenac (Votaren), piroxicam (Feldene) and oxaprozin (Daypro), each of which may be used for all types of swelling, according to Dr. Corman.

All of the NSAIDs are effective, although some people will improve more with one drug than another, says Dr. Knodel. This means that you may have to try several NSAIDs before you find the one that's right for you.

AT A GLANCE

CORTISONE

Brand name: Cortone

How taken: Injection, tablet

Prescription: Yes

	YES	NO
Generic substitutes	✓	
Potentially addicting		✓
May cause drowsiness		✓
Alcohol discouraged		✓

Possible drug interactions include: Taking this drug may decrease the effects of diabetes drugs.

Possible side effects include: Lowered resistance to infection, weight gain, indigestion, mood changes, insomnia and increased appetite.

CAUTION: May be dangerous when taken with vaccines.

DEXAMETHASONE

Brand names: AK-Dex, Dexasone, Hexadrol

How taken: Tablet, liquid, injection

Prescription: Yes

	YES	NO
Generic substitutes	✓	
Potentially addicting	✓	
May cause drowsiness		✓
Alcohol discouraged	✓	

Possible drug interactions include: Taking this drug may increase or decrease the effects of anti-clotting drugs.

Possible side effects include: Weight gain, mood changes, increased appetite, indigestion, insomnia, retention of salt and water and lowered resistance to infection.

CAUTION: Discontinue this medication 72 hours before vaccination and do not resume it for at least 14 days afterward.

The Top Guns

For heavy-duty inflammation, drugs called corticosteroids—steroids for short—can't be beat. These drugs, which are available in many forms, start to work within minutes but, depending on the degree of inflammation, the benefits may not be apparent for up to 24 hours. These drugs are potent enough to subdue virtually all types of swelling, says Dr. Knodel.

Don't confuse anti-inflammatory steroids with *anabolic* steroids, those muscle-building drugs that are sometimes abused by athletes and bodybuilders. Instead, anti-inflammatory steroids such as prednisone (Deltasone), cortisone (Cortone) and dexamethasone (Ak-Dex, Dexasone, Hexadrol) work by blocking the body's production of inflammation-causing prostaglandins, thus reducing swelling.

How effective are steroids? In one study, people suffering from an inflammation in their "trigger" fingers were given a series of injections of triamcinolone (Aristospan-40, Kenalog). Researchers found that the steroid injections worked as well as surgery, with fewer complications.

Steroids can be used for the inflammation that often accompanies asthma, too. In one study, people were treated either with terbutaline, a standard asthma drug, or with budesonide, a type of prescription steroid that they took through an inhaler. Researchers found that those who used budesonide breathed easier than those using terbutaline.

The problem with steroids, particularly those taken orally, is side effects. When taken in large doses for long periods of time (more than a week), they may cause suppressed immune function, poor wound healing, increased susceptibility to infection, acne, mood changes, osteoporosis or high blood pressure. "Steroids do require careful supervision," Dr. Knodel says.

Anti-itch Drugs

Soothing the Scratchies

Go up the middle . . . a little to the left . . . now up . . . over . . . ahhh!

Few things feel better than scratching—and relieving—an irritating itch. But some itches won't go away no matter how much you scratch. The result can be miserable days, sleepless nights and sometimes infected skin.

Prolonged itching doesn't just happen. It could be a sign that you have dry skin. Or perhaps you strayed past a mosquito swarm or through a poison ivy patch. It even could indicate more serious problems, such as eczema or, in rare cases, diabetes.

"The best thing for an itch is to treat the underlying problem," says Debra L. Breneman, M.D., associate professor of dermatology at the University of Cincinnati. The next best thing is to treat the symptoms. There are many anti-itch drugs—some treat the underlying

NATURAL ALTERNATIVES

It's Sunday night, the pharmacy is closed and the kids apparently tiptoed through poison ivy earlier in the day. Now they're crying like sirens. What do you do?

Relax, says Charles H. Banov, M.D., clinical professor of medicine and microbiology-immunology at the Medical University of South Carolina College of Medicine in Charleston. Quick relief may be just a cool bath away. "Put the kids in cool baths, or put cool compresses on," he says. "I find these soaks to be of benefit. They tend to have soothing qualities." Adding baking soda to the bathwater also can relieve minor skin irritation, says Dr. Banov.

In the morning you can pick up stronger help from your doctor or pharmacist.

---

problem, others focus only on that miserable itch. Let's take a look at both kinds.

Spread-on Relief

The skin is the largest organ of the body. It's an easy target for mosquitoes, thorns, poison ivy and other itch-causing rascals.

Regardless of the culprit, non-prescription medicated creams may be all you need. At Pennsylvania's Camp Echo Ridge, for example, Girl Scouts regularly have close encounters with insects and poison ivy, says camp director Alison Fulmer. "When they get into poison ivy, we use calamine lotion. Of course," she adds, "the girls complain because it makes their legs pink."

Regardless of its unfashionable staining, calamine lotion's cooling, soothing ability makes it useful for controlling minor itching.

Some drug manufacturers mix calamine with other anti-itch ingredients. One example is Caladryl, a mixture of calamine and a topical antihistamine. Exercise caution, however, whenever you use an antihistamine lotion. Unlike antihistamine tablets, topical antihistamines can sometimes make itching worse. Should this happen to you, discontinue use.

For minor itchy rashes, such as mild poison ivy, many doctors prefer over-the-counter creams containing hydrocortisone (Bactine Brand Hydrocortisone Anti-Itch Cream, Cortaid, Cortizone-10). Absorbed by the skin, these drugs quell inflammation in a number of ways.

For more serious problems—for example, extensive poison ivy or a bad case of eczema—your doctor may prescribe a potent

AT A GLANCE

HYDROCORTISONE

Brand names: Bactine Brand Hydrocortisone Anti-Itch Cream, Caldecort, Cortaid, Cortizone-10, Lanacort 10

How taken: Cream, lotion, ointment, solution, spray

Prescription: Sometimes, depending on strength

	YES	NO
Generic substitutes	✓	
Potentially addicting		✓
May cause drowsiness		✓
Alcohol discouraged		✓

Possible drug interactions include: Interactions are unlikely.

Possible side effects include: Mild stinging when applied.

AZATADINE

Brand names: Optimine, Trinalin

How taken: Tablet

Prescription: Yes

	YES	NO
Generic substitutes		✓
Potentially addicting		✓
May cause drowsiness	✓	
Alcohol discouraged	✓	

Possible drug interactions include: Taking this drug may increase the effects of anticholinergics (used for stomach cramps), sedatives, painkillers and muscle relaxants.

Possible side effects include: Dryness of the mouth, nose, throat or vagina.

steroid cream containing triamcinolone (Aristocort A, Kenalog, Mytrex) or betamethasone (Betatrex, Celestone, Selestoject). These are very effective for easing itching and inflammation, Dr. Breneman says.

However, when steroids are used for long-term relief, they may cause rashes, thinning of the skin and other problems. So talk with your doctor about the relative pros and cons of using these potent drugs for any length of time.

Also effective against most itching are over-the-counter topical anesthetics containing benzocaine (Anbesol, Dermoplast, Lanacane) or lidocaine (Mycitracin Plus Pain Reliever, Neosporin Plus, Xylocaine). Available in creams, ointments and sprays, anesthetics numb nerve endings in the skin, thus stopping the itch. The problem with topical anesthetics is that some people become sensitive and can't use them again, warns Charles H. Banov, M.D., clinical professor of medicine and microbiology-immunology at the Medical University of South Carolina College of Medicine in Charleston. "Then when you need them for something more serious, they won't work."

Moisture Solutions

For many people, itching merely means dry skin, says Dr. Breneman. This is particularly true during the winter months, when the one-two punch of cold outside air and central heating robs your skin of protective moisture.

A moisturizer may be all you need to scratch the itch. You can put moisture back where it belongs with a variety of over-the-counter creams. Some contain lactic acid (LactiCare Lotion) or urea (Aqua Care Lotion, Carmol 10, Eucerin Plus), says Dr. Breneman. Other helpful emollients contain camphor and menthol. For best results, apply them soon after bathing, then three to four times a day as needed, says Dr. Banov. He adds,

however, "If the itching is getting out of hand, then go to the doctor."

Working from Within

For itching from allergies or skin sensitivities, you may find relief with antihistamine tablets, creams or liquids. Drugs such as azatadine (Optimine, Trinalin) and diphenhydramine (Benadryl, Benylin, Caladryl) help block "itch" messages from traveling from your skin to the brain. The oral types also cause drowsiness, which further reduces itching, Dr. Banov says.

AT A GLANCE

BENZOCAINE

Brand names: Anbesol, BiCozene, Dermoplast, Lanacane, Orajel

How taken: Cream, gel, ointment, spray

Prescription: No

	YES	NO
Generic substitutes	✓	
Potentially addicting		✓
May cause drowsiness		✓
Alcohol discouraged		✓

Possible drug interactions include: Taking this drug may increase the effects of anticholinergics (used for stomach cramps).

Possible side effects include: Redness, rash and swelling at application site.

LIDOCAINE

Brand names: Mycitracin Plus Pain Reliever, Neosporin Plus, Xylocaine

How taken: Ointment

Prescription: Sometimes, depending on strength

	YES	NO
Generic substitutes	✓	
Potentially addicting		✓
May cause drowsiness		✓
Alcohol discouraged		✓

Possible drug interactions include: Taking this drug may increase the effects of anticholinergics (used for stomach cramps).

Possible side effects include: Anxiety and restlessness.

AT A GLANCE

DIPHENHYDRAMINE

Brand names: Benadryl, Benylin, Caladryl

How taken: Capsule, tablet, cream, liquid

Prescription: Sometimes, depending on strength

	YES	NO
Generic substitutes	✓	
Potentially addicting		✓
May cause drowsiness	✓	
Alcohol discouraged	✓	

Possible drug interactions include: Taking this drug may increase the effects of anticholinergics (used for stomach cramps).

Possible side effects include: Dryness of the mouth, nose, throat or vagina.

CAUTION: Do not take if you have bronchitis, pneumonia or active bronchial asthma.

TERFENADINE

Brand name: Seldane

How taken: Tablet

Prescription: Yes

	YES	NO
Generic substitutes		✓
Potentially addicting		✓
May cause drowsiness		✓
Alcohol discouraged		✓

Possible drug interactions include: This drug taken in combination with erythromycin (an antibiotic) or keto-conazole (an antifungal drug) may result in heart problems.

Possible side effects include: Loss of appetite, blurred vision and dryness of the mouth, nose, throat or vagina.

Some people, however, can't take antihistamines because they make them feel *too* drowsy. If this is the case with you, ask your doctor about "non-sedating" antihistamines. Prescription drugs such as terfenadine (Seldane) and astemizole (Hismanal) don't make you dopey the way older antihistamines do. Unfortunately, says Dr. Banov, these newer antihistamines may be less effective as well.

Anti-psychotic Drugs

Gateways to the World of Reality

For people with mental illness, the world can seem a very frightening place. They may see people who aren't there . . . hear voices no one else can hear . . . believe things that can't possibly be true.

In the past, people with serious mental illnesses such as paranoia and schizophrenia often were locked away in institutions, says Robert D. Kerns, Ph.D., chief of the psychology service at the West Haven Veterans Administration Medical Center in Connecticut and associate professor of psychiatry at Yale University. Today, these people can sometimes lead fairly normal lives with the help of anti-psychotic drugs. These medications don't cure mental illness, but they can relieve some of the terrible—and terrifying—symptoms.

Mental Rescue

With some types of mental illness, or psychosis, receptors in the brain take in too much dopamine, a chemical that carries messages from cell to cell. Anti-psychotic medications, by blocking the access of dopamine to these receptors, frequently can eliminate delusions, hallucinations and other symptoms of mental illness, says Steven C. Dilsaver, M.D., professor of psychiatry and behavioral sciences at the University of Texas Medical School at Houston.

Not everyone with mental illness needs drugs, he adds. "But if someone has had two or three nasty episodes of psychosis in five years, then treatment with medication might be acceptable."

The oldest of the anti-psychotic medications is a prescription drug called chlorpromazine (Ormazine, Thoradol, Thorazine). First used to treat mental illness in the early 1950s, this drug, taken orally, rectally or by injection, remains the drug of choice for many types of psychosis, says Dr. Dilsaver. Similar drugs are perphenazine (Trilafon) and trifluoperazine (Stelazine, Suprazine). Another prescription anti-psychotic is haloperidol (Haldol, Haloperon). Taken orally or by injection, it's more potent than chlorpromazine. This means it can be taken in lower doses, which often can reduce the sometimes-severe side effects of the drug.

Most recently, a novel anti-psychotic drug called clozapine (Clorazil), taken orally, has been shown to be effective in even the toughest cases of mental illness, says Dr. Kerns.

Regardless of which drug is used, symptoms aren't relieved all at once. Imaginary voices, for example, may be silenced within a week. Irrational thoughts, on the other hand—"I know they're trying to poison me"—may take longer to eliminate.

This is why doctors often prescribe sedatives to be taken along with anti-psychotic drugs during the first weeks of treatment. Then, when the anti-psychotic medications are fully effective, the sedatives can be discontinued.

AT A GLANCE

CHLORPROMAZINE

Brand names: Ormazine, Thoradol, Thorazine

How taken: Capsule, injection, liquid, tablet, suppository, syrup

Prescription: Yes

	YES	NO
Generic substitutes	✓	
Potentially addicting		✓
May cause drowsiness	✓	
Alcohol discouraged	✓	

Possible drug interactions include: Taking this drug may increase the effects of sedatives and atropine-like drugs (used for asthma); taking it may decrease the effects of guanethidine (a blood pressure drug).

Possible side effects include: Dizziness, blurred vision, shaking and other Parkinson's-like symptoms.

PERPHENAZINE

Brand name: Trilafon

How taken: Tablet, liquid, injection

Prescription: Yes

	YES	NO
Generic substitutes	✓	
Potentially addicting		✓
May cause drowsiness	✓	
Alcohol discouraged	✓	

Possible drug interactions include: Taking this drug may increase the effects of sedatives and atropine-like drugs (used for asthma); taking it may decrease the effects of guanethidine (a blood pressure drug).

Possible side effects include: Dizziness, blurred vision, dry mouth, shaking and other Parkinson's-like symptoms.

AT A GLANCE

TRIFLUOPERAZINE

Brand names: Stelazine, Suprazine

How taken: Injection, liquid, tablet

Prescription: Yes

	YES	NO
Generic substitutes	✓	
Potentially addicting		✓
May cause drowsiness	✓	
Alcohol discouraged	✓	

Possible drug interactions include: Taking this drug may increase the effects of sedatives and atropine-like drugs (used for asthma); taking it may decrease the effects of guanethidine (a blood pressure drug) and lithium (used for manic depression).

Possible side effects include: Dizziness, blurred vision and rash.

HALOPERIDOL

Brand names: Haldol, Haloperon

How taken: Liquid, tablet, injection

Prescription: Yes

	YES	NO
Generic substitutes	✓	
Potentially addicting		✓
May cause drowsiness	✓	
Alcohol discouraged	✓	

Possible drug interactions include: Taking this drug may decrease the effects of guanethidine (a blood pressure drug). This drug taken in combination with sedatives may result in excessive drowsiness.

Possible side effects include: Low blood pressure, blurred vision, dry mouth, shaking and other Parkinson's-like symptoms.

Common Problems

Even though anti-psychotic drugs have revolutionized the treatment of mental illness, they require careful handling, says Dr. Kerns.

One "problem" with these drugs is that they work so well. "People will stop hearing voices, or some of the delusional thoughts may clear, and they'll convince themselves that they're no longer ill and don't require medication," says Dr. Kerns. The result of this can be a rapid return of symptoms.

Some people, however, do improve so much that they eventually do not need medications, adds Dr. Dilsaver. Because of potential side effects, "we like to get people off the drugs as soon as intelligently possible," he says.

One troublesome side effect is a neurological condition called tardive dyskinesia, which is characterized by involuntary movements of the lips, jaw, tongue and eyelids. In some cases, it can become a permanent problem, persisting even after the drug has been discontinued.

Other potential side effects include faintness, dry mouth and a condition called orthostatic hypotension—dizziness while standing up or changing position. In addition, many people feel tired and listless. "In many cases the drugs may leave patients feeling unable to experience pleasure," Dr. Dilsaver says.

If you're taking one of these drugs, be sure to tell your doctor about any side effects that you may be experiencing, says Dr. Dilsaver. He may decide to change the dose or, in some cases, change the drug. He can provide much-needed moral support as well.

If you're always forgetting to take your medication, your doctor may give you long-lasting injections instead. These remain active for one to four weeks, depending on the preparation, says Dr. Dilsaver.

Antiseptics and Antibiotic Creams

Putting Nasty Germs under Arrest

Pity the scraped knee of antiquity. However painful the injury, the treatments—ranging from simple neglect to sprinklings of powdered "unicorn's horn"—were likely to make things worse. Not only did bacteria flourish, but the "ouch" factor when applying the remedy was something to be reckoned with.

Today's antiseptic soaps, sprays and liquids still can sting, though they're considerably more effective than, say, preparations of unicorn. Better still are antibiotic creams, which not only fight infection but are essentially ouchless.

Although antiseptics and antibiotics both prevent infection, they're used for different jobs, says James J. Leyden, M.D., professor of dermatology at the University of Pennsylvania in Philadelphia. Let's first take a look at antibiotics, relative newcomers to the war on germs.

Germ Warfare

Antibiotics usually are substances produced by bacteria that have the ability to kill other bacteria, explains Dr. Leyden.

HYDROGEN PEROXIDE: GOOD BUBBLES . . . OR NOT WORTH THE TROUBLE?

Because of its low cost and safe reputation, hydrogen peroxide is often thought to be a first-aid star. Poured on a wound, it bubbles, it hisses, it goes *Snap! Crackle! Pop!*

Hydrogen peroxide is water with an extra atom of oxygen. (The chemical symbol is H_2O_2.) When it comes into contact with catalase, an enzyme found in blood and tissues, it fizzes like Alka-Seltzer. You can actually see (and hear) it working.

But while it's killing germs, it's potentially irritating to the skin, says James J. Leyden, M.D., professor of dermatology at the University of Pennsylvania in Philadelphia. "These days, we don't really prescribe hydrogen peroxide for anything," he says. "You're much better off treating your small cuts and scrapes with an antibiotic ointment."

There are dozens of antibiotic creams and lotions from which to choose. Your doctor or pharmacist can help you decide which is best for you.

For example, prescription creams containing silver sulfadiazine (Flint SSD, Sildimac, Silvadene) often are used to kill the bacteria that colonize burns. Nonprescription preparations such as bacitracin (Baciguent) and neomycin (Myciguent), on the other hand, are effective at fighting bacteria inside cuts and scrapes.

For small abrasions of any kind, doctors often recommend nonprescription antibiotic ointments that contain several active ingredients. For example, a combination of neomycin, polymyxin B and bacitracin can zap many types of bacteria at once, says Debra L. Breneman, M.D., associate professor of dermatology at the University of Cincinnati.

In fact, multiple-ingredient antibiotics do more than prevent infection; they may promote faster wound healing as well. In a study at the University of Pennsylvania, researchers treated blister wounds with antibiotic creams or with antiseptics such as tincture of iodine. People treated with a triple antibiotic (neomycin–polymyxin B–bacitracin) healed in approximately 9 days, compared to 13 to 14 days for those treated with the other drugs.

"The best way to care for a wound is to gently cleanse it with soap and water to remove dirt and then treat it with topical antibiotics," says Dr. Leyden. Apply the antibiotic ointment one to three times a day until the wound is healed.

AT A GLANCE

BACITRACIN

Brand name: Baciguent

How taken: Ointment

Prescription: Sometimes, depending on strength

	YES	NO
Generic substitutes	✓	
Potentially addicting		✓
May cause drowsiness		✓
Alcohol discouraged		✓

Possible drug interactions include: Interactions are unlikely.

Possible side effects include: Itching, rash and swelling of the skin.

NEOMYCIN

Brand name: Myciguent

How to take: Cream, ointment

Prescription: No

	YES	NO
Generic substitutes	✓	
Potentially addicting		✓
May cause drowsiness		✓
Alcohol discouraged		✓

Possible drug interactions include: Interactions are unlikely.

Possible side effects include: Itching, rash, redness and swelling of the skin.

Broad Attacks

If antibiotics are the sharpshooters of germ warfare, antiseptics are the shotguns.

When poured on a wound, antiseptics such as isopropyl alcohol or tincture of iodine will kill virtually all of the bacteria present, says Dr. Leyden. But the sting, as many an unhappy patient will report, is not soon forgotten.

Indeed, antiseptics can be more than painful, Dr. Leyden says. He found that blisters treated with tincture of iodine or a camphorphenol solution took longer to heal than blisters treated with antibiotics. They even healed more slowly than blisters that weren't treated at all, possibly because these harsh solutions actually damaged the skin.

Does this mean that all antiseptics should be swept into the medical trash? Not at all, says Dr. Leyden. Doctors use these solutions constantly—not to treat open wounds, but to disinfect the skin *before* opening it.

Before surgery, for example, surgeons may apply chlorhexidine or tincture of iodine to the surgical area. These potent antiseptics make the skin virtually germ-free. Similarly, the skin is swabbed with alcohol before shots are given or blood is drawn.

Even common deodorant soaps may contain mild antiseptics, which can help eliminate odor-causing bacteria.

AT A GLANCE

SILVER SULFADIAZINE

Brand names: Flint SSD, Sildimac, Silvadene

How to take: Cream

Prescription: Yes

	YES	NO
Generic substitutes		✓
Potentially addicting		✓
May cause drowsiness		✓
Alcohol discouraged		✓

Possible drug interactions include: Using this drug may decrease the effects of enzymes used to treat various skin conditions.

Possible side effects include: Burning, itching, rash and discoloration of the skin.

NEOMYCIN–POLYMYXIN B–BACITRACIN

Brand names: Bactine First Aid Antibiotic Plus Anesthetic Ointment, Maximum Strength Mycitracin Triple Antibiotic First Aid Ointment, Campho-Phenique Triple Antibiotic Ointment Plus Pain Reliever

How to take: Ointment

Prescription: Sometimes, depending on strength

	YES	NO
Generic substitutes	✓	
Potentially addicting		✓
May cause drowsiness		✓
Alcohol discouraged		✓

Possible drug interactions include: Interactions are unlikely.

Possible side effects include: Itching, swelling, rash and redness of the skin.

But for treating cuts and scrapes at home, Dr. Leyden says you should stick with antibiotic creams or ointments. "I can't think of too many circumstances when people at home need to be using antiseptics."

Antiviral Drugs

Protection from Little Invaders

At the very bottom of the evolutionary ladder, below the mammals, reptiles, insects and even the lowly paramecium, you will find the viruses. These microscopic organisms, which are anywhere from 10 to 1,000 times smaller than bacteria, are so primitive that they lack even the basic machinery that is needed for reproduction.

When viruses get inside your body, however, reproduce they do, using material from inside your cells. With enough numbers, they can cause flu, herpes, chicken pox and many other viral infections. In general, viruses are tougher to kill than bacteria—and antibiotics won't do the job. But there are

---

NATURAL ALTERNATIVES

It's impossible to avoid all colds and flu, but there are things you can do to ease the aches—or even, in some cases, switch on the infection protection.

Use a humidifier. Winter air is dry air. As your nose and throat lose moisture, they also lose some of their germ-trapping ability. Adding humidity to the air can keep them "sticky" all year long.

Have a long soak. When you're sick and achy, a soothing bath or shower can give welcome relief. At the same time, the steam can help moisten your airways and break up nasal congestion.

Try some soup. Doctors have found that eating soup or drinking hot liquids—and inhaling the steam—can further humidify your airways and help break up congestion.

Eat lots of oranges. In one study healthy volunteers given vitamin C produced 40 percent less histamine. Histamine is a body chemical that can contribute to runny noses and other flu symptoms.

---

medications that may. Antiviral drugs, taken in time, can sometimes halt a viral takeover, knocking days or even weeks off your sick time.

Halting the Herpesvirus

Some of the most common viral infections are caused by the herpesvirus. This family of troubles includes genital herpes, oral herpes, encephalitis and certain eye infections, says Joshua Hoffman, M.D., an internist and assistant clinical professor of medicine at the University of California, Davis, Medical Center in Sacramento.

For people with genital herpes, a sexually transmitted disease that can cause painful sores on or near the genitals, doctors often prescribe acyclovir (Zovirax). Taken orally for seven to ten days, acyclovir "will shorten the length of the attack and diminish the symptoms of the initial outbreak," says Dr. Hoffman. This drug is not a cure, however. When you stop taking the drug, symptoms may return.

That's why people who have frequent outbreaks of herpes—six or more a year, for example—may take acyclovir every day to prevent problems. Studies show that acyclovir, taken once a day, can prevent attacks in up to 90 percent of cases.

Acyclovir is also effective against outbreaks of oral herpes—a condition that causes the painful sores, usually on the lips, known as cold

---

AT A GLANCE

ACYCLOVIR

Brand name: Zovirax

How taken: Capsule, injection, liquid, ointment

Prescription: Yes

	YES	NO
Generic substitutes		✓
Potentially addicting		✓
May cause drowsiness		✓
Alcohol discouraged		✓

Possible drug interactions include: The effects of this drug may increase if taken with probenecid (used for gout). The side effects of this drug may increase if taken with cyclosporine (an immunosuppressant), penicillamine (used for arthritis) and some cancer drugs. Taking this drug in combination with interferon and methotrexate (used for psoriasis, cancer and rheumatoid arthritis) may affect the nervous system.

Possible side effects include: Itching or burning of the skin, nausea, headache and dizziness.

---

sores. For battling cold sores doctors prescribe acyclovir in ointment form. "The topical preparation may be helpful for very mild cold sores on the lip," says Peter Axelrod, M.D., an infectious disease specialist and assistant professor of medicine at Temple University School of Medicine in

WIPING OUT WARTS

Folklore is jam-packed with remedies for warts. One gypsy remedy calls for applying wild garlic juice under a full moon.

Sir Francis Bacon tried pork fat. Huckleberry Finn recommended dead cats. His pal Tom Sawyer preferred stagnant water taken from the crotch of a dead tree.

The truth is, these unsightly little growths, caused by an infectious organism called human papilloma virus, usually disappear whether you treat them or not. Unfortunately, this can take months or even years.

If you're in a hurry, warts can be frozen with liquid nitrogen, burned with lasers or cut out with surgery. Or, if you're patient, they can be dissolved with over-the-counter medications, says Bruce Bart, M.D., clinical professor of dermatology at the University of Minnesota and chief of dermatology at Hennepin County Medical Center in Minneapolis.

Most wart-removal preparations contain a substance called salicylic acid (Salactic Film Topical Solution, Wart-off Topical Solution). This is roughly the same stuff that is in aspirin, says Dr. Bart. "When used in low concentrations, it has a very mild peeling effect."

Sold as a cream, ointment or patch, salicylic acid helps loosen layer after layer of skin cells. Eventually, says Dr. Bart, "it probably exposes the cells that contain the viral package." Without its protective wart, the virus is exposed to your body's immune system, which steps in to finish the job.

To be effective, however, wart removers must be used correctly. For example:

- Soak the wart in warm water for five minutes before applying the medication. This will help the acid penetrate the skin.

- Gently rub off dead skin cells with a washcloth or pumice stone between applications.

- Don't put the medication on healthy skin surrounding the wart. It can cause painful irritation.

- Be patient. It may take weeks or months before the wart disappears. "Warts are *very* unpredictable," says Dr. Bart.

Philadelphia. "But it's clearly not as good as the oral form."

A more serious infection caused by the herpesvirus is a brain inflammation called encephalitis. This condition may also be treated with acyclovir. Under unusual circumstances doctors treat herpes encephalitis with a prescription drug called vidarabine (Vira-A). But vidarabine taken by injection can cause serious side effects, including nausea, vomiting, diarrhea, confusion and hallucinations, says Dr. Axelrod. In the majority of cases, he says, "acyclovir is very clearly superior."

Antiviral medications such as vidarabine, idoxuridine (Herplex, Liquifilm, Stoxil) and trifluridine (Viroptic) are used for treating viral eye infections such as herpes keratitis.

Fighting Flu, Fighting AIDS

Flu is one viral disease that usually is best treated by resting, drinking plenty of fluids and taking mild pain relievers. But for some people—the elderly, for example, or those with serious health problems—influenza can cause a life-threatening illness. That's when antiviral drugs can help.

A prescription drug called amantadine (Symadine, Symmetrel), taken orally, can help prevent a virulent type of flu called influenza A.

AT A GLANCE

VIDARABINE

Brand name: Vira-A

How taken: Injection, ophthalmic ointment

Prescription: Yes

	YES	NO
Generic substitutes		✓
Potentially addicting		✓
May cause drowsiness		✓
Alcohol discouraged		✓

Possible drug interactions include: Interactions are unlikely.

Possible side effects include: Tearing, stinging or burning eyes; may make eyes more light sensitive.

IDOXURIDINE

Brand names: Herplex, Liquifilm, Stoxil

How taken: Ointment, eyedrops

Prescription: Yes

	YES	NO
Generic substitutes		✓
Potentially addicting		✓
May cause drowsiness		✓
Alcohol discouraged		✓

Possible drug interactions include: Interactions are unlikely (unless using boric-acid-containing eye products).

Possible side effects include: Eye pain or inflammation; may make the eyes more light sensitive.

CAUTION: May be dangerous when used with eye products containing boric acid.

AT A GLANCE

AMANTADINE

Brand names: Symadine, Symmetrel

How taken: Capsule, liquid

Prescription: Yes

	YES	NO
Generic substitutes	✓	
Potentially addicting		✓
May cause drowsiness	✓	
Alcohol discouraged	✓	

Possible drug interactions include: Taking this drug may increase the effects of drugs used to treat Parkinson's disease. Taking this drug in combination with amphetamines or other stimulants may result in excessive stimulation.

Possible side effects include: Nausea and dizziness.

CAUTION: May be dangerous when taken by people with epilepsy or certain heart problems.

ZIDOVUDINE (AZT)

Brand name: Retrovir

How taken: Capsule, injection, liquid

Prescription: Yes

	YES	NO
Generic substitutes		✓
Potentially addicting		✓
May cause drowsiness		✓
Alcohol discouraged	✓	

Possible drug interactions include: The effects of this drug may increase if taken with acetaminophen, acyclovir (another antiviral drug), aspirin, sedatives or indomethacin (an anti-inflammatory drug).

Possible side effects include: Insomnia, headache, nausea, dizziness and muscle soreness.

"If one resident in a nursing home gets the flu and physicians suspect influenza A, it might be appropriate to give amantadine to the other residents and staff to prevent them from getting it," says Dr. Axelrod.

The drug can be used to treat as well as prevent influenza A. To be effective, however, it must be taken within two days after symptoms begin, says Dr. Hoffman. If you wait more than 48 hours, it probably won't work.

Unfortunately, amantadine may cause side effects—such as anxiety, dizziness and insomnia—that may be severe enough to force patients to prematurely stop taking it, says Dr. Axelrod.

Not all antiviral drugs are designed to fight the herpes and flu bugs. For relatively rare infections caused by a potent type of respiratory virus, for example, the prescription drug ribavirin (Virazol) can help. Taken by aerosol inhaler for up to 18 hours a day, this drug is primarily used to treat seriously ill infants.

And for those afflicted with the AIDS virus, the powerful prescription drug zidovudine, or AZT (Retrovir) can help treat some of the infections that occur along with the disease. But zidovudine often causes side effects, including headache and fever. It also seems to become less effective the longer it's used, as the AIDS virus often becomes resistant over time, doctors say.

The alarming spread of AIDS has prompted scientists worldwide to work on developing new, more effective medications for battling viruses. Someday we may be better able to put them in their place.

Arthritis Drugs

Counterpoints to Achy Joints

Everywhere in the body where bone meets bone there's a joint. And for people with arthritis, every one of these joints is a potential hot spot for pain, stiffness and inflammation.

Although there isn't yet a cure for arthritis—the word literally means "inflammation of the joint"—there are many drugs that can relieve painful swelling. And for rheumatoid arthritis, which is the most debilitating form of the disease, there are drugs that can stop its progression, or sometimes even reverse the condition.

Stop the Swelling

For the majority of people who have arthritis, medications called NSAIDs—nonsteroidal anti-inflammatory drugs—do an excellent job of quelling flare-ups, says

---

NATURAL ALTERNATIVES

You don't have to take arthritis sitting down. In fact, don't be surprised if your doctor wants you to keep moving.

"Exercise is very important," says Carey Dachman, M.D., director of rheumatology at Edgewater Hospital in Chicago. "It builds muscle, which increases the ability to move. It also stimulates bone growth. Most important, exercise increases your production of endorphins, your natural painkillers."

Endorphins provide dual benefits, he adds. Not only do they relieve pain directly, they also may reduce the amount of substance P present in your body. Substance P is a pain- and inflammation-causing chemical that seems to accumulate in arthritic joints, says Dr. Dachman.

Experts agree that swimming and walking are among the best exercises for people with arthritis. (Some people combine the two by walking in water.) Both will help keep your muscles toned and your joints limber. They also can boost your heart rate, which, over time, may further decrease your levels of substance P.

Carey Dachman, M.D., director of rheumatology at Edgewater Hospital in Chicago, a lecturer in medicine at the University of Health Sciences/The Chicago Medical School and a rheumatologist in Schaumburg, Illinois.

There are many NSAIDs. You can buy over-the-counter drugs such as aspirin (Anacin, Genuine Bayer Aspirin) and ibuprofen (Advil, Motrin IB, Nuprin), or your doctor can prescribe drugs like ketoprofen (Orudis) and indomethacin (Indocin). NSAIDs work, at least in part, by blocking the production of prostaglandins, chemicals that cause pain and inflammation.

Because NSAIDs are rapidly absorbed from the digestive system, they quickly go to work, sometimes relieving pain and swelling within a few hours.

Unfortunately, virtually all of the NSAIDs can cause stomach upset. If this becomes a problem, says Dr. Dachman, you might want to try buffered aspirin or talk to your doctor about other, less irritating anti-inflammatories. Possible choices may include prescription salicylates (Disalcid, Mono-Gesic) and nonprescription magnesium salicylate (Doan's, Maximum Pain Relief Pamprin, Mobigesic).

When NSAIDs don't bring relief, your doctor may recommend steroids instead. Taken orally or by injection, prescription drugs such as prednisone (Deltasone, Meticorten, Orasone) and prednisolone (Hydeltrasol, Hydeltra-T.B.A.,

Pediapred) are the gold standard for beating arthritis inflammation, says Dr. Dachman.

Like the NSAIDs, however, steroids, particularly the oral forms, can cause side effects. These include mood changes, increases in blood pressure and a greater susceptibility to infection. "However, a doctor can give injections right into a joint without the side effects that oral steroids sometimes cause," says Leroy C. Knodel, Pharm.D., director of the Drug Information Service and associate professor of pharmacology at the University of Texas Health Science Center at San Antonio.

Still, oral steroids can sometimes be very helpful, particularly when used in conjunction with other, slower-acting arthritis drugs. "With steroids you can control the inflammation almost immediately," says Dr. Knodel.

Along with NSAIDs and steroids,

AT A GLANCE

IBUPROFEN

Brand names: Advil, Motrin IB, Nuprin

How taken: Capsule, liquid, tablet

Prescription: Sometimes, depending on strength

	YES	NO
Generic substitutes	✓	
Potentially addicting		✓
May cause drowsiness	✓	
Alcohol discouraged		✓

Possible drug interactions include: This drug taken in combination with aspirin, acetaminophen, digitalis (a heart medicine), anti-clotting drugs, colchicine (used for gout) and many other drugs may cause serious side effects.

Possible side effects include: Rash, stomach cramps, diarrhea, dizziness, headache, heartburn and nausea.

CAUTION: Do not take if you are allergic to aspirin.

KETOPROFEN

Brand name: Orudis

How taken: Capsule

Prescription: Yes

	YES	NO
Generic substitutes		✓
Potentially addicting		✓
May cause drowsiness	✓	
Alcohol discouraged	✓	

Possible drug interactions include: This drug taken in combination with aspirin, acetaminophen, digitalis (a heart medicine), anti-clotting drugs, colchicine (used for gout) and many other drugs may cause serious side effects.

Possible side effects include: Rash, stomach cramps, diarrhea, dizziness, headache, heartburn and nausea.

CAUTION: Do not take if you are allergic to aspirin.

your doctor may give you pain-killing drugs to further ease discomfort. Prescription drugs such as phenytoin (Dilantin), clonazepam (Klonopin) or imipramine (Tofranil) often work very well, with few side effects, says Dr. Dachman.

It's important to remember that while all of these drugs can ease arthritis flare-ups, they won't eliminate the problem or alter the course of the disease. There are other drugs to do that.

Rheumatic Rescuers

Doctors call them disease-modifying anti-rheumatic drugs, or DMARDs for short. These drugs can slow or even stop the progress of rheumatoid arthritis (they don't work for osteoarthritis).

AT A GLANCE

PREDNISONE

Brand names: Deltasone, Meticorten, Orasone

How taken: Liquid, tablet

Prescription: Yes

	YES	NO
Generic substitutes	✓	
Potentially addicting		✓
May cause drowsiness		✓
Alcohol discouraged	✓	

Possible drug interactions include: The effects of this drug may decrease if taken with antacids, antibiotics and antifungal drugs. Taking this drug may decrease the effects of diuretics (water pills) and digitalis (a heart medication).

Possible side effects include: Acne, weight gain, stomach upset and insomnia.

CAUTION: See your doctor if you experience unusual bruising or irregular heartbeat. Avoid vaccines such as the polio vaccine.

GOLD

Brand names: Myochrysine, Ridaura, Solganal

How taken: Capsule, injection

Prescription: Yes

	YES	NO
Generic substitutes	✓	
Potentially addicting		✓
May cause drowsiness		✓
Alcohol discouraged	✓	

Possible drug interactions include: Taking this drug may increase the effects of phenytoin (an anti-seizure drug). This drug taken in combination with antimalarials and penicillamine (other arthritis drugs) may cause side effects.

Possible side effects include: Diarrhea, loss of appetite or a metallic taste in the mouth, skin rash and soreness of the mouth.

AT A GLANCE

METHOTREXATE

Brand names: Mexate, Rheumatrex

How taken: Injection, tablet

Prescription: Yes

	YES	NO
Generic substitutes	✓	
Potentially addicting		✓
May cause drowsiness		✓
Alcohol discouraged	✓	

Possible drug interactions include: Interactions are unlikely (unless also taking aspirin, ibuprofen or other nonsteroidal anti-inflammatory drugs).

Possible side effects include: Diarrhea, stomach pain, flushing, nausea and sores in the mouth or on the lips.

CAUTION: Avoid vaccines such as the polio vaccine. May be dangerous if taken with aspirin, ibuprofen or other nonsteroidal anti-inflammatory drugs.

HYDROXYCHLOROQUINE

Brand name: Plaquenil

How taken: Tablet

Prescription: Yes

	YES	NO
Generic substitutes		✓
Potentially addicting		✓
May cause drowsiness		✓
Alcohol discouraged		✓

Possible drug interactions include: Taking this drug may increase the effects of digitalis (a heart medicine) and penicillamine (another arthritis drug).

Possible side effects include: Headache or difficulty reading, itching, loss of appetite, stomach cramps, diarrhea, nausea and vomiting.

Doctors aren't sure how DMARDs work, but prescription drugs such as gold, methotrexate and hydroxychloroquine put the brakes on pain, sometimes for years at a time.

The oldest of the DMARDs, gold (Myochrysine, Ridaura, Solganal), has been used for decades, says Lourdes C. Corman, M.D., a rheumatologist and associate professor of medicine at the University of Florida College of Medicine in Gainesville. Generally taken by injection, gold—yes, the same metal you wear on your fingers—suppresses the immune system and relieves arthritis pain. Doctors estimate that about two-thirds of people taking gold injections enjoy some relief.

The problem with gold isn't the scarcity of the metal. A full year's supply of the medication wouldn't contain enough gold to forge even a thin wedding band. The real problem with gold is that it's better at masking damage than preventing it: Joint damage may silently continue even while symptoms are absent. Gold is also not recommended for long-term use because it can cause serious side effects, including liver and kidney problems.

A prescription drug used for treating inflammatory bowel disease, sulfasalazine (Azulfidine), also can be helpful, says Dr. Corman. Taken orally, sulfasalazine works quickly (by the slow standards of DMARDs), often eliminating symptoms within about two months.

Rheumatologists also prescribe a drug called methotrexate (Mexate, Rheumatrex), available as tablets or injections. Used to treat psoriasis and some cancers as well as arthritis, "methotrexate has an 80 percent chance of inducing true remission for people with rheumatoid arthritis," says Dr. Dachman.

A managing editor at the *Albuquerque Journal* newspaper, Frankie McCarty, said methotrexate made a big difference in her life. "Before, I was limping and I had trouble getting out of a chair," she remembers. "At news meetings, I'd have to put my hands down on the table and lift myself up. That is not the case now. I pop right out of my chair."

Her case isn't unusual. In fact, rheumatologists speculate that methotrexate not only can stop rheumatoid arthritis from progressing but also may reverse disease by helping joints to heal. It also works more quickly than other DMARDs,

sometimes relieving symptoms within a month.

Unfortunately, methotrexate, like gold, can cause serious side effects, including liver and lung damage, increased risk for infections and, if taken by pregnant women, birth defects.

Other DMARDs are the antimalarials—prescription drugs originally used to treat malaria. Usually taken orally, drugs such as chloroquine (Aralen) and hydroxychloroquine (Plaquenil) can relieve rheumatoid arthritis symptoms and may slow the progress of the disease. Once again, however, potentially dangerous side effects limit their usefulness.

In fact, because DMARDs so often cause side effects, doctors traditionally prescribed them only when milder drugs—aspirin, for instance—were no longer effective. "But the longer you wait, the less joint there is to save," says Dr. Corman. "Many rheumatologists today, when they have a patient with clear-cut rheumatoid arthritis, will use disease-modifying drugs right away."

A possible alternative to the DMARDs is a relatively new class of medications called biologicals. Unlike drugs that suppress the entire immune system, the biologicals "may be capable of targeting that part of the immune system that is aberrant or overreactive," says Dr. Dachman. Researchers hope they will be more effective (and cause fewer side effects) than the DMARDs used today.

Asthma Drugs

Airway Expanders

For people with asthma, it doesn't take much: Drifting pollen, a fast walk or even a blast of cold air can cause airways inside the lungs to suddenly narrow or shut down. In an instant, the precious flow of oxygen can be reduced or, in serious cases, stopped entirely.

Asthma affects approximately 5 percent of Americans, and many of these people depend, at least occasionally, on breath-restoring asthma medications, says Robert B. Mellins, M.D., a council member of the American Lung Association and director of the pediatric pulmonary division at Columbia University College of Physicians and Surgeons in New York City.

There are two types of asthma drugs: anti-inflammatories, which reduce swelling in the airways, and bronchodilators, which relax the muscles that surround the airways. Both types work well and, in many cases, says Dr. Mellins, both are needed.

Increasing Airflow

Traditionally, bronchodilators have been the mainstay of asthma therapy, says Anthony Rooklin, M.D., an asthma expert in the Division of Allergy and Clinical Immunology at Crozer-Chester Medical Center in Chester, Pennsylvania. These drugs may be taken daily to prevent problems or used only "as needed" to stop attacks already in progress.

The bronchodilators that are most in use today are called beta-adrenergic agents, or beta agonists, Dr. Rooklin says. Usually taken orally or by inhaler, prescription drugs like albuterol (Proventil, Ventolin) and terbutaline (Brethaire) and over-the-counter agents such as epinephrine (AsthmaHaler, Bronkaid Mist, Primatene Mist) can help keep the airways open.

In general, beta agonists are best for short-term relief, Dr. Rooklin adds. "For people who need medication intermittently— to prevent attacks while they exer-

NATURAL ALTERNATIVES

There are many things you can do to ward off asthma attacks, says Robert B. Mellins, M.D., director of the pediatric pulmonary division at Columbia University College of Physicians and Surgeons in New York City. For example:

Observe what makes you sick—then avoid it. Suppose you wheeze every time you visit your neighbor and her 14 cats. Presumably it's the cats (and not the neighbor) that are causing your problems. Instead of going to her house, let her visit you.

Create an allergen-free environment. Wash the bed linen in hot water at least once a week to eliminate dust mites. Vacuum your carpets thoroughly and often.

Time your outings. Airborne pollen typically takes flight between 5:00 and 10:00 A.M. If you often have morning attacks, consider staying inside during this high-risk time.

Sip hot soup. Drinking warm liquids can relax the bronchial tubes inside your lungs.

Avoid dehydration. Drinking four to six glasses of water a day may thin mucus in your lungs, which will help keep air flowing.

Keep your lungs warm. Try staying inside on cold days. Or, if you do venture out, cover your nose and mouth with a scarf to warm incoming air.

Stay calm. Stress doesn't cause asthma, but it can make it worse. Ask your doctor about biofeedback, self-hypnosis and other relaxation techniques.

cise, for example—the beta agonists work beautifully."

Unfortunately, beta agonists can be dangerous when overused, Dr. Rooklin adds. "If you're using up more than one prescription a month," he says, "you may be using too much."

One of the oldest bronchodilators is the prescription drug atropine. Taken orally, atropine prevents a natural chemical in the body called acetylcholine from causing asthma-sensitive airways to shut down.

But atropine has many potential side effects, including an accelerated heart rate and dryness of the nose and mouth. To provide the benefits of atropine without the side effects, your doctor may recommend instead the prescription drug ipratropium bromide (Atrovent). Taken by inhaler, it may help to slowly open the airways and keep them open for up to six hours, according to Dr. Mellins.

Another asthma warhorse is theophylline (Aerolate, Theo-Dur). Chemically related to caffeine, this prescription drug, usually taken orally once or twice a day, acts longer than beta-agonist- and atropine-like drugs. "It controls symptoms so you can sleep through the night and have a clear chest when you wake up in the morning," says Dr. Rooklin.

Clearing Inflammation

Although muscle spasms in the lungs play a big part in asthma, so, too, does inflammation. Anti-inflammatory drugs, by reducing swelling, can restore easy breathing very quickly.

The most potent of these drugs are corticosteroids, or steroids for short. If there is such a thing as a miracle drug available today for treating asthma, it's the steroids,

---

AT A GLANCE

ALBUTEROL

Brand names: Proventil, Ventolin

How taken: Spray, liquid, tablet

Prescription: Yes

	YES	NO
Generic substitutes		✓
Potentially addicting		✓
May cause drowsiness	✓	
Alcohol discouraged		✓

Possible drug interactions include: This drug taken in combination with monoamine oxidase (MAO) inhibitors (used for depression) may result in high blood pressure and changes in heart rhythm.

Possible side effects include: Nervousness, trembling and lightheadedness.

EPINEPHRINE

Brand names: Adrenalin, Asthma-Haler, Bronkaid Mist, Primatene Mist

How taken: Spray, injection

Prescription: Sometimes, depending on strength

	YES	NO
Generic substitutes	✓	
Potentially addicting		✓
May cause drowsiness	✓	
Alcohol discouraged		✓

Possible drug interactions include: The effects of this drug may decrease if taken with beta-blockers (used for blood pressure problems). Taking this drug may increase the effects of monoamine oxidase (MAO) inhibitors (used for depression).

Possible side effects include: Nervousness, restlessness and trembling.

AT A GLANCE

IPRATROPIUM BROMIDE

Brand name: Atrovent

How taken: Inhaler

Prescription: Yes

	YES	NO
Generic substitutes		✓
Potentially addicting		✓
May cause drowsiness	✓	
Alcohol discouraged		✓

Possible drug interactions include: May increase the effects of atropine-like drugs (other asthma drugs).

Possible side effects include: Cough, headache and dryness of the nose, mouth or throat.

THEOPHYLLINE

Brand names: Aerolate, Theo-Dur

How taken: Capsule, liquid, tablet

Prescription: Yes

	YES	NO
Generic substitutes		✓
Potentially addicting		✓
May cause drowsiness		✓
Alcohol discouraged		✓

Possible drug interactions include: Taking this drug may decrease the effects of phenytoin (an anti-seizure drug). This drug taken in combination with beta-blockers (used for high blood pressure) may prevent either medication from working properly.

Possible side effects include: Nervousness, nausea, restlessness and burning or irritation of the rectum.

BECLOMETHASONE DIPROPIONATE

Brand names: Beclovent, Vanceril

How taken: Spray

Prescription: Yes

	YES	NO
Generic substitutes		✓
Potentially addicting		✓
May cause drowsiness	✓	
Alcohol discouraged		✓

Possible drug interactions include: Interactions are unlikely.

Possible side effects include: Cough, mild abdominal pain, a bloated feeling, constipation, diarrhea and dizziness.

CROMOLYN SODIUM

Brand name: Intal

How taken: Inhaler

Prescription: Yes

	YES	NO
Generic substitutes	✓	
Potentially addicting		✓
May cause drowsiness	✓	
Alcohol discouraged		✓

Possible drug interactions include: Interactions are unlikely.

Possible side effects include: Throat irritation or dryness, cough, wheezing, nausea and a bad taste in the mouth.

GETTING THE MOST FROM YOUR INHALER

In order for an inhaler to be effective, you need to use it properly. Here's how.

- Put the mouthpiece on the inhaler canister and shake well.

- Hold it with the mouthpiece on the bottom and the canister above, one to two inches in front of your mouth.

- Tilt your head back slightly, open your mouth wide and breathe out.

- Press down on the inhaler to release the medicine and inhale slowly for three to five seconds, then hold your breath for about ten seconds.

- Two puffs usually are recommended. The first puff opens the airways. The second, taken three to five minutes later, penetrates deep inside the lungs where it can do the most good.

says Dr. Rooklin. Prescription drugs such as prednisone (Deltasone, Orasone 1-50), which are taken orally, can relieve or even eliminate air-blocking inflammation. At the same time, they can help make the airways less sensitive to asthma "triggers"—cold air, for example—that often cause attacks.

The problem with taking steroids orally, says Dr. Rooklin, is side effects, which may include cataracts, weight gain, high blood pressure and bone and hormonal changes.

To get the benefits of oral steroids without the side effects, your doctor may recommend inhaled steroids instead, which contain drugs such as beclomethasone dipropionate (Beclovent, Vanceril), flunisolide (AeroBid) or triamcinolone acetonide (Azmacort). "With inhalers you can put the drug right where you want it without having to worry as much about side effects," says Dr. Rooklin.

A nonsteroidal inhaled drug called cromolyn sodium (Intal) is also very effective for preventing inflammation. And like the steroids, it has the extra benefit of making the airways less reactive as well.

Baldness Drugs

A Hair-Raising Discovery

When Delilah stealthily snipped a sleeping Samson's locks, she removed more than just his hair. She cut away his strength and masculinity as well.

The average man, of course, has little to fear from impromptu haircuts. What he may worry about, however, is hair loss of a more gradual kind. Approximately 35 million American men (and some women) have what is called androgenic alopecia, or male pattern baldness.

Beginning at puberty and continuing throughout life, hair follicles, under the influence of male hormones called androgens, gradually stop producing hair. (Men produce more androgens than women, so they lose more hair.) Until recently, the only "remedies" for hair loss were of the snake-oil variety. They did more to line manufacturers' pockets than to restore thinning hair.

Today, however, there really is a medicine that makes hair grow. Doctors agree it doesn't work for everybody. But for some men, it will put hair in places that previously were bare.

A Useful Side Effect

In the 1980s, the Upjohn Company introduced a new blood pressure medication called minoxidil. Taken orally, the drug had a curious side effect: It caused hair to grow on the forehead, cheeks and elsewhere on the body.

Minoxidil never really caught on as a blood pressure drug. Yet this side effect didn't go unnoticed. The company quickly reformulated it as a liquid (Rogaine) and began testing it on bald men. In studies, 5 to 8 percent of men who applied minoxidil to their scalps showed noticeable hair growth in four months. After a year, 39 percent got results.

"About two out of ten men who are balding or recently bald who put minoxidil on twice a day for a year or so will grow enough hair to look different," says Guy Webster, M.D., Ph.D., assistant professor of dermatology at Jefferson Medical College of Thomas Jefferson University in Philadelphia.

Realistic Expectations

As exciting as minoxidil is, it is not a miracle drug. "People have expectations that often aren't realistic," explains Dr. Webster. "Somebody will come in for a prescription and expect to start hearing popping sounds as hairs start thrusting out of his head. That just doesn't happen."

What does happen is that minoxidil appears to enlarge some hair follicles and helps protect others from the destructive effects of male hormones. This slows the rate at which hair falls out while encouraging new hairs to grow.

Minoxidil is most effective for young men who have small bald spots on the tops of their heads. It doesn't work as well for baldness on the forehead or the sides or back of the head. Nor will it restore hair to men who are totally bald.

In short, the drug isn't for everyone. It must be applied twice a day, every day, says Dr. Webster. It also can cost upward of $500 a year. That's $500 *every* year: As soon as you stop applying it, you'll start losing hair again.

Minoxidil currently is the only drug approved by the Food and Drug Administration for growing hair. Yet the potential market is enormous. Several companies are investigating other compounds, but so far the results have been disappointing, says Dr. Webster.

Still, the days of ridiculing hair-loss remedies are gone for good. "Fifteen years ago, if you said there would be a cream that would make hair grow, you would have been laughed out of medicine," says Dr. Webster. "Minoxidil really works."

AT A GLANCE

MINOXIDIL

Brand name: Rogaine

How taken: Cream, spray

Prescription: Yes

	YES	NO
Generic substitutes		✓
Potentially addicting		✓
May cause drowsiness		✓
Alcohol discouraged		✓

Possible drug interactions include: Interactions are unlikely.

Possible side effects include: Mild skin irritation.

Birth Control Medications

Freedom from Worry

It wasn't so many years ago that a woman who didn't want to become pregnant had few choices but to abstain from sex entirely or put up with birth control methods that were inconvenient, ineffective or both.

Today, however, there are many forms of contraception that are both reliable and easy to use. Birth control pills, for example, are among the most widely used prescription medications in the world. There is also a wide variety of contraceptive foams, injections, creams and even implants. Choosing the one that's right for you can be a confusing process. So let's take a look at the benefits—and drawbacks—of some commonly used birth control medications.

The Number-One Choice

No other contraceptive is as effective or as popular as the birth control pill—the Pill, for short—which is used by approximately 60 million women worldwide. All birth control pills contain one or more synthetic hormones. Taken orally, these hormones very slightly disrupt a woman's natural chemical balance. This prevents conception for as long as she takes the medication.

Most oral contraceptives contain not one but two synthetic hormones: estrogen and a progestin (progestins are manufactured versions of progesterone). As a result, they are called combination pills. "We almost always use combination pills," says Jacqueline Gutmann, M.D., a fertility specialist with the Philadelphia Fertility Institute and assistant clinical associate at the University of Pennsylvania. "They really work very well."

Sold by prescription, combination pills are considered 97 to 100 percent effective in preventing pregnancy when used regularly, says Dr. Gutmann. There are many brands available, including Demulen, Nordette, Ovcon, Triphasil and Norquest.

These pills are used for more than just contraception, adds Dr. Gutmann. Doctors also may prescribe them for treating conditions such as menstrual cramps or irregular periods.

When oral contraceptives came on the scene in the 1960s, there were alarming reports that women taking them were at increased risk for stroke, blood clots, high blood pressure and other serious conditions. But these problems occurred most often when the drugs were used in high doses and in women already at risk for these conditions, says Dr. Gutmann. Today, the Pill is prescribed in much smaller doses and serious complications are rare.

Still, there remains a slightly increased risk of stroke and other cardiovascular diseases in women who use the Pill. The risk is highest in women over the age of 35, particularly those who smoke. As a result, some doctors won't prescribe the Pill unless a woman agrees to give up smoking first.

Other problems that may be caused by the Pill include fatigue, weight gain, bloating or mild breast tenderness. In such cases, says Dr. Gutmann, your doctor may recommend you switch to a different drug. One possibility is the "mini-pill."

The Single-Ingredient Mini-Pill

Mini-pills is the name given to oral contraceptives that contain progestin but no estrogen, says Phillip C. Galle, M.D., an infertility and reproductive special-ist in private practice in Springfield, Illinois. Prescription mini-pills like norgestrel (Micronor, Ovrette), taken orally, are about 97 to 98 percent effective. This makes them slightly less effective than the Pill, but still very effective, says Dr. Galle.

Unlike combination pills, however, progestin-only mini-pills often cause midcycle, or breakthrough, bleeding. "Some patients find that's really unacceptable," says Dr. Galle. In fact, mini-pills usually are recommended only for women who, because of side effects or underlying medical conditions, can't take the combination pills, he says.

Under-the-Skin Protection

Despite being very effective, oral contraceptives have one serious drawback: They don't work if you forget to take them. This isn't a problem with some newer medicinal options, which remain active in the body for months or even years at a time.

For example, many women have begun using prescription progestins (Curretab, Depo-Provera, Medroxyprogesterone). Given by injection, the progestins can prevent pregnancy for three months, says Dr. Gutmann. "I think it's a good choice for women who are unlikely to remember to take the Pill," she says. Like the mini-pills, they are 99 to 100 percent effective.

Yet another birth control option is to have tiny medicated capsules implanted under the skin of the arm. Once in place, the capsules (Norplant) remain active for up to five years, slowly releasing a progestin called levonorgestrel into the bloodstream, says Dr. Galle.

As with the mini-pills, however, progestin implants and injections may cause side effects such as fatigue, weight gain or, more commonly, breakthrough bleeding. "About 25 percent of people on Depo-Provera will have irregular bleeding," says Dr. Galle.

One study found that 95 percent of women using Norplant reported side effects. Despite this, most of the women also said the implants were an acceptable form of birth control.

AT A GLANCE

ETHYNODIOL DIACETATE and ETHINYL ESTRADIOL

Brand name: Demulen

How taken: Tablet

Prescription: Yes

	YES	NO
Generic substitutes		✓
Potentially addicting		✓
May cause drowsiness		✓
Alcohol discouraged		✓

Possible drug interactions include: The effects of this drug may decrease if taken with antibiotics, anti-seizure drugs, sedatives or anti-inflammatory steroids.

Possible side effects include: Cramps, bloating, blood clots, acne, mood changes, breast tenderness and midcycle bleeding.

CAUTION: Cigarette smokers taking this medication may have an increased risk of dangerous heart and circulation problems, including blood clots.

LEVONORGESTREL and ETHINYL ESTRADIOL

Brand names: Nordette, Triphasil

How taken: Tablet

Prescription: Yes

	YES	NO
Generic substitutes		✓
Potentially addicting		✓
May cause drowsiness		✓
Alcohol discouraged		✓

Possible drug interactions include: The effects of this drug may decrease if taken with antibiotics, anti-seizure drugs, sedatives or anti-inflammatory steroids.

Possible side effects include: Cramps, bloating, acne, fatigue, blood clots, mood changes, breast tenderness and midcycle bleeding.

CAUTION: Cigarette smokers taking this medication may have an increased risk of dangerous heart and circulation problems, including blood clots.

AT A GLANCE

NORETHINDRONE and ETHINYL ESTRADIOL

Brand names: Ovcon, Norquest

How taken: Tablet

Prescription: Yes

	YES	NO
Generic substitutes		✓
Potentially addicting		✓
May cause drowsiness		✓
Alcohol discouraged		✓

Possible drug interactions include:
The effects of this drug may decrease if taken with antibiotics, anti-seizure drugs, sedatives or nonsteroidal anti-inflammatory drugs.

Possible side effects include:
Cramps, bloating, acne, fatigue, blood clots, mood changes, breast tenderness and midcycle bleeding.

CAUTION: Cigarette smokers taking this medication may have an increased risk of dangerous heart and circulation problems, including blood clots.

NORGESTREL

Brand name: Micronor, Ovrette

How taken: Tablet

Prescription: Yes

	YES	NO
Generic substitutes		✓
Potentially addicting		✓
May cause drowsiness		✓
Alcohol discouraged		✓

Possible drug interactions include:
The effects of this drug may decrease if taken with some antibiotics. Taking this drug may decrease the effects of anti-clotting, anti-seizure, blood pressure and diabetes drugs.

Possible side effects include:
Cramps, acne, fatigue, blood clots, mood changes, breast tenderness and midcycle bleeding.

CAUTION: This drug may cause birth defects if taken during pregnancy.

Over-the-Counter Protection

Although many women prefer prescription contraceptives, there are a number of over-the-counter products available as well. Most of these products (including some condoms) include a spermicidal chemical called nonoxynol 9, which kills sperm on contact, says E. Don Nelson, Pharm.D., professor of clinical pharmacology at the University of Cincinnati College of Medicine.

The advantage of spermicides is that they're relatively low in cost, easy to use and available without a prescription. Their disadvantage, says Dr. Nelson, is that they're not

AT A GLANCE

PROGESTIN

Brand names: Curretab, Depo-Provera, Medroxyprogesterone

How taken: Tablet, injection

Prescription: Yes

	YES	NO
Generic substitutes	✓	
Potentially addicting		✓
May cause drowsiness		✓
Alcohol discouraged		✓

Possible drug interactions include: The effects of this drug may decrease if taken with drugs to treat tuberculosis. Taking this drug may decrease the effects of insulin and bromocriptine (used to treat menstrual problems).

Possible side effects include: Cramps, bloating, fatigue, blood clots, mood changes, breast tenderness and midcycle bleeding.

CAUTION: May cause birth defects if taken during pregnancy.

LEVONORGESTREL

Brand name: Norplant

How taken: Implant

Prescription: Yes

	YES	NO
Generic substitutes		✓
Potentially addicting		✓
May cause drowsiness		✓
Alcohol discouraged		✓

Possible drug interactions include: The effects of this drug may decrease if taken with anti-seizure drugs such as phenytoin and carbamazepine.

Possible side effects include: Nausea, dizziness, cramps, bloating, acne, blood clots, mood changes, breast tenderness and midcycle bleeding.

CAUTION: Cigarette smokers taking this medication may have an increased risk of dangerous heart and circulation problems, including blood clots.

particularly effective unless they're used in combination with barrier forms of birth control. When used alone under ideal circumstances— that is, they're applied at the right time *every* time—spermicides are thought to be about 97 percent effective. In real life, however, in which people sometimes are forgetful, the number may be as low as 79 percent.

One popular form of spermicide is contraceptive foam (Delfen, Emko). When used alone, foams are thought to be slightly more effective than other vaginal contraceptives such as jellies, possibly because they are more likely to adhere to the cervix and vaginal walls. Their greatest advantage is convenience. Foams are very easy to use, and the applicators may be filled up to a week in advance.

Vaginal suppositories (Encare, Intercept), which are inserted high into the vagina, gradually release their spermicide as they dissolve. To be most effective, they should be inserted 10 to 15 minutes before intercourse. Although these are easy to use, they may not completely dissolve, causing a gritty sensation during intercourse.

Vaginal jellies and creams (Koromex, Ortho-Creme), which typically contain low amounts of spermicide, can be used alone but are most effective when used in combination with barrier forms of birth control, such as a diaphragm.

Less messy than jellies and creams is the contraceptive sponge (Today). Impregnated with spermicide, these small, disposable sponges are inserted into the vagina against the cervix. They're easy to use and remain effective for up to 24 hours. But some experts say that the sponge is less effective in women who have had children because it may not form as tight a fit against the cervix.

Regardless of the type, spermicides are unlikely to cause side effects. In rare cases, women (or their partners) may get a genital rash or itching, and some women may become more prone to urinary tract infections. If this happens to you, ask your doctor or pharmacist about other choices, suggests Dr. Nelson.

Blood Pressure Medications

Policing Your Heart and Arteries

With every heartbeat, your blood courses through 60,000 *miles* of arteries, veins and capillaries. To work efficiently, this incredibly complex system requires precise amounts of pressure. Too little pressure, and the blood won't circulate. Too much, and you have a serious condition called high blood pressure, or hypertension.

Some 60 million Americans suffer from high blood pressure, although "suffer" isn't quite the right word, because this condition rarely causes symptoms. What it does is silently go about its dirty work, sometimes causing strokes, heart attacks and other serious problems. So even when high

NATURAL ALTERNATIVES

Of the millions of Americans who have high blood pressure, approximately 70 percent can keep it under control just by making some simple lifestyle changes. Here's what the experts recommend.

Try to stay trim. People who are overweight are far more likely to have high blood pressure.

Give up cigarettes. Smoking itself doesn't cause long-term increases in blood pressure, but it can cause temporary increases and can significantly boost your risk for heart disease. The sooner you quit, the better.

If you drink, do so in moderation. Drinking one or more alcoholic beverages a day can cause your blood pressure to creep upward.

Moderate your salt intake. In the past, doctors often warned people to shake the salt habit—for good. Today it's believed that only those sensitive to salt need abstain. Others can have up to four to six grams of salt a day, about one level teaspoonful—which you usually get naturally through food.

Exercise more often. People who are physically active typically have lower blood pressures. Aerobic exercise is best. Of course, if you have high blood pressure, check with your doctor before beginning an exercise program.

blood pressure is "silent," doctors say, it should never be ignored.

Watch the Numbers

Chances are your doctor checks your blood pressure whenever you visit. There are two numbers he looks at. The higher number, taken while the heart contracts, is called systolic pressure. The lower number, called diastolic, is taken while the heart relaxes.

Normal blood pressure is approximately 120 (systolic) over 80 (diastolic). In real life, however, blood pressure is constantly changing. It goes up when you exercise. It goes down when you relax. Some people get high blood pressure just from having their blood pressure checked—a condition doctors humorously refer to as white-coat hypertension.

If your blood pressure on average runs as high or higher than 140 over 90, you may need medical treatment, says Norman M. Kaplan, M.D., a blood pressure expert at the University of Texas

Health Science Center at Dallas. This usually means losing weight, exercising, reducing sodium intake and, in some cases, cutting back on alcohol. When these simple measures aren't sufficient, your doctor probably will recommend medications.

Flush Away Fluids

The drugs most commonly used to relieve high blood pressure are called diuretics, or water pills. These prescription drugs work by causing people to urinate more often. This reduces the amount of

---

AT A GLANCE

INDAPAMIDE

Brand name: Lozol

How taken: Tablet

Prescription: Yes

	YES	NO
Generic substitutes		✓
Potentially addicting		✓
May cause drowsiness	✓	
Alcohol discouraged	✓	

Possible drug interactions include: The effects of this drug may decrease if taken with antihistamines. Taking this drug may increase the effects of lithium (used to treat manic depression) and other blood pressure medications; taking it may decrease the effects of oral diabetes drugs.

Possible side effects include: Dry mouth, fatigue, irregular heartbeat and changes in blood sugar levels.

FUROSEMIDE

Brand name: Lasix

How taken: Tablet, liquid, injection

Prescription: Yes

	YES	NO
Generic substitutes	✓	
Potentially addicting		✓
May cause drowsiness		✓
Alcohol discouraged	✓	

Possible drug interactions include: The effects of this drug may decrease if taken with antihistamines. Taking this drug may increase the effects of lithium (used to treat manic depression), heart drugs and other blood pressure medications; taking it may decrease the effects of oral diabetes drugs.

Possible side effects include: Dizziness, increase in blood sugar and uric acid levels and decrease in potassium levels, which can cause muscle cramps.

CAUTION: May cause intense sensitivity to sunlight. To prevent painful rash or sunburn, be sure to wear sunscreen and protective clothing whenever going outside.

447

AT A GLANCE

NIFEDIPINE

Brand names: Adalat, Procardia

How taken: Tablet, capsule

Prescription: Yes

	YES	NO
Generic substitutes	✓	
Potentially addicting		✓
May cause drowsiness	✓	
Alcohol discouraged	✓	

Possible drug interactions include: The effects of this drug may decrease if taken with medications containing antihistamines. Taking this drug may increase the effects of beta-blockers such as atenolol (another blood pressure drug) or heart medications such as digitalis.

Possible side effects include: Dizziness, headache, weakness, nausea, rapid heart rate, sweating and swelling of the feet and ankles.

ENALAPRIL

Brand name: Vasotec

How taken: Tablet

Prescription: Yes

	YES	NO
Generic substitutes		✓
Potentially addicting		✓
May cause drowsiness		✓
Alcohol discouraged	✓	

Possible drug interactions include: The effects of this drug may decrease if taken with medications containing antihistamines. This drug taken in combination with diuretics (water pills) or potassium supplements may result in an increased amount of potassium in the bloodstream, which can lead to heart rhythm problems.

Possible side effects include: Dizziness, fainting and dry cough.

fluid in the bloodstream, which in turn lowers blood pressure, says Dr. Kaplan.

Usually taken orally, prescription medications such as chlorothiazide (Diuril), indapamide (Lozol) and furosemide (Lasix), can lower blood pressure within two to four weeks. "They're very inexpensive and very effective medications," says John F. Setaro, M.D., director of the Cardiovascular Disease Prevention Center at Yale University School of Medicine.

For people who have mild hypertension, diuretics alone may do the trick. In more serious cases, they may be combined with other medications, says Dr. Setaro. Although diuretics are quite safe, they aren't without problems. Many people get tired of having to urinate so frequently. In addition, some diuretics leach potassium from the body, which can cause weakness or confusion.

One solution to this problem is to replace the lost mineral with supplements. Or your doctor may prescribe a potassium-sparing diuretic instead. A combination diuretic such as triamterene and hydrochlorothiazide (Dyazide, Maxzide), taken orally, can help lower blood pressure without depleting potassium, says Dr. Kaplan. A diuretic such as spironolactone (Aldactone), also taken orally, is another option.

Open the Pipes

Another way to lower high blood pressure is to increase the diameter of the blood vessels. This is very efficiently done with medications called calcium channel blockers, says Alan D. Forker, M.D., professor of medicine at the

---

AT A GLANCE

PRAZOSIN

Brand names: Hypovase, Minipress

How taken: Capsule
Prescription: Yes

	YES	NO
Generic substitutes	✓	
Potentially addicting		✓
May cause drowsiness	✓	
Alcohol discouraged	✓	

Possible drug interactions include: The effects of this drug may increase if taken with diuretics (water pills) or beta-blockers such as atenolol (another blood pressure drug); effects of this drug may decrease if taken with medications containing antihistamines.

Possible side effects include: Dizziness, dry mouth, stuffy nose and constipation.

CLONIDINE

Brand name: Catapres

How taken: Tablet, patch
Prescription: Yes

	YES	NO
Generic substitutes	✓	
Potentially addicting		✓
May cause drowsiness	✓	
Alcohol discouraged	✓	

Possible drug interactions include: The effects of this drug may decrease if taken with some antidepressants. Taking this drug may decrease the effects of levodopa (used for Parkinson's disease). This drug taken in combination with other blood pressure medications may cause rebound high blood pressure.

Possible side effects include: Fatigue, dizziness, constipation and dryness of the nose and mouth.

AT A GLANCE

PROPRANOLOL

Brand names: Inderal, Inderal LA

How taken: Tablet, capsule, liquid, injection

Prescription: Yes

	YES	NO
Generic substitutes	✓	
Potentially addicting		✓
May cause drowsiness	✓	
Alcohol discouraged	✓	

Possible drug interactions include: The effects of this drug may decrease if taken with monoamine oxidase (MAO) inhibitors (used for depression) or anti-inflammatory drugs such as indomethacin. Taking this drug may increase the effects of other blood pressure medications. This drug taken in combination with clonidine (another blood pressure drug) may cause rebound high blood pressure.

Possible side effects include: Fatigue, dizziness, slow heart rate, cold hands and feet and insomnia.

ATENOLOL

Brand name: Tenormin

How taken: Tablet, injection

Prescription: Yes

	YES	NO
Generic substitutes		✓
Potentially addicting		✓
May cause drowsiness	✓	
Alcohol discouraged	✓	

Possible drug interactions include: The effects of this drug may decrease if taken with monoamine oxidase (MAO) inhibitors (used for depression) or anti-inflammatory drugs such as indomethacin. Taking this drug may increase the effects of other blood pressure medications. This drug taken in combination with clonidine (another blood pressure drug) may cause rebound high blood pressure.

Possible side effects include: Dizziness, fatigue, slow heart rate, cold hands and feet and insomnia.

University of Missouri–Kansas City School of Medicine and chief of cardiology at the Truman Medical Center in Kansas City. Prescription drugs such as nifedipine (Adalat, Procardia), diltiazem (Cardizem) and verapamil (Calan, Isoptin, Verelan), usually taken orally, work by preventing calcium atoms from slipping inside muscle cells in the blood vessels. Without calcium, blood vessels expand. This causes blood pressure to go down, says Dr. Forker.

These drugs can be very effective, although they may cause constipation, dizziness or other side effects, says Dr. Kaplan. They're also considerably more expensive than the diuretics.

A class of drugs called angiotension-converting enzyme (or ACE) inhibitors work in a similar fashion to the calcium blockers, while causing fewer side effects. In fact, prescription medications such as captopril (Capoten), enalapril (Vasotec) and lisinopril (Prinivil, Zestril), usually taken orally, actually can reduce side effects—such as the dip in potassium levels—that may be caused by diuretics. Some doctors prescribe ACE inhibitors together with diuretics for added effectiveness. Both types of drugs are available in combination products such as Capozide and Vaseretic.

Yet another class of drugs used to relax blood vessels is called alpha-adrenergic blocking agents, or alpha-blockers. Prescription medications such as prazosin (Hypovase, Minipress) and terazosin (Hytrin), taken orally, can help lower both blood pressure and cholesterol, while rarely causing side effects. However, adds Dr. Setaro, they're frequently less effective than the other drugs.

Old-Fashioned Help

Perhaps the oldest drugs used for treating high blood pressure are those that act directly on the brain. Called centrally acting agents, these medications help lower blood pressure by "turning off" specialized receptors (nerve endings) in the brain. This causes blood vessels to expand.

Prescription medications such as clonidine (Catapres), guanfacine (Tenex) and methyldopa (Aldomet), usually taken orally, have been a mainstay of blood pressure therapy for decades, says Dr. Kaplan. Yet these drugs are generally less effective than modern medications. They also may cause pronounced side effects, including a dry mouth, drowsiness and fatigue.

Easing the Force

So far, we've looked at medications that either make blood vessels larger or, in the case of diuretics, remove fluids from the system. But there's another way to lower blood pressure: by making the heart pump less forcefully.

A class of drugs called beta-adrenergic blocking agents, or beta-blockers, work by preventing a body chemical called norepinephrine from stimulating the heart muscle. This causes the heart to beat more slowly and with less force, lowering blood pressure.

Prescription medications such as propranolol (Inderal, Inderal LA), atenolol (Tenormin) and metoprolol (Lopressor), usually taken orally, can be very effective, says Dr. Forker. They may be used by themselves but frequently are combined with diuretics, he says.

Unfortunately, adds Dr. Forker,

"beta-blockers can have worrisome side effects, including fatigue, insomnia and depression." They can cause a mild increase in cholesterol, which in time can *raise* blood pressure by narrowing arteries. They may also cause serious breathing problems in people with asthma.

But, says Dr. Forker, there are some newer beta-blockers—for example, acebutolol (Sectral)—that can lower blood pressure without raising cholesterol.

Cancer Drugs

Tumor Battlers

Every year more than one-and-a-half million people will be diagnosed with cancer. About one in three Americans will have cancer at some time in their lives, and approximately half a million will die from it. Frightening though these numbers are, doctors have developed some powerful weapons for fighting back. Among these weapons is chemotherapy, the use of potent prescription drugs.

"With chemotherapy we've been able to increase cure rates from zero in the 1950s to, for testicular cancer, about 90 percent," says Irwin H. Krakoff, M.D., head of the Division of Medicine at M. D. Anderson Cancer Center at the University of Texas in Houston. For Hodgkin's disease, the cure rate also approaches 90 percent; for lymphocytic leukemia, about 70 percent; for some lymphomas, about 50 percent.

Drugs don't always bring a cure, of course. But in many cases they can at least help slow down the progression of the disease and perhaps prevent the cancer from spreading.

Chemical Weapons

Cancer cells don't act like normal cells. They not only divide and reproduce very rapidly, they live longer, too. It's this out-of-control growth that causes tumors and metastasis—the spread of cancer cells to different parts of the body.

"Even when we see a cancer that appears to be localized—in the breast, for example—there may be cancer cells also circulating in the

452

NATURAL ALTERNATIVES

Women with breast cancer often are anxious, depressed and in pain. So researchers at Stanford University School of Medicine asked some of these women to attend support groups for 90 minutes a week. At the very least, thought the researchers, the weekly meetings would help the women make friends, cope with their illness and develop a sense of emotional well-being.

As they expected, many of the women did start feeling better. What took the doctors by surprise was that many of their patients lived longer—on average, 18 months longer—than women who didn't attend the meetings.

In the study, 86 women with advanced breast cancer were divided into two groups. Women in one group received standard medical care. Those in the other group received similar care, plus they met weekly with fellow patients and a psychiatrist or social worker. In the meetings they swapped stories, practiced self-hypnosis and encouraged each other to be more assertive and to help other patients and their families.

The support groups may have helped in two ways, says Stanford's Jim Spira, Ph.D., a fellow and instructor in the Department of Psychiatry and Behavioral Sciences. First, people who feel stronger emotionally can often tolerate more rigorous medical treatment. Second, "social support and improved mood impacts the immune system, especially the natural killer cells, which, in turn, regulate the spread of cancer," says Dr. Spira.

bloodstream," explains Gary Fishbein, M.D., an oncologist (cancer specialist) and clinical assistant professor of medicine at Thomas Jefferson University Hospital in Philadelphia.

Prescription cancer drugs, usually taken orally or by injection, primarily target these circulating cells. They can also affect the body's normal cells, but these effects are usually temporary, says Dr. Fishbein.

Finding the Right Combination

Cancer cells are not all alike. In fact, two people with the same disease may have many different types of cells. That's why doctors usually prescribe two or more cancer drugs during the course of treatment.

For example, someone with Hodgkin's disease might be given mechlorethamine (Mustargen), vin-

AT A GLANCE

MECHLORETHAMINE

Brand name: Mustargen

How taken: Injection

Prescription: Yes

	YES	NO
Generic substitutes		✓
Potentially addicting		✓
May cause drowsiness		✓
Alcohol discouraged		✓

Possible drug interactions include: The effects of this drug may decrease if taken with oral contraceptives. Taking this drug may increase the effects of other cancer medications; taking it may decrease the effects of probenecid and sulfinpyrazone (both used for gout).

Possible side effects include: Black stools, pain or redness at site of injection, bleeding, bruising, blood in urine, fever, chills, cough or hoarseness, painful or difficult urination, pinpoint-size red spots on skin and lower back or side pain.

VINCRISTINE

Brand names: Oncovin, Vincasar PFS, Vincrex

How taken: Injection

Prescription: Yes

	YES	NO
Generic substitutes	✓	
Potentially addicting		✓
May cause drowsiness		✓
Alcohol discouraged		✓

Possible drug interactions include: Taking this drug may increase the effects of other cancer medications; taking it may decrease the effects of probenecid and sulfinpyrazone (both used for gout). This drug taken in combination with vaccines may increase the risk of infection.

Possible side effects include: Fever, chills, cough, hoarseness, red spots on skin, black stools, pain or redness at site of injection, stomach cramps, constipation, nausea, vomiting and hair loss.

cristine (Oncovin, Vincasar PFS, Vincrex) and procarbazine (Matulane), as well as with the anti-inflammatory drug prednisone. "Let's say any one of these drugs may have a 33 percent chance of creating a positive response," says Dr. Fishbein. "When you combine them all together, greater than three-fourths of patients will have a very meaningful response to the treatment."

There are dozens of cancer drugs available. Some of the most common include fluorouracil (Adrucil, Efudex), bleomycin (Blenoxane) and cisplatin (Platinol, Platinol-AQ). Which drugs your doctor chooses to use will depend on the kind of cancer you have, the extent of its growth and how well you respond to the treatment.

Chemotherapy will in some cases be used in combination with other treatments, such as radiation therapy or surgery.

Upcoming Treatments

Although some of the most effective cancer drugs have been in use since the 1950s, others are still in their infancy.

AT A GLANCE

PROCARBAZINE

Brand name: Matulane

How taken: Capsule

Prescription: Yes

	YES	NO
Generic substitutes		✓
Potentially addicting		✓
May cause drowsiness	✓	
Alcohol discouraged	✓	

Possible drug interactions include: Taking this drug may increase the effects of diabetes drugs, antihistamines, insulin, ipratropium (used for asthma), meclizine (a nausea drug) and promethazine (an antihistamine). This drug taken in combination with amphetamines, dextromethorphan (a cough medicine), methyldopa (a blood pressure drug), cold or asthma medications or narcotics may result in high blood pressure; taking it with vaccines may increase the risk of infection.

Possible side effects include: Stiff or sore neck, irregular heartbeat, dilated pupils, headache, hair loss, high blood pressure and muscle or joint pain; may make eyes more light sensitive.

FLUOROURACIL

Brand names: Adrucil, Efudex, 5-FU, Fluoroplex

How taken: Injection, cream

Prescription: Yes

	YES	NO
Generic substitutes	✓	
Potentially addicting		✓
May cause drowsiness		✓
Alcohol discouraged		✓

Possible drug interactions include: Taking this drug, by injection, may increase the effects of antifungal drugs, anti-thyroid drugs, azathioprine (an immunosuppressant), chloramphenicol (an antibiotic), colchicine (a gout drug), flucytosine (an antifungal drug), zidovudine (used to treat AIDS) and plicamycin (another cancer drug). This drug taken in combination with vaccines may increase the risk of infection.

Possible side effects include: Diarrhea, heartburn, sores in mouth, black stools, nausea, vomiting, difficult or painful urination, stomach cramps, fever and chills.

CAUTION: May increase sensitivity to sunlight, possibly resulting in serious burns.

AT A GLANCE

CISPLATIN

Brand names: Platinol, Platinol-AQ

How taken: Injection

Prescription: Yes

	YES	NO
Generic substitutes		✓
Potentially addicting		✓
May cause drowsiness		✓
Alcohol discouraged	✓	

Possible drug interactions include: Taking this drug may increase the effects of antifungal drugs, antithyroid drugs, azathioprine (an immunosuppressant), chloramphenicol (an antibiotic), colchicine (used for gout), plicamycin (another cancer drug) and zidovudine (used to treat AIDS). This drug taken in combination with vaccines may increase the risk of infection.

Possible side effects include: Black stools, blood in urine or stools, redness or pain at the injection site, coughing, hoarseness, fever, chills and joint or lower back pain.

TAMOXIFEN

Brand name: Nolvadex

How taken: Tablet

Prescription: Yes

	YES	NO
Generic substitutes		✓
Potentially addicting		✓
May cause drowsiness		✓
Alcohol discouraged		✓

Possible drug interactions include: The effects of this drug may decrease if taken with oral contraceptives.

Possible side effects include: Increased fertility, headache, nausea, vomiting, hot flashes, weight gain and bone pain.

One of the most promising treatments is the experimental drug taxol. In one study, researchers at Johns Hopkins Oncology Center in Baltimore gave injections of taxol every 22 days to women with a drug-resistant type of ovarian cancer. In 30 percent of the cases, tumor size was reduced for 3 to 15 months, a performance researchers summarized as remarkable.

Another promising prescription drug is tamoxifen (Nolvadex). Taken orally, it works by preventing the hormone estrogen from fueling the growth of some breast cancers. Researchers in the United States and Canada have embarked on an extensive study to determine if ta-moxifen, taken daily, actually can help prevent breast cancer for women with a high risk of con-tracting the disease.

Some drugs in the cancer war are copies of chemicals already in your body. In experiments, high doses of interferons, interleukins and other naturally occurring pro-teins have been found to stimulate the immune system, which in turn may destroy cancerous cells, says Dr. Krakoff. He adds, however, that this therapy is still experimental. It may be many more years before "biological" therapy joins chemo-therapy on the cancer front.

Coping with Chemotherapy

The ideal drug would destroy every cancer cell in your body without making you sick in the process. Unfortunately, that drug doesn't yet exist. Chemotherapy often causes pain, nausea, hair loss, fatigue and other troublesome side effects.

To reduce the problems (and boost the benefits) of chemother-apy, cancer drugs usually are given in cycles. "People may get treat-ment every three to four weeks for six to eight months," says Dr. Fish-bein. This allows the drugs to de-stroy cancer cells without over-whelming healthy cells.

There are many things you can do to make yourself more comfort-able during chemotherapy. For ex-ample:

- Eat small meals throughout the day. This can help reduce the nausea you may experience before and during treatments. In general, it's best not to eat for at least a few hours before taking the drugs.

- Get plenty of rest. Because can-cer drugs reduce the number of oxygen-carrying red blood cells in the bloodstream, you may feel tired and fatigued. Con-serve your energy, doctors say. Try to sleep more at night and take naps during the day.

- Watch out for infections. Can-cer drugs also reduce the num-ber of infection-fighting white blood cells in the body. As a result, infections are common. Be sure to wash your hands often during the day. Use sani-tary napkins instead of tam-pons. Trim your nails carefully, and, to avoid nicks, shave with an electric razor instead of a blade; small wounds like these are open doors for germs.

Cholesterol-Lowering Drugs

Potential Lifesavers

Cholesterol is the goo that everybody loves to hate—with good reason. If you have gobs of cholesterol lollygagging about in your arteries, they could possibly block the movement of blood. When that happens, you could find yourself in a race-through-the-streets visit to the coronary care unit of your local hospital . . . and you won't be in the driver's seat.

Fortunately, cholesterol-lowering drugs could save you the trip. Studies have shown that for every *1 percent* reduction in cholesterol, you can reduce your risk for heart disease by *2 percent* or more. There are a number of cholesterol-lowering drugs available, and they work very well, says Simeon Margolis, M.D., Ph.D., professor of medicine at Johns Hopkins University School of Medicine in Baltimore. These drugs are generally used, he says, as a last resort when dietary changes, such as shunning fatty foods and eating more fiber, have

been tried and have failed to lower a high cholesterol count. For some people who have been dealt a bad hereditary hand, even the strictest of diets may not be enough.

Drug treatment for high cholesterol is not a short-term affair. Most people who take these drugs take them forever.

Sticky Solutions

For dangerously high cholesterol, doctors often prescribe drugs called bile acid resins, or sequestrants. Medications such as cholestyramine (Cholybar, Questran) and colestipol (Colestid), taken orally, cause the body to withdraw cholesterol from the bloodstream and to excrete it. As a result, LDL cholesterol (the dangerous kind) may plummet 15 to 30 percent.

Because these drugs aren't absorbed by the body—they do all their work in the intestine—they're safe for long-term use. "They are the standard-bearers for the treatment of high cholesterol," says James M. McKenney, Pharm.D., professor of pharmacy at Virginia Commonwealth University/Medical College of Virginia in Richmond.

The bile acid resins do have drawbacks, however. One, they stick not only to cholesterol but also to other medications, blocking their effects. And they often come in powder form, with a gritty texture many people dislike, says Dr. Margolis. Finally, they can cause uncomfortable side effects, including constipation and cramping.

To reduce side effects, doctors usually begin treatment with low doses, slowly increasing them as the body adjusts. In addition, drinking lots of water can help prevent constipation, says Dr. McKenney.

A Victorious Vitamin

The B vitamin nicotinic acid, or niacin, also is very effective for lowering cholesterol. Taken orally, this over-the-counter and prescription drug (Niacor, Nicobid) can lower LDL cholesterol by about 25 percent, while boosting the protective HDL cholesterol by roughly 30 percent. It has the added benefit of being the least expensive of all the cholesterol-lowering drugs, says Dr. Margolis.

Still, niacin therapy requires a

NATURAL ALTERNATIVES

Doctors agree that most people can lower high cholesterol just by watching what they eat. So before embarking on drug therapy, here are some things to try.

Trim fat from your diet. Foods high in saturated fats, such as cheeseburgers, pork chops, french fries, chocolate shakes and doughnuts, can drive your cholesterol to artery-clogging levels.

Cut fat from your meat. Instead of buying fatty cuts like prime rib, shop for lean meats like top round. And be sure to trim visible fat from meat before you start cooking.

Fill up on fiber. Fiber-rich foods such as vegetables, fruit and grains ferry cholesterol from the body. They also fill you up, leaving less room for fatty foods.

Have some extra C. Researchers have found that vitamin C, abundant in many fruits and vegetables, can help boost the amounts of protective HDL cholesterol in the bloodstream.

Don't forget to exercise. Researchers have also found that losing weight and adding muscle may knock a few points off a high cholesterol count.

doctor's supervision. To be effective, it must be taken in very large doses, usually between one and three grams a day. These amounts can cause severe redness and itching of the face and neck. More rarely, it can cause liver inflammation and gastrointestinal problems. "A lot of people can't tolerate niacin," says Dr. Margolis.

An alternative is slow-release niacin (Slo-Niacin), which is less likely to cause flushing. Yet slow-release niacin may have a greater risk of causing liver problems, says Dr. McKenney. It's also more expensive. As a result, most doctors prefer the older forms of the drug.

Enzyme Blockers

A group of prescription drugs called reductase inhibitors act directly on the liver. Medications such as lovastatin (Mevacor), pravastatin (Pravachol) and simvastatin (Zocor), taken orally, work

---

AT A GLANCE

CHOLESTYRAMINE

Brand names: Cholybar, Questran

How taken: Powder, chewable bar

Prescription: Yes

	YES	NO
Generic substitutes		✓
Potentially addicting		✓
May cause drowsiness		✓
Alcohol discouraged		✓

Possible drug interactions include: Taking this drug may decrease the effects of warfarin (an anti-clotting drug), chlorothiazide (a blood pressure drug), propranolol (used for heart and blood pressure problems), tetracycline (an antibiotic) and phenobarbital (used for seizures).

Possible side effects include: Cramping, bloating and constipation.

COLESTIPOL

Brand name: Colestid

How taken: Powder

Prescription: Yes

	YES	NO
Generic substitutes		✓
Potentially addicting		✓
May cause drowsiness		✓
Alcohol discouraged		✓

Possible drug interactions include: Taking this drug may decrease the effects of the mineral iron, acetaminophen, digitoxin and digoxin (both used for heart problems) and phenobarbital (used for seizures).

Possible side effects include: Constipation, nausea and bloating.

AT A GLANCE

NIACIN		
Brand names: Niacor, Nicobid		
How taken: Capsule, liquid, tablet		
Prescription: Sometimes, depending on strength		
	YES	**NO**
Generic substitutes	✓	
Potentially addicting		✓
May cause drowsiness	✓	
Alcohol discouraged		✓

Possible drug interactions include: Taking this drug may increase the effects of some blood pressure medications, causing low blood pressure.

Possible side effects include: Diarrhea, darkening of urine, flushing, dizziness and itching and tingling of the face and neck.

SLOW-RELEASE NIACIN		
Brand name: Slo-Niacin		
How taken: Capsule, tablet		
Prescription: Sometimes, depending on strength		
	YES	**NO**
Generic substitutes	✓	
Potentially addicting		✓
May cause drowsiness	✓	
Alcohol discouraged		✓

Possible drug interactions include: Taking this drug may increase the effects of some blood pressure medications, causing low blood pressure.

Possible side effects include: Headache, indigestion, flushing and itching and tingling of the face and neck.

by blocking an enzyme called HMG CoA reductase. This, in turn, helps stem the liver's output of cholesterol.

Lovastatin and the other reductase inhibitors appear to be extremely safe, although they may cause minor liver inflammation. Also, some people may experience gas, nausea and other minor side effects. Still, lovastatin and its cousins are rapidly becoming the drugs of choice for lowering cholesterol. Not only are they the most effective, but they are convenient. There are no gritty powders as with the resins. These drugs are taken as tablets. "It's so much easier to take a reductase inhibitor than some of the other drugs," comments Dr. Margolis.

Other Options

If a single drug doesn't do the trick, your doctor may combine drugs for better results. For example, niacin combined with a resin will slow cholesterol production while speeding its excretion. In one study, this combination lowered total cholesterol by 45 percent,

AT A GLANCE

LOVASTATIN

Brand name: Mevacor

How taken: Tablet

Prescription: Yes

	YES	NO
Generic substitutes		✓
Potentially addicting		✓
May cause drowsiness		✓
Alcohol discouraged	✓	

Possible drug interactions include: This drug taken in combination with gemfibrozil (another cholesterol-lowering drug) or cyclosporine (an immunosuppressant) may result in muscle problems.

Possible side effects include: Stomach pain, diarrhea, skin rash and headache.

GEMFIBROZIL

Brand name: Lopid

How taken: Capsule, tablet

Prescription: Yes

	YES	NO
Generic substitutes		✓
Potentially addicting		✓
May cause drowsiness	✓	
Alcohol discouraged		✓

Possible drug interactions include: Taking this drug may increase the effects of warfarin (an anti-clotting drug); taking it may decrease the effects of chenodiol (a gallstone-dissolving drug).

Possible side effects include: Gas, stomach pain, diarrhea and increases in blood sugar.

while increasing the protective HDL by a similar amount.

Yet another option is a class of drugs called fibric acid derivatives. Taken orally, medications such as gemfibrozil (Lopid) and clofibrate (Atromid-S) can be very effective. They're primarily prescribed to people who have both high cholesterol levels and high levels of triglycerides, another type of blood fat, says Dr. Margolis.

It's important to remember that none of these drugs cures high cholesterol. You have to take them for life, says Dr. Margolis. Stop taking them, and once again the goo will start building up in your arteries.

Cold Remedies

Quick Relief for Stubborn Symptoms

In the last 50 years medical science has made incredible progress in battling disease. Conditions such as smallpox and polio have virtually been eradicated, and dozens of other diseases are prevented with vaccines. Other infections are treated by antibiotics.

Unfortunately, there is one infectious disease that modern medicine, with all its technology and drugs, can't stop: the common cold.

Caused by dozens of different viruses, the most common being the rhinovirus, this miserable condition descends on the average adult two to four times a year. When it hits, it causes coughs, sneezes, sniffles and other uncomfortable symptoms. Viruses are extremely adaptable and hard to kill, which is why there still isn't a cure for the common cold. There are, however, a number of medications that can help make its seasonal visits easier to bear.

NATURAL ALTERNATIVES

To turn the tables on sniffles and help bring out the smiles, try the following:

Stir up some chicken soup. Some researchers believe there really is something special about Grandma's favorite remedy. Whether it's the heat from the broth, the aromatic smell or some "secret" ingredient, hot chicken soup does humidify the airways and help break up nasal congestion.

Take a soothing bath. Experts agree there's nothing quite like soaking in a hot bath to ease a cold's aches and steam the airways open.

Fill up on liquids. It's important to drink six to eight glasses of water, juice or tea every day to replace lost fluids and keep your nose and throat comfortably lubricated until the cold has finally run its course.

AT A GLANCE

OXYMETAZOLINE

Brand names: Dristan Long Lasting Nasal Spray, Vicks Sinex Long-Acting 12-Hour Nasal Spray

How taken: Nasal spray, nose drops

Prescription: No

	YES	NO
Generic substitutes	✓	
Potentially addicting		✓
May cause drowsiness		✓
Alcohol discouraged		✓

Possible drug interactions include: Taking this drug may decrease the effects of some heart and blood pressure medications; taking it may increase the effects (and side effects) of antihistamines and bronchodilators. This drug taken in combination with methyldopa (a blood pressure drug) may result in high blood pressure.

Possible side effects include: Burning, dryness and stinging of the nose, sneezing and a runny nose.

CAUTION: When used for more than three days, rebound congestion may occur. May be extremely dangerous when taken with monoamine oxidase (MAO) inhibitors (used for depression).

PSEUDOEPHEDRINE

Brand names: Afrinol Repetabs, Halofed, Sudafed

How taken: Tablet, capsule, liquid

Prescription: Sometimes, depending on strength

	YES	NO
Generic substitutes	✓	
Potentially addicting		✓
May cause drowsiness		✓
Alcohol discouraged		✓

Possible drug interactions include: Taking this drug may decrease the effects of atenolol, betaxolol, propanolol and other beta-blocking drugs (used for high blood pressure). This drug taken in combination with monoamine oxidase (MAO) inhibitors (used for depression) may result in high blood pressure.

Possible side effects include: Restlessness and insomnia.

Choosing the Right Drug

Although there are more than 800 cold remedies on pharmacy shelves, all contain one (or more) of just a handful of medications commonly used to relieve cough, congestion and other cold symptoms, says Michael L. Macknin, M.D., head of the Section of General Pediatrics at the Cleveland Clinic in Ohio.

In the belief that if one is good, more must be better, many drug companies include several ingredients in each remedy—a practice

464

doctors refer to as the shotgun approach. Typical "shotguns" are Robitussin Night Relief, NyQuil Nighttime Colds Medicine and Tylenol Cold Medication, which contain drugs for pain, cough, congestion and a runny nose.

The advantage of shotgun remedies is that, like their namesake, they're almost certain to hit *something*. On the other hand, some doctors say, why take medications to relieve symptoms you may not even have? "It doesn't make sense to take an antihistamine, a decongestant and an expectorant when all you want to do is suppress your cough," says Dr. Macknin.

Rather than taking multiple-ingredient products, he says, it makes more sense to match the medication with your symptoms.

AT A GLANCE

DEXTROMETHORPHAN

Brand names: Benylin DM, Mediquell, Pertussin CS

How taken: Tablet, liquid, lozenge

Prescription: No

	YES	NO
Generic substitutes	✓	
Potentially addicting		✓
May cause drowsiness	✓	
Alcohol discouraged	✓	

Possible drug interactions include: The effects of this drug may increase if taken with antihistamines, antidepressants, sedatives or narcotics. This drug taken in combination with furazolidone (an antibiotic) or monoamine oxidase (MAO) inhibitors (used for depression) may result in high blood pressure.

Possible side effects include: Side effects are unlikely.

CAUTION: If you have asthma, talk to your doctor before taking this drug.

ASPIRIN

Brand names: Anacin, Genuine Bayer Aspirin, Empirin

How taken: Tablet, capsule, chewing gum, suppository

Prescription: No

	YES	NO
Generic substitutes	✓	
Potentially addicting		✓
May cause drowsiness		✓
Alcohol discouraged	✓	

Possible drug interactions include: Taking this drug may increase the effects of methotrexate (used for psoriasis, cancer and rheumatoid arthritis) and some oral diabetes medications. This drug taken in combination with anti-clotting drugs may increase the risk of bleeding.

Possible side effects include: Nausea, indigestion and stomach cramps. Long-term use may cause internal bleeding.

AT A GLANCE

ACETAMINOPHEN

Brand names: Actamin, Datril Extra-Strength, Maximum Strength Panadol, Tylenol

How taken: Tablet, capsule, liquid

Prescription: No

	YES	NO
Generic substitutes	✓	
Potentially addicting		✓
May cause drowsiness		✓
Alcohol discouraged	✓	

Possible drug interactions include: This drug taken in combination with zidovudine (used to treat AIDS) may increase the risk of side effects, such as fatigue and weakness.

Possible side effects include: Side effects are unlikely.

IBUPROFEN

Brand names: Advil, Haltran, Motrin IB, Nuprin

How taken: Capsule, tablet, liquid

Prescription: Sometimes, depending on strength

	YES	NO
Generic substitutes	✓	
Potentially addicting		✓
May cause drowsiness	✓	
Alcohol discouraged		✓

Possible drug interactions include: This drug taken in combination with anti-clotting and anti-inflammatory medications may increase the risk of bleeding.

Possible side effects include: Nausea, diarrhea, dizziness, mild stomach cramps, fluid retention (weight gain) and discoloration of urine.

CAUTION: Do not take if you are allergic to aspirin.

Suppose you have a stuffy nose. For short-term relief, your best bet would be to use a fast-acting, over-the-counter decongestant spray containing oxymetazoline (Dristan Long Lasting Nasal Spray, Vicks Sinex Long-Acting 12-Hour Nasal Spray). For long-term relief, you're better off with an oral decongestant such as pseudoephedrine (Afrinol Repetabs, Halofed, Sudafed).

When your cold is accompanied by a rib-wracking, sleep-disturbing cough, you may want an over-the-counter cough suppressant called dextromethorphan (Benylin DM, Mediquell, Pertussin CS). Taken orally, this medication puts a damper on the cough center inside the brain, relieving coughs without, in most cases, causing side effects.

Many cold remedies contain an over-the-counter oral antihistamine called diphenhydramine (Diphen Cough, Nordryl Cough). This medication may be somewhat helpful in drying a runny nose, although doctors agree it's likely to be more effective for allergies than for colds.

For short-term relief of a sore throat, over-the-counter lozenges or sprays containing an anesthetic such as benzocaine (Spec-T Sore Throat) or menthol (Luden's Original Menthol Throat Drops) can be a big help. Be sure not to inhale while applying the spray, which can make it less effective. Also, lozenges should be allowed to slowly dissolve—chewing them doesn't count!

Finally, nearly everyone with a cold will have headaches or miscel-laneous aches and pains. For adults, the easiest (and cheapest) way to relieve cold aches is with over-the-counter painkillers such as aspirin (Anacin, Genuine Bayer Aspirin, Empirin), acetaminophen (Actamin, Datril Extra-Strength, Tylenol) or ibuprofen (Advil, Motrin IB, Nuprin).

For children, however, aspirin shouldn't be used because of the slight risk of Reye's syndrome, an extremely dangerous liver and neurological problem, says Dr. Macknin. To be safe, he says, give them only aspirin substitutes such as acetaminophen.

Cough Medicines

Promoters and Inhibitors

It always happens at the worst of times—at church services, for example, or during the hushed opening movement of *Bolero*. First your throat feels a little dry. Then there's an itch . . . a tickle . . . an irrepressible urge. Then you explode with a hacking, wracking, thunderous cough.

Although coughing can be terribly annoying (just ask your neighbors at the symphony), it's an important part of your body's lung-cleaning mechanism. "I tell people to go ahead and cough," says Michael L. Macknin, M.D., head of the Section of General Pediatrics at the Cleveland Clinic in Ohio. "You need to keep your airways clear, and that's what a cough is designed to do."

At least, that's what *productive* coughs—those that bring up phlegm—are designed to do. Dry coughs, on the other hand, come up empty, says Dr. Macknin. There are different medicines for each type of cough: those that encourage coughing, and those that stop it.

Phlegm Fighters

When you're suffering from a cold, bronchitis or allergies, a thick, sticky mucus called phlegm often begins to accumulate in the lungs and airways. Phlegm, like the last bit of honey in a jar, can be tough to budge, even with the most vigorous cough.

To get phlegm moving, doctors say, expectorants can help. These over-the-counter and prescription drugs help liquefy or thin phlegm in much the same way that hot water dissolves honey in a jar. Essentially, these drugs help coughs to clear your system of mucus, says Michael Benninger, M.D., chairman of the Department of Otolaryngology–Head and Neck Surgery at Henry Ford Hospital in Detroit.

The leading expectorant in cold and cough remedies is a drug called guaifenesin (Amonidrin, Anti-Tuss, Robitussin), available over the counter. "We frequently use guaifenesin to help keep mucus thinner," says Dr. Benninger.

Another oral expectorant is the prescription drug iodinated glycerol (Iophen, Organic-1, Organidin). In one study, people with

---

NATURAL ALTERNATIVES

There are many effective cough remedies not found in drugstores. For example:

Drink plenty of fluids. Choose warm fluids such as soup or hot tea with lemon. This helps thin mucus so it flows more readily. It also increases moisture in your respiratory tract, which can help mucus slide right out.

Get hot. Fiery foods like chili peppers and garlic get mucus flowing, which can help your lungs cough it up and out. Any slowly dissolving hard candy (go for sugar-free, of course) may help relieve cough-causing tickles in your throat. (Chomping doesn't help.)

Get steamed. Taking a hot shower or bath will fill your lungs with soothing steam. It probably won't cure your cough, but it may provide some temporary relief.

Give up the cigs. Doctors agree that smoking is a leading cause of coughs in this country. When you kick the butts, you may kick your cough, too.

AT A GLANCE

GUAIFENESIN

Brand names: Amonidrin, Anti-Tuss, Glytuss, Humibid L.A., Humibid Sprinkle, Robitussin

How taken: Capsule, liquid, tablet

Prescription: No

	Yes	No
Generic substitutes	✓	
Potentially addicting		✓
May cause drowsiness		✓
Alcohol discouraged		✓

Possible drug interactions include: Taking this drug may increase the effects of sedatives and drugs used for depression, particularly the monoamine oxidase (MAO) inhibitors.

Possible side effects include: Side effects are unlikely.

IODINATED GLYCEROL

Brand names: Iophen, Organic-1, Organidin

How taken: Liquid, tablet

Prescription: Yes

	Yes	No
Generic substitutes	✓	
Potentially addicting		✓
May cause drowsiness		✓
Alcohol discouraged		✓

Possible drug interactions include: Taking this drug may increase the effects of lithium (used for manic depression) and drugs taken for thyroid problems.

Possible side effects include: Side effects are unlikely.

bronchitis were given either iodinated glycerol or a placebo. After eight weeks, people treated with the active drug had "improved cough frequency, cough severity and chest discomfort," according to the researchers.

Dry Up Dry Coughs

Few things are more uncomfortable than dry, bone-rattling coughs. They expel no mucus and provide no benefits. Worse, they can be painful. People even have injured ribs during severe attacks.

"If the cough is keeping you up at night, then it's very reasonable to take something," Dr. Macknin says. That usually means an antitussive or cough suppressant. These are drugs that dampen electrical signals in the brain, thus blunting the urge to cough.

Many prescription and over-the-counter cough suppressants, taken orally, contain codeine (Actifed with Codeine, Anatuss with Codeine,

Dimetapp-C). Codeine is very effective, but it can cause drowsiness, constipation and other side effects, says Leonard Rybak, M.D., Ph.D., professor of surgery and pharmacology at Southern Illinois University School of Medicine in Springfield. "I prefer to stay away from potentially addicting drugs and drugs that may be sedating," he says.

Dr. Rybak says the drug of choice for dry coughs is dextromethorphan (Benylin DM, Delsym, Pertussin CS). Taken orally, this over-the-counter drug is chemically related to codeine. But it's less likely to cause side effects, says Dr. Rybak.

Some dextromethorphan preparations are effective for four hours. Others last all night. Ask your doctor or pharmacist which type is right for you.

Yet another common cough suppressant is diphenhydramine (Compoz, Nytol with DPH, Sominex Formula 2). As with codeine and dextromethorphan, this over-the-counter and prescription antihistamine, usually taken orally, acts directly on the cough center in the brain. As a result, it can cause drowsiness and other central nervous system side effects. It shouldn't be taken before driving or in situations where mental alertness is required, says Dr. Rybak.

To help relieve cough-causing tickles in the throat, many people use over-the-counter lozenges containing cooling ingredients such as menthol (Robitussin Cough Drops, Ricola Cherry Mint Herb Throat Drops). Although there's little scientific evidence that these lozenges are effective, many people say they help.

AT A GLANCE

DIPHENHYDRAMINE

Brand names: Benadryl, Compoz, Excedrin P.M., Nytol with DPH, Sominex Formula 2

How taken: Capsule, injection, liquid, tablet

Prescription: Sometimes, depending on strength

	YES	NO
Generic substitutes	✓	
Potentially addicting		✓
May cause drowsiness	✓	
Alcohol discouraged	✓	

Possible drug interactions include: The effects of this drug may increase if taken with monoamine oxidase (MAO) inhibitors (used for depression). Taking this drug may increase the effects of sedatives and atropine and related drugs used for intestinal spasms and other conditions.

Possible side effects include: Constipation, thickened mucus and dryness of the nose, mouth and throat.

CAUTION: Do not take if you have bronchitis, pneumonia or active bronchial asthma.

AT A GLANCE

CODEINE

Brand names: Actifed with Codeine, Anatuss with Codeine, Dimetapp-C

How taken: Injection, liquid, tablet

Prescription: Sometimes, depending on strength

	YES	NO
Generic substitutes	✓	
Potentially addicting	✓	
May cause drowsiness	✓	
Alcohol discouraged	✓	

Possible drug interactions include: Taking this drug may increase the effects of sedatives and atropine and related drugs used for intestinal spasms and other conditions.

Possible side effects include: Urine retention, nausea, vomiting, constipation and dryness of the mouth, nose or throat.

CAUTION: May cause thickened mucus and breathing difficulties when taken by people with asthma, bronchitis or emphysema.

DEXTROMETHORPHAN

Brand names: Benylin DM, Delsym, Mediquell, Pertussin CS, St. Joseph for Children

How taken: Liquid, lozenge, tablet

Prescription: No

	YES	NO
Generic substitutes	✓	
Potentially addicting		✓
May cause drowsiness	✓	
Alcohol discouraged	✓	

Possible drug interactions include: Taking this drug may increase the effects of sedatives. This drug taken in combination with monoamine oxidase (MAO) inhibitors (used for depression) may result in disorientation or other problems.

Possible side effects include: Side effects are unlikely.

CAUTION: If you have asthma, talk to your doctor before taking this drug.

Decongestants

Offering a Breath of Fresh Air

The average adult gets two to four colds a year, while young children may have six to ten. That's a lot of sniffly, stuffy, unhappy noses. In most cases a stuffy nose will get un- stuffed within a few days to a week. But in the meantime, you can't breathe, you can't sleep and you sound like Elmer Fudd. That's when decongestants can come to your nose's defense.

NATURAL ALTERNATIVES

You may not have to go to the drugstore to get a decongestant. Here are some things you can do at home to help relieve conges- tion.

Heat your palate. Eating spicy foods such as curry, hot peppers and horseradish can get your nose running in a hurry. Or, if you're not up to a full meal, try mixing half a dozen drops of Tabasco sauce in a cup of warm water.

Drink up. By drinking plenty of fluids—anything from water or orange juice to broth—you may help thin the sticky secretions that are clogging you up.

Call tea time. Perhaps it's the steam that helps, but many people say that drinking hot tea laced with honey and lemon helps relieve minor congestion. Others swear by hot chicken soup.

Get clean. A relaxing way to possible short-term relief may be a hot bath or shower. Or heat up a pot of water, turn off the stove, drape a towel over your head and the pot, and inhale the steam. Make sure that you keep your face at least 18 inches from the pot so you don't burn yourself.

Nose Plugs

Before talking about *decongestants*, let's take a look at congestion. Nasal congestion is a buildup of mucus and the swelling of blood vessels in the nasal tissues. It may feel awful, but it's nature's way of protecting your delicate schnozz when things like cold viruses, pollen and tobacco smoke are on the attack.

But what's good for the nose isn't so good for you. The more swollen and inflamed your nasal tissues get, the harder it is to breathe, eat or sleep, explains Michael Benninger, M.D., chairman of the Department of Otolaryngology–Head and Neck Surgery at Henry Ford Hospital in Detroit.

Enter the decongestants. These fast-acting drugs cause tiny blood vessels inside the nose to constrict. This helps shut the door on swelling and open the door to breathing, says Dr. Benninger.

A Spritz in Time

The fastest relief from nasal congestion comes in a bottle. Decongestant nose sprays or drops put nose-clearing action right where it's needed. Used as directed, they can help relieve nasal congestion within minutes and remain active for up to 12 hours, says Leonard Rybak, M.D., Ph.D., professor of surgery and pharmacology at Southern Illinois University School of Medicine in Springfield.

AT A GLANCE

OXYMETAZOLINE

Brand names: Afrin Nasal Spray, Dristan 12-Hour Nasal Spray Decongestant, Neo-Synephrine 12-Hour Nasal Spray

How taken: Nose drops, nasal spray

Prescription: No

	YES	NO
Generic substitutes	✓	
Potentially addicting		✓
May cause drowsiness		✓
Alcohol discouraged		✓

Possible drug interactions include: Taking this drug may decrease the effects of some heart and blood pressure medications; taking it may increase the effects (and side effects) of antihistamines and bronchodilators. This drug taken in combination with methyldopa (a blood pressure drug) may result in high blood pressure.

Possible side effects include: Burning, dryness and stinging of the nose, sneezing and a runny nose.

CAUTION: When used for longer than three days, rebound congestion may occur. May be extremely dangerous when taken with monoamine oxidase (MAO) inhibitors (used for depression).

There are dozens of over-the-counter and prescription decongestant nose sprays and drops. Most contain drugs such as oxymetazoline (Afrin Nasal Spray, Dristan 12-hour Nasal Spray Decongestant, Neo-Synephrine 12-Hour Nasal Spray), phenylephrine (Dristan Nasal Decongestant Spray, Nostril, Novahistine Elixir) and xylometa-

---

AT A GLANCE

PHENYLEPHRINE

Brand names: Dristan Nasal Decongestant Spray, Nostril, Novahistine Elixir

How taken: Tablet, nose drops, liquid, nasal spray

Prescription: No

	YES	NO
Generic substitutes	✓	
Potentially addicting		✓
May cause drowsiness		✓
Alcohol discouraged		✓

Possible drug interactions include: Taking this drug may decrease the effects of sedatives and beta-blockers and other heart and blood pressure drugs. This drug taken in combination with some antidepressants may result in increased blood pressure; taking it with asthma drugs or amphetamines may result in nervousness.

Possible side effects include: Burning, dryness and stinging inside the nose or an increase in runny nose.

CAUTION: May be extremely dangerous when taken with monoamine oxidase (MAO) inhibitors (used for depression).

XYLOMETAZOLINE

Brand names: Chlorohist-LA, Neo-Synephrine II Long Acting Nasal Spray, Otrivin

How taken: Nose drops, nasal spray

Prescription: No

	YES	NO
Generic substitutes	✓	
Potentially addicting		✓
May cause drowsiness		✓
Alcohol discouraged		✓

Possible drug interactions include: Taking this drug may decrease the effects of some heart and blood pressure medications; taking it may increase the effects of antihistamines and bronchodilators. This drug taken in combination with some antidepressants or methyldopa (a blood pressure drug) may result in high blood pressure.

Possible side effects include: Sneezing and burning, dryness and stinging of the nose.

CAUTION: When used for longer than three days, rebound congestion may result. May be extremely dangerous when taken with monoamine oxidase (MAO) inhibitors (used for depression).

AT A GLANCE

PHENYLPROPANOLAMINE

Brand names: Prolamine, Propagest, Rhindecon

How taken: Capsule, chewing gum, tablet

Prescription: Sometimes, depending on strength

	YES	NO
Generic substitutes	✓	
Potentially addicting		✓
May cause drowsiness		✓
Alcohol discouraged		✓

Possible drug interactions include: This drug taken in combination with amantadine (an antiviral drug), amphetamines, caffeine or heart or asthma drugs may result in nervousness, irritability or irregular heartbeat; taking it with monoamine oxidase (MAO) inhibitors (used for depression) may result in high blood pressure.

Possible side effects include: Nervousness, dizziness, headache, high blood pressure, nausea, insomnia and dryness of the nose and mouth.

PSEUDOEPHEDRINE

Brand names: Afrinol Repetabs, Halofed, Sudafed

How taken: Capsule, liquid, tablet

Prescription: Sometimes, depending on strength

	YES	NO
Generic substitutes	✓	
Potentially addicting		✓
May cause drowsiness		✓
Alcohol discouraged		✓

Possible drug interactions include: Taking this drug may decrease the effects of atenolol, betaxolol, propranolol and other beta-blocking drugs (used for high blood pressure). This drug taken in combination with monamine oxidase (MAO) inhibitors (used for depression) may result in high blood pressure.

Possible side effects include: Nervousness, restlessness and insomnia.

zoline (Cholorhist-LA, Neo-Synephrine II Long Acting Nasal Spray, Otrivin). If you aren't sure which drug is right for you, ask your doctor or pharmacist for guidance.

Although decongestant sprays are extremely safe, they aren't meant for long-term use. If you use them for more than three to five days, you may develop a condition called rebound congestion. This means your nose will be more stuffed up than it was in the first place.

One spray that can be used regularly is saline (Ocean Mist). You can buy saline sprays over the counter or, if you prefer, you can make your own solution at home. Just mix ½ teaspoon salt in a pint of water, then pour the solution into a spray bottle. Inhale as you spray. "It's a chicken-soup kind of remedy," says Dr. Benninger. "It usually will help and it absolutely can't hurt." (Homemade solutions should be replaced every few days.)

Long-Term Relief

Oral decongestants can provide the benefits of sprays without causing rebound congestion. This means they can be taken for longer periods of time, says Dr. Rybak.

Most oral decongestants contain drugs such as phenylpropanolamine (Prolamine, Propagest, Rhindecon) and pseudoephedrine (Afrinol Repetabs, Halofed, Sudafed). These over-the-counter and prescription drugs also help shrink swollen nasal tissues but, unlike sprays, oral decongestants may take up to an hour to be effective, says Dr. Rybak.

Oral decongestants may also cause side effects such as shakiness and high blood pressure and can be dangerous when taken by people with diabetes or heart problems. If you have these or other medical problems, check with your doctor before taking them, advises Dr. Benninger.

Diabetes Drugs

Glucose Couriers

In Greek mythology, Tantalus, a son of Zeus, was condemned for eternity to Hades. There he was tormented by luscious fruit he couldn't reach, refreshing water he couldn't drink.

Like Tantalus, people who have diabetes are *tantalized* by something they crave but can't get enough of—not fruit or water but glucose, a simple sugar that the body demands for fuel.

It's not that glucose is scarce. Any time you eat fruit, vegetables and many other foods, glucose is released in the bloodstream. But in order for glucose to be transported into hungry cells, it requires the presence of a hormone called insulin. People with diabetes don't produce enough insulin or are insensitive to its effects. This means that glucose accumulates in the bloodstream, creating a dangerous

NATURAL ALTERNATIVES

Of the 12 million Americans with non-insulin-dependent, or Type II, diabetes, 80 percent could get by fine without drugs if they would "diet, exercise and lose weight," says Richard Guthrie, M.D., director of Mid-America Diabetes Associates and Diabetes Treatment Center at St. Joseph's Hospital in Wichita, Kansas.

Here are the experts' top recommendations for natural diabetes control.

Try to lose weight. The majority of people with Type II diabetes are overweight. As the pounds add up, blood sugar problems mount, Dr. Guthrie says. In many cases, you can substantially control blood sugar levels by losing as little as ten pounds.

Cut back on sugar. If you do indulge your sweet tooth, choose desserts that are fat-free or contain no more. than three grams of fat per four-ounce serving. Sugar-free, nonfat frozen yogurt or frozen fruit juice bars with less than 70 calories and no cream or coconut are some alternatives.

Cut back on fat of all kinds. The less fat you eat, the easier it is to lose weight. Also, foods that are high in fat often are high in sugar, too.

Exercise several times a week. Whether you enjoy walking, swimming or dancing, exercising will help you lose weight and help control blood sugar.

condition called hyperglycemia, or high blood sugar. At the same time, their cells, like poor Tantalus, are hungry amidst plenty.

When Insulin Is Missin'

Diabetes strikes between 2 and 4 percent of all Americans, although among certain groups—the Pima Indians in Arizona, for example—it may affect 35 percent. Untreated, this condition can lead to blindness, nerve damage and other serious health problems.

There are two main types of diabetes, explains Richard Guthrie, M.D., director of Mid-America Diabetes Associates and Diabetes Treatment Center at St. Joseph's Hospital in Wichita, Kansas. Insulin-dependent, or Type I, diabetes occurs when the pancreas gland produces little or no insulin. More common is non-insulin-dependent, or Type II, diabetes, in which the pancreas continues to produce insulin, but not enough to

AT A GLANCE

TOLBUTAMIDE

Brand names: Oramide, Orinase
How taken: Tablet
Prescription: Yes

	YES	NO
Generic substitutes	✓	
Potentially addicting		✓
May cause drowsiness	✓	
Alcohol discouraged	✓	

Possible drug interactions include:
This drug taken in combination with aspirin, monoamine oxidase (MAO) inhibitors (used for depression), sulfa medicines, beta-blockers (used for heart and blood pressure problems) and appetite suppressants may result in low blood sugar.

Possible side effects include:
Changes in taste, constipation, headache, heartburn and chest pain.

CHLORPROPAMIDE

Brand names: Diabinese, Glucamide
How taken: Tablet
Prescription: Yes

	YES	NO
Generic substitutes	✓	
Potentially addicting		✓
May cause drowsiness	✓	
Alcohol discouraged	✓	

Possible drug interactions include:
This drug taken in combination with aspirin, monoamine oxidase (MAO) inhibitors (used for depression), sulfa medications, beta-blockers (used for heart and blood pressure problems) and appetite suppressants may result in low blood sugar.

Possible side effects include: Constipation, water retention, breathing difficulty, headache, heartburn, chest pain and sensitivity to sunlight.

meet the body's needs.

For both types, watching your weight and sticking to a healthy diet are important parts of therapy, says Dr. Guthrie. In addition, many people with Type II diabetes—and everyone with Type I—require drugs to keep their blood sugar under control.

Oral Options

Type II diabetes often is treated with prescription drugs called sulfonylureas. Taken orally, the sulfonylureas work primarily by stimulating the pancreas gland to make more insulin, says Dr. Guthrie.

The so-called first-generation

sulfonylureas have been in use since the 1950s and include drugs such as tolbutamide (Oramide, Orinase), tolazamide (Tolamide, Tolinase) and chlorpropamide (Diabinese, Glucamide). The drugs have similar effects, although they differ in how long they last, says Mary Korytkowski, M.D., director of the Pittsburgh Diabetes Center and assistant professor of medicine at the University of Pittsburgh School of Medicine.

These drugs aren't without problems. For example, they may prevent other medications from working. Also, they primarily affect the output of insulin. Newer drugs, on the other hand, not only boost insulin output but also seem to make the body more sensitive to its effects. Doctors are phasing out the use of the first-generation drugs, according to Dr. Guthrie.

The newer drugs, called second-

AT A GLANCE

GLYBURIDE

Brand names: DiaBeta, Micronase

How taken: Tablet

Prescription: Yes

	YES	NO
Generic substitutes		✓
Potentially addicting		✓
May cause drowsiness	✓	
Alcohol discouraged	✓	

Possible drug interactions include: This drug taken in combination with aspirin, monoamine oxidase (MAO) inhibitors (used for depression), sulfa medicines, beta-blockers (used for heart and blood pressure problems) and appetite suppressants may result in low blood sugar.

Possible side effects include: Constipation, diarrhea, dizziness, headache and heartburn.

GLIPIZIDE

Brand name: Glucotrol

How taken: Tablet

Prescription: Yes

	YES	NO
Generic substitutes		✓
Potentially addicting		✓
May cause drowsiness	✓	
Alcohol discouraged	✓	

Possible drug interactions include: This drug taken in combination with aspirin, monoamine oxidase (MAO) inhibitors (used for depression), sulfa medicines, beta-blockers (used for heart and blood pressure problems) and appetite suppressants may result in low blood sugar.

Possible side effects include: Constipation, dizziness, headache, heartburn and chest pain.

AT A GLANCE

SYNTHETIC HUMAN INSULIN

Brand names: Humulin R, Novolin R

How taken: Injection

Prescription: No

	YES	NO
Generic substitutes	✓	
Potentially addicting		✓
May cause drowsiness		✓
Alcohol discouraged	✓	

Possible drug interactions include: The effects of this drug may decrease if taken with adrenocorticoids (used to treat allergies or skin problems). This drug taken in combination with beta-blockers (used for heart and blood pressure problems) may result in high or low blood pressure.

Possible side effects include: Redness, itching and swelling at the site of the injection.

CAUTION: May cause low or high blood sugar.

EXTENDED INSULIN ZINC

Brand name: Ultralente

How taken: Injection

Prescription: No

	YES	NO
Generic substitutes	✓	
Potentially addicting		✓
May cause drowsiness		✓
Alcohol discouraged	✓	

Possible drug interactions include: The effects of this drug may decrease if taken with adrenocorticoids (used to treat allergies or skin problems). This drug taken in combination with beta-blockers (used for heart and blood pressure problems) may result in high or low blood pressure.

Possible side effects include: Redness, itching and swelling at the site of the injection.

CAUTION: May cause low or high blood sugar.

---

generation sulfonylureas, are 100 to 150 times more powerful than their predecessors. This means that prescription drugs such as glyburide (DiaBeta, Micronase) and glipizide (Glucotrol) can be taken in lower doses, sometimes just once a day. And they are less likely to block the effects of other medications, says Dr. Guthrie.

A Shot in Time

While most people with Type II diabetes still produce insulin, those with Type I produce virtually none. They need insulin injections. "If you take insulin for Type I diabetes, you take it for life," says Dr. Guthrie.

Some insulin is derived from animal organs, although synthetic human insulin (Humulin R, Novolin R) now is produced in the laboratory. They are equally effective, although synthetic insulin is slightly less likely to cause allergic reactions, says Dr. Korytkowski.

In most cases, it's not important where the insulin comes from. What matters is how quickly it takes effect and how long it lasts. A type of insulin, called regular insulin taken just before meals, may kick in within 15 to 30 minutes. By contrast, an insulin called extended insulin zinc (Ultralente) can be taken once a day (but it must be supplemented with regular insulin before meals).

Insulin therapy varies from person to person. A few people need only one daily injection, while others need many. Many doctors now believe that insulin injections work best when given frequently. Giving insulin frequently, Dr. Guthrie explains, "is really an attempt to give the insulin the way the body normally delivers it."

Planning Your Treatment

Thanks to insulin, many people who have diabetes now live long and productive lives. Yet insulin therapy is not without complications.

First, there is the inconvenience of taking daily injections. Researchers have been trying for years to develop nasal sprays, implantable pumps and other, less pointed ways of giving the drug, but with limited success.

Occasionally, insulin injections will cause a rash, itching and other uncomfortable skin reactions. In most cases, symptoms will disappear once you get used to the shots, says Dr. Guthrie. In the meantime, taking an antihistamine can help quell the discomfort.

Far more serious is the risk of hypoglycemia, dangerously low blood sugar levels that can be caused by taking too much insulin. Hypoglycemia can lead to coma, seizures and brain damage. That's why it's so important to stick to a routine and take injections and blood sugar tests regularly.

Your doctor also may advise you to carry glucagon. This fast-acting prescription injection blocks insulin and pumps glucose into the bloodstream, quickly interrupting hypoglycemic attacks. In a pinch, eating something sweet also can help short-circuit problems, says Dr. Guthrie.

Ear Drugs

Hearing Protectors

Ears—be they big, medium or small—sometimes attract all sorts of troublesome things, including fungi, bacteria and pent-up air pressure.

"Ear problems can be very painful," says James Donaldson, M.D., an ear specialist at the Seattle Ear Clinic and professor emeritus of otolaryngology at the University of Washington School of Medicine. But in most cases, he adds, they're easily treated with tablets or drops.

Infection Correction

Few conditions are more painful—or, for parents awakened at midnight by a child's tears, more frightening—than ear infections. Called otitis media, these infections of the middle ear often occur at the same time as colds and other respiratory tract infections. They are caused by bacteria that take up residence in the ear canal.

In the days before antibiotics, ear infections could be very dangerous. Today, however, they're treated with oral prescription antibiotics. (Eardrops won't work because the infection actually is *behind* the eardrum, says Dr. Donaldson.)

Antibiotics such as penicillin G (Bicillin, Wycillin) or amoxicillin (Amoxil, Trimox, Wymox) usually will begin relieving symptoms within 12 to 24 hours, says Orval E. Brown, M.D., associate professor of otorhinolaryngology (ear, nose and throat problems) and chairman of the Division of Pediatric Otorhinolaryngology at the University of Texas Southwestern Medical Center at Dallas.

In most cases, the antibiotics are taken for ten days to two weeks to make sure all the tiny troublemakers are eradicated, adds Dr. Donaldson. Antibiotics are very safe, although they may cause some mild diarrhea. If this is a serious problem, tell your doctor.

Poolside Help

Despite the fact that our bodies are made up of a high percentage of water, it can, unfortunately, sometimes cause trouble.

Waterborne bacteria that swim into the ear canal—and stay

there—can cause extremely painful infections called swimmer's ear.

But with a little attention to your ears, swimmer's ear can be prevented with over-the-counter eardrops, says Dr. Donaldson. These usually contain mild antiseptics such as acetic acid and aluminum acetate (Star-Otic) or isopropyl alcohol (Swim-Ear). Dropped into the ears soon after leaving the pool, these can eliminate any unwanted visitors that may have swum in (four drops in each ear would be adequate). In addition, isopropyl alcohol absorbs moisture from the ear, making it a less attractive breeding ground, says Dr. Donaldson.

You can make your own drops at home by mixing one part white vinegar with one part rubbing alcohol, says Dr. Brown. "Several drops (three or four drops) in each ear should prevent swimmer's ear," he says.

Should swimmer's ear develop into a full-blown infection, then you'll probably need antibiotics, says Dr. Donaldson. Unlike middle ear infections, however, swimmer's ear can be treated with topical pre-

---

NATURAL ALTERNATIVES

There are times when terrible ear pain seems to come out of the blue—actually, the wild blue yonder.

This condition, called otitic barotrauma, or airplane ear, is caused by changes in airplane cabin pressure on descent, says James Donaldson, M.D., an ear specialist at the Seattle Ear Clinic and professor emeritus of otolaryngology at the University of Washington School of Medicine.

But airplane ear can be prevented. Here's what the experts recommend.

Don't fly cold. Colds often cause blocked eustachian tubes—canals from the back of the throat to the middle ear—which are very sensitive to changes in air pressure.

Decongest. If you have a cold but must fly, take a decongestant before boarding. This will help keep your eustachian tubes wide open.

Exercise your jaw. Swallowing and yawning are both effective tricks for opening blocked eustachian tubes. Chewing gum when you fly also will keep you swallowing, which is one more way to keep the tubes open.

Take a deep breath. You can further equalize pressure in your ears by taking a deep breath, then, while covering your nose and mouth, puffing out your cheeks and blowing gently but firmly.

scription antibiotic steroid drops combining neomycin, polymyxin B and hydrocortisone (Cortisporin, Pediotic). Again, however, you may be required to use the medication for a week to ten days to make sure the infection is entirely cleared up, he adds.

Helping Wax Wane

When you wear earplugs, it's amazing how silent the world seems. The same thing occurs when you have a buildup of earwax—except it's a lot more difficult to remove wax when you want to start hearing again!

Earwax itself isn't a problem. In fact, it's your ears' way of keeping dust and debris from piling up inside. Unfortunately, many people try to remove earwax with fingers or cotton swabs. As a result of all this prodding, says Dr. Donaldson, a dense little wax plug may lodge next to the eardrum. This can make music—and telephones and doorbells—sound like they're coming from under water.

There are many over-the-counter products that can help remove

---

AT A GLANCE

PENICILLIN G

Brand names: Bicillin, Wycillin

How taken: Injection, liquid, tablet

Prescription: Yes

	YES	NO
Generic substitutes	✓	
Potentially addicting		✓
May cause drowsiness		✓
Alcohol discouraged		✓

Possible drug interactions include: Taking this drug may decrease the effects of oral contraceptives.

Possible side effects include: Yeast infections in women.

CAUTION: Seek immediate medical care if you develop an allergic reaction, which can include wheezing, hives and rash.

AMOXICILLIN

Brand names: Amoxil, Trimox, Wymox

How taken: Capsule, liquid, tablet

Prescription: Yes

	YES	NO
Generic substitutes	✓	
Potentially addicting		✓
May cause drowsiness		✓
Alcohol discouraged		✓

Possible drug interactions include: Taking this drug may decrease the effects of oral contraceptives, antibiotics like tetracycline, erythromycin or chloramphenicol, and antacids.

Possible side effects include: Yeast infections in women.

AT A GLANCE

ACETIC ACID and ALUMINUM ACETATE		
Brand name: Star-Otic		
How taken: Eardrops		
Prescription: No		
	Yes	No
Generic substitutes		✓
Potentially addicting		✓
May cause drowsiness		✓
Alcohol discouraged		✓

Possible drug interactions include: Interactions are unlikely.

Possible side effects include: Side effects are unlikely.

CARBAMIDE PEROXIDE		
Brand names: Debrox Drops, Murine Ear Drops		
How taken: Eardrops		
Prescription: No		
	YES	NO
Generic substitutes	✓	
Potentially addicting		✓
May cause drowsiness		✓
Alcohol discouraged		✓

Possible drug interactions include: Interactions are unlikely.

Possible side effects include: Side effects are unlikely, but read the entire label carefully before using.

compacted earwax. Most contain ingredients such as glycerin and mineral oil, which help soften wax and make it easier to dislodge. "Doctors hesitate to use products containing carbamide peroxide (Debrox Drops, Murine Ear Drops) due to possible sensitization of the ear canal; it could turn red, become itchy and swell up. These products might be used upon a doctor's advice," according to Dr. Brown.

"I recommend mineral oil, three to four drops, put in the ear two to three times a day for several days," says Dr. Brown. "It's very cheap, very easy, and it usually works."

After the wax has been thoroughly softened, however, it won't necessarily fall out on its own. To help it along, suggests Dr. Donaldson, fill a rubber bulb syringe (called an ear syringe and available in drugstores) with warm (body temperature) water and gently squirt it into the ear, hanging your head over the bathroom sink. This can help remove the softened wax so you can hear your favorite music again.

Eye Drugs

Visionary Treatments

The eyes have been called windows to the soul. Unfortunately, they're also *open* windows to everything from bacteria and viruses to blazing sunshine.

Eye specialists see a lot of red, dry, itching eyes, says Alan Sugar, M.D., professor of ophthalmology at W. K. Kellogg Eye Center at the University of Michigan School of Medicine at Ann Arbor. They also see infected eyes and, less often, eyes with a serious condition called glaucoma.

Many common eye disorders can be treated with prescription and over-the-counter medications. As you might expect, many of these are put directly into the eye in the form of drops. Which drugs you need— antibiotics, beta-blockers or artificial tears, to name just a few— depends on your condition.

Infection Fighters

The eyes are warm, moist and open to the environment— nearly perfect for wandering viruses and bacteria looking for a place to perch. As a result, eye infections are very common, says Dr. Sugar. They have many names, depending on the part of the eye that's infected. An infection of the cornea is called keratitis; an infection of the membrane covering the eye is conjunctivitis.

Most bacterial infections can be treated with prescription eyedrops or ointments containing antibiotics such as sulfonamide (Bleph-10, Ophthacet, Sulfair Forte) or erythromycin (Ilotycin). In the majority of cases, Dr. Sugar says, the infection "will begin to clear up within a couple of days."

Unlike oral drugs, which may cause diarrhea or yeast infections, antibiotic drops rarely cause side effects, says Gilbert Smolin, M.D., clinical professor of ophthalmology at the University of California, San Francisco. But for eye infections that don't respond to drops, your doctor may prescribe oral drugs.

Bacteria aren't the only cause of painful eye infections, he adds. In many cases, viral infections also are treated with eyedrops—not antibiotics, of course, but antiviral drugs.

For example, your doctor may prescribe drops containing vidarabine (Vira-A) or trifluridine (Viroptic), which often begin relieving symptoms within two days. "They're very effective," says Dr. Smolin. They're also quite safe, because most of the drug stays right in the eye. The amount absorbed by the body isn't likely to cause problems, he says.

But for more serious eye infections, your doctor may want a drug that has systemic, or whole-body, effects. A prescription drug called acyclovir (Zovirax) can be very helpful. Taken orally, it doesn't actually kill viruses but prevents them from multiplying, giving your immune system a chance to get the upper hand. Acyclovir causes few side effects, says Dr. Smolin.

Righting the Reds

During a famous battle several hundred years ago, American soldiers were ordered not to shoot until they saw the "whites of their eyes." If this same battle had taken place in a modern city filled with car fumes, factory pollution and hot, stagnant air, the soldiers would still be waiting.

All too often our poor, tired eyes turn as red as a matador's cape. Often triggered by dryness, irritation or allergies, the redness occurs when delicate blood vessels inside the eyes become enlarged, explains Dr. Sugar.

Antihistamines can relieve redness that is caused by allergies.

NATURAL ALTERNATIVES

When your eyes feel as dry and itchy as an old, stale bread crust, it may be time to wet them down. For relief in a blink:

Try a warm compress. Dip a small towel or washcloth in warm water. Lightly wring it out, then gently drape it across your dry eyes. This will direct moisture where it can do the most good.

Turn on the humidifier. Adding moisture to the air can help keep moisture in your eyes, too.

Try to get enough sleep. A good night's shut-eye can go a long way toward refreshing dry, tired eyes.

Think blink. Studies have shown that people watching television or computer screens blink less often, which can cause dryness as well as fatigue and irritation. Simply reminding yourself to blink can help keep your eyes lubricated.

AT A GLANCE

ERYTHROMYCIN

Brand name: Ilotycin

How taken: Ointment

Prescription: Yes

	YES	NO
Generic substitutes	✓	
Potentially addicting		✓
May cause drowsiness		✓
Alcohol discouraged		✓

Possible drug interactions include: Interactions are unlikely.

Possible side effects include: Side effects are unlikely.

TRIFLURIDINE

Brand name: Viroptic

How taken: Eyedrops

Prescription: Yes

	YES	NO
Generic substitutes		✓
Potentially addicting		✓
May cause drowsiness		✓
Alcohol discouraged		✓

Possible drug interactions include: Interactions are unlikely.

Possible side effects include: Temporary stinging or burning of the eye.

Many of these medications are available over the counter, although your doctor may recommend a prescription variety, which is frequently stronger. Commonly used antihistamines, usually taken orally, are chlorpheniramine (Chlor-Trimeton Allergy-Sinus Tablets, Coricidin, Sine-off Sinus Medicine) and diphenhydramine (Actifed Sinus Daytime/Nighttime, Benadryl Decongestant).

One problem with many antihistamines is side effects. They commonly cause drowsiness and dryness of the mouth and throat. For the benefits of antihistamines without these problems, your doctor may recommend a non-sedating antihistamine instead. There are two: terfenadine (Seldane) and astemizole (Hismanal). These oral prescription drugs can help ease allergy discomfort with fewer side effects than many over-the-counter drugs.

Yet another way to temporarily take the red out, with virtually no side effects, is with prescription and over-the-counter eyedrops containing oxymetazoline (OcuClear, Visine L.R.) or naphazoline (Allerest, Clear Eyes). These drugs very quickly shrink blood vessels in the eye, which takes out the red and brings back the whites, says Dr. Sugar.

These drugs shouldn't be used for more than several days or a week without a doctor's supervision, he adds. If your eyes stay red longer than that, there may be an underlying condition that needs medical attention. Another reason not to use medicated eyedrops long-term is that your eyes can become dependent on them. "Then, when you stop taking them, your blood vessels will be more dilated than they were before," says Dr. Sugar.

Lubricate the Lenses

Your body is nearly two-thirds water, which should be enough to keep your eyes moist and lubricated. But sometimes your eyes do, in fact, dry out. This can be caused by dry weather or by eye conditions such as kerato-conjunctivitis sicca—dry-eye syndrome, for short. But in many cases, dry eyes are a condition brought on by years. "Dry eyes are very common among the elderly, particularly in women," says Dr. Sugar.

Usually, dry eyes are treated easily with over-the-counter drops known as artificial tears. These gentle solutions contain mild medications such as carboxymethylcellulose (Cellufresh, Celluvisc), glycerin (Clear Eyes ACR) or polyvinyl alcohol (Murine, Tears Plus).

For heavy-duty protection from dry eyes, some artificial tears contain white petrolatum and mineral oil (Lacri-Lube, Refresh P.M.). These preparations are much thicker, so they remain active twice as long. But they're usually used only at bedtime, says Dr. Smolin. "It

OXYMETAZOLINE

Brand names: OcuClear, Visine L.R.

How taken: Eyedrops

Prescription: No

	YES	NO
Generic substitutes		✓
Potentially addicting		✓
May cause drowsiness		✓
Alcohol discouraged		✓

Possible drug interactions include: Interactions are unlikely.

Possible side effects include: Increased redness and irritation of the eye when used for long periods.

CARBOXYMETHYLCELLULOSE

Brand names: Cellufresh, Celluvisc

How taken: Eyedrops

Prescription: No

	YES	NO
Generic substitutes	✓	
Potentially addicting		✓
May cause drowsiness		✓
Alcohol discouraged		✓

Possible drug interactions include: Interactions are unlikely.

Possible side effects include: Side effects are unlikely.

AT A GLANCE

TIMOLOL

Brand name: Timoptic

How taken: Eyedrops

Prescription: Yes

	YES	NO
Generic substitutes		✓
Potentially addicting		✓
May cause drowsiness		✓
Alcohol discouraged		✓

Possible drug interactions include: Interactions are unlikely.

Possible side effects include: Burning or stinging of the eyes.

PILOCARPINE

Brand names: Akarpine, Pilocar, Spectro-Pilo

How taken: Eyedrops, gel

Prescription: Yes

	YES	NO
Generic substitutes	✓	
Potentially addicting		✓
May cause drowsiness		✓
Alcohol discouraged	✓	

Possible drug interactions include: Interactions are unlikely.

Possible side effects include: Poor nighttime vision and temporary blurred vision.

would cause blurring in your vision if you used them during the day," he says.

Artificial tears are generally very safe and free of side effects, says Dr. Smolin. If dry eyes are a constant problem, however, you should check with your doctor.

Beating the Pressure

Although many eye problems are only mildly annoying, some can be quite serious. One of the most common of these is a condition called glaucoma, in which pressure inside the eye increases to abnormally high levels. Without treatment, glaucoma can reduce blood supply to vital nerves inside the eye, causing nerve damage or possibly even blindness.

If you have glaucoma, your doctor may give you prescription eyedrops that will help reduce the pressure. Drugs commonly used for this condition are called beta-adrenergic blocking agents, or beta-blockers. These include drugs such as timolol (Timoptic), betaxolol (Betoptic) and levobunolol (Betagon). They work by blocking the release of fluids in the eye, which helps keep pressure down.

Although beta-blockers generally are safe for most people, they do slow the heart rate and lower blood pressure, says Dr. Smolin. They also can cause blurred vision, and some people eventually become allergic to them.

When beta-blockers aren't effective or cause too many side effects, a doctor may prescribe drops called miotics. These work by improving the flow of fluids in the eye, which helps keep the pressure down.

Miotic drops and gels such as pilocarpine (Akarpine, Pilocar, Spectro-Pilo) and carbachol (Isopto carbachol, Miostat) can be very effective. Unfortunately, Dr. Sugar adds, they must be taken four times a day, which many people find inconvenient. And because they narrow the pupils, seeing at night may be difficult.

On the other hand, adds Dr. Smolin, "They don't affect the heart and people don't become allergic to them."

Other prescription drugs that can relieve glaucoma are acetazolamide (Dazamide, Diamox), epinephrine (Epifrin, L-Epinephrine) or iso-flurophate (Floropryl). But some of these drugs may cause side effects such as fatigue or depression, so they're primarily used only when other drugs don't work.

Female Hormones

A Key to Chemical Balance

Beginning with puberty and continuing until meno-pause, women produce powerful chemicals, female hormones, that help to make them so distinctly different from men.

Under the influence of estrogen, a woman develops sexually: The breasts develop, the vagina becomes elastic and the pelvis widens in preparation for childbirth. A second hormone, progesterone, regulates the uterine lining, preparing it for pregnancy or, conversely, causing it to shed during the menstrual period.

Should levels of these hormones go awry—during menopause, for example, or because of problems with the pituitary gland—hormone supplements can help put a woman's chemistry back on track.

Midlife Changes

When a woman reaches meno-pause, the ovaries begin producing less estrogen. Menstrual periods become increasingly irregular, then stop altogether. The vagina often becomes dry and less elastic. At the same time, many women experience estrogen "withdrawal" in the form of nausea, dizziness and searing hot flashes.

The lack of estrogen may have other consequences, too. "As soon as women lose their estrogen, they are at increased risk for heart disease and osteoporosis," says Deborah Metzger, M.D., Ph.D., assistant professor of obstetrics and gynecology and director of the Endometriosis and Pelvic Pain Center at the University of Connecticut Health Center in Farmington.

To help prevent problems, doctors often recommend that women who are past menopause take hormone supplements. This treatment is called hormone-replacement therapy, or HRT, says Michael K. Rees, M.D., an internist and clinical instructor of medicine at Harvard University School of Medicine.

Taken in low doses, prescription estrogen supplements such as estradiol (DepGynogen, Estrace, Estraderm), estropipate (Ogen) and conjugated estrogens (Premarin) act very much like the body's natural estrogen, says Dr. Rees.

The medications are available in many forms, including tablets, capsules, creams, suppositories, patches and injection. Estrogen may be given alone, but more often it is combined with other female hormones called progestins (Amen, Depo-Provera, Medroxyprogesterone).

Ideally, HRT will completely eliminate symptoms such as hot

NATURAL ALTERNATIVES

Hot flashes—those volcanic surges of heat that can raise your temperature seven to eight degrees in just a few seconds—affect up to 70 percent of women in menopause. To help put out the fire:

Dress up by dressing down. Be prepared for hot flashes by wearing clothes in layers. When hot flashes loom, you can peel off unneeded layers until you feel cool again.

Fan the flames. Keeping a fan nearby—either a traditional fold-up kind or a battery-powered model—will allow you to direct cooling breezes right where they're needed.

Be prepared. Keep moist towelettes in your purse, desk or glove compartment. Then, when hot flashes hit, you can mop your brow for quick relief.

Be cool—even when you're hot. Hot flashes rarely last more than a minute or two. Remind yourself that what you're feeling is normal and will soon be over. Keeping a positive attitude will help make these temporary discomforts easier to stand.

AT A GLANCE

ESTRADIOL

Brand names: DepGynogen, Estrace, Estraderm, Valergen-10

How taken: Patch, cream, tablet

Prescription: Yes

	YES	NO
Generic substitutes	✓	
Potentially addicting		✓
May cause drowsiness		✓
Alcohol discouraged		✓

Possible drug interactions include: Taking this drug may decrease the effects of bromocriptine (used for menstrual problems). This drug taken in combination with anabolic steroids, gold (used for arthritis) or very large doses of acetaminophen may result in liver damage.

Possible side effects include: Nausea, bloating, weight gain and breast tenderness.

CONJUGATED ESTROGENS

Brand name: Premarin

How taken: Cream, tablet

Prescription: Yes

	YES	NO
Generic substitutes		✓
Potentially addicting		✓
May cause drowsiness		✓
Alcohol discouraged		✓

Possible drug interactions include: Taking this drug may decrease the effects of bromocriptine (used for menstrual problems). This drug taken in combination with anabolic steroids, gold (used for arthritis) or extremely large doses of acetaminophen may result in liver damage.

Possible side effects include: Nausea, bloating, weight gain and breast tenderness.

flashes. At the same time, the incidence of heart disease can drop by 30 to 40 percent, and the incidence of osteoporosis-related bone fractures can drop by half. "I think the majority of postmenopausal women can benefit from HRT," says Dr. Metzger.

HRT Isn't for Everyone

It's been suggested that long-term HRT may increase a woman's risk for breast cancer.

"The general feeling is that taking estrogen replacement therapy for more than seven to ten years may be inappropriate," says Dr. Rees.

In the short run, some women taking HRT will experience mild side effects, such as fluid retention, nausea and breast tenderness. In most cases, however, the drugs are given in such low doses—as little as one-fifth to one-tenth of the body's "normal" levels—that side effects aren't a serious problem.

"Side effects are easy to avoid,"

AT A GLANCE

PROGESTIN

Brand names: Amen, Cycrin, Depo-Provera, Medroxypro-gesterone

How taken: Injection, tablet

Prescription: Yes

	YES	NO
Generic substitutes	✓	
Potentially addicting		✓
May cause drowsiness		✓
Alcohol discouraged		✓

Possible drug interactions include: Taking this drug may decrease the effects of bromocriptine (used for menstrual problems).

Possible side effects include: Weight gain, bloating and changes in menstrual bleeding.

CAUTION: May cause birth defects if taken during pregnancy.

---

says Dr. Metzger. "There are many different estrogen preparations and several progestins. Women who have a problem with one will usually do just fine with another."

Restoring Balance

Menopause isn't the only condition that can cause hormone levels to go helter-skelter. Some women have ovarian or pituitary disorders that alter the balance of hormones secreted from the ovary. This can cause symptoms ranging from acne outbreaks, excess facial hair and weight gain to painful menstrual periods, a condition doctors call dysmenorrhea.

In many cases, these conditions are easily treated with prescription hormones that may contain estrogens, progestins or a combination of the two. Often taken orally or in suppository form, these drugs can restore the body's hormone balance to healthy levels. When taken for menstrual pain, they work by inhibiting ovulation, which often (but not always) stops the cramps, says Dr. Metzger.

Endometriosis, which occurs when tissue from inside the uterus spreads to nearby tissues, also can be treated with female hormones, usually prescription progestins such as norethindrone (Micronor, Norlutin) or medroxyprogesterone.

Endometriosis also can be controlled with medications called gonadotropin-releasing hormone (GnRH) agonists (Lupron, Synarel, Zoladex), which shut down estrogen production, says Dr. Metzger. "When you deprive the endometrium of its growth stimulus, it gets very inactive." About half the women who take this drug for six to nine months will remain symptom-free for up to six years, she adds.

Fertility Drugs

Prescription Storks

Having a baby is one of life's most exciting events. But for the approximately 4.5 million American couples who struggle with infertility, even getting pregnant can be a long, arduous, frustrating process.

There are many conditions—endometriosis, for example—that can cause infertility. (Experts define infertility as being unable to get pregnant after a year of try-ing.) Occasionally, surgical repairs are needed. But in many cases, fertility medications alone can help put an eager couple on the baby track.

Aid for Egg Production

Infertility may occur because a woman's pituitary gland doesn't produce enough of the hormones needed for ovulation. This prob-

---

NATURAL ALTERNATIVES

Sometimes getting pregnant requires more than time and patience. You may need a few simple tricks as well. For example:

Aim for midcycle. Ovulation usually occurs in the middle of a woman's menstrual cycle, and that's when the odds for getting pregnant are highest. So, if your normal cycle is 28 days, the most fertile time for intercourse will occur around day 14.

Get examined. Make doctors' appointments for you *and* your spouse. It takes two to tango—and make babies. About 40 percent of infertility occurs because of male problems like blocked ducts or a low sperm count.

Keep your man cool. Men who spend a lot of time in whirlpools or hot tubs may lower their sperm counts. In fact, the average man produces enough extra sperm that this shouldn't be a problem. But when you're trying to get pregnant, every bit helps.

AT A GLANCE

HUMAN CHORIONIC GONADOTROPIN (HCG)

Brand names: A.P.L., Pregnyl, Profasi

How taken: Injection

Prescription: Yes

	YES	NO
Generic substitutes	✓	
Potentially addicting		✓
May cause drowsiness	✓	
Alcohol discouraged	✓	

Possible drug interactions include: Interactions are unlikely.

Possible side effects include: Bloating, headache, fluid retention, mood changes, fatigue, skin irritation at the injection site and stomach or pelvic pain.

lem often can be corrected with a prescription drug called clomiphene (Clomid, Milophene, Serophene). Taken orally, clomiphene increases the levels of hormones—specifically, luteinizing hormone (LH) and follicle-stimulating hormone (FSH)—that trigger the ovaries to release their eggs.

"You would generally expect to ovulate about a week after finishing the pills," says Jacqueline Gutmann, M.D., a fertility expert at the Philadelphia Fertility Institute and assistant clinical associate at the University of Pennsylvania. For women who don't ovulate during their first menstrual cycle on the drug, the dosage is slowly raised in subsequent cycles, she says.

About 80 percent of women given clomiphene will ovulate, and about half of those will eventually become pregnant, Dr. Gutmann says. The drug also can be given to men to stimulate sperm production, although this is rarely done, says Roger P. Smith, M.D., chief of the Section of General Obstetrics and Gynecology at the Medical College of Georgia in Augusta.

Clomiphene is an effective drug—sometimes *very* effective: About 6 to 8 percent of women taking clomiphene will have multiple births, usually twins. Some women will have side effects such as hot flashes, nausea and breast discomfort.

High-Powered Help

If clomiphene doesn't trigger ovulation, your doctor may recommend a combination of prescription hormones—menotropins (Pergonal) plus human chorionic gonadotropin (A.P.L., Pregnyl, Profasi). Given by injection, these hormones work by stimulating eggs to ripen and then causing them to be released from the ovaries at the appropriate time.

These hormone injections are extremely effective, causing ovulation usually within several menstrual cycles in up to 90 percent of

AT A GLANCE

CLOMIPHENE

Brand names: Clomid, Milophene, Serophene

How taken: Tablet

Prescription: Yes

	YES	NO
Generic substitutes		✓
Potentially addicting		✓
May cause drowsiness		✓
Alcohol discouraged	✓	

Possible drug interactions include: Interactions are unlikely.

Possible side effects include: Bloating, dizziness, blurred vision, hot flashes and pelvic pain.

CAUTION: May cause birth defects if taken after pregnancy occurs.

MENOTROPINS

Brand name: Pergonal

How taken: Injection

Prescription: Yes

	YES	NO
Generic substitutes		✓
Potentially addicting		✓
May cause drowsiness		✓
Alcohol discouraged	✓	

Possible drug interactions include: Interactions are unlikely.

Possible side effects include: Diarrhea, bloating, dizziness, weight gain, stomach or pelvic pain and heart rhythm irregularities.

cases. And, like clomiphene, they can be given to men, although this isn't commonly done, says Dr. Smith.

Pergonal and Pregnyl are used fairly often in women, Dr. Gutmann adds. But 10 to 20 percent of the women who take them will have multiple births. In addition, they cause the ovaries to enlarge. In rare cases, this can develop into a potentially dangerous condition.

Gallstone Medications

The Stone Dissolvers

The gallbladder is a small, pear-shaped organ that's just waiting to make trouble. For approximately 25 million Americans, that means gallstones. Over time, these stones—sometimes one, sometimes a hundred—can make the gallbladder bulge and ache.

The gallbladder is a storage sac for bile, a digestive fluid produced by the liver. Bile normally contains an abundance of dissolved cholesterol and other liquid substances. Occasionally, however, these substances form into tiny solid particles, which, over time, begin to grow, like pearls in an oyster. The result is gallstones.

Gallstones usually are "silent," causing no symptoms at all, says Keith Lillemoe, M.D., associate professor of surgery at Johns Hopkins University School of Medicine in Baltimore. But sometimes they cause severe abdominal pain, nausea, vomiting and other problems. When that happens, it's time to remove the stones—either with surgery or, in some cases, with stone-dissolving drugs.

Oral Options

One drug that has been used to eliminate, or at least shrink, gallstones is chenodiol (Chenix). Sold by prescription and taken orally, chenodiol works by reducing the amount of cholesterol present in the bile. In time, this makes gallstones slowly dissolve.

Chenodiol has three serious drawbacks, says Dr. Lillemoe. It's not particularly effective, dissolving stones completely only in about 15 percent of cases. It can cause side effects, including diarrhea, liver problems and increases in blood cholesterol. Finally, its benefits are short lived. When people stop taking chenodiol, the stones frequently come back.

A newer prescription drug, also taken orally, is ursodiol (Actigall). Studies show ursodiol often can relieve gallbladder pain within several weeks. As with chenodiol, however, it's not without problems. It dissolves stones at the glacial pace of one millimeter per month. This can mean years of expensive therapy. Furthermore, when people stop taking the drug, the stones often return. "In 50 percent of cases, the stones come back within five to seven years," says Dr. Lillemoe.

An experimental drug, called methyl tert-butyl ether, or MTBE, appears to be very effective. In one study, it completely dissolved gallstones in 95 percent of cases. But unlike the other drugs, MTBE isn't taken orally. Instead, treatments are done in the hospital, where the drug is infused directly into the gallbladder for one to three days. Doctors agree this treatment is still too complicated—and potentially dangerous—for common use.

A Kinder Cut

In fact, none of these drugs is ideal, if only because gallstones so frequently return. So why do doctors use them? They don't very often. The reason is simple: Surgery is faster, more efficient and, for most people, not terribly uncomfortable, says Dr. Lillemoe.

It was different ten years ago. Then, surgery required a large incision, a lengthy hospital stay and many weeks to recover. Stone-dissolving drugs were an important breakthrough.

But in the late 1980s, surgeons were perfecting a technique called

---

AT A GLANCE

CHENODIOL

Brand name: Chenix

How taken: Tablet

Prescription: Yes

	YES	NO
Generic substitutes		✓
Potentially addicting		✓
May cause drowsiness		✓
Alcohol discouraged	✓	

Possible drug interactions include: The effects of this drug may decrease if taken with antacids, estrogens, oral contraceptives or some cholesterol-lowering drugs.

Possible side effects include: Diarrhea, constipation, gas, indigestion and loss of appetite.

URSODIOL

Brand name: Actigall

How taken: Capsule

Prescription: Yes

	YES	NO
Generic substitutes		✓
Potentially addicting		✓
May cause drowsiness		✓
Alcohol discouraged	✓	

Possible drug interactions include: The effects of this drug may decrease if taken with antacids, estrogens, oral contraceptives or cholesterol-lowering drugs.

Possible side effects include: Mild diarrhea.

---

laparoscopic cholecystectomy, or "keyhole" gallbladder surgery. This allowed them to remove the gallbladder through a small puncture in the abdomen. People often went home the following day and were largely healed within a week.

"With drugs you treat a person for the rest of his life with an expensive medication," says Dr.

Lillemoe. With surgery, "he comes in for an overnight stay in the hospital and is free of his problems once and for all."

This isn't to say that everyone with gallbladder problems wants, needs or is a good candidate for surgery. When surgery, for whatever reason, isn't an option, it may be time for gallstone medications.

Gout Drugs

Putting the Brakes on Aches

In the past, those suffering from gout were advised to forgo rich foods such as anchovies and organ meats and to abstain from beer and other spirits. There was little more they could do.

While temperance may be helpful in preventing flare-ups of this agonizing form of arthritis, it won't stop attacks already in progress. But today there are many drugs that can ease gout pain and, in some cases, stop it entirely, says Mary Ann Spadaro Antonelli, M.D., a rheumatologist and associate professor of medicine at West Virginia University School of Medicine in Morgantown. What's more, some of the drugs that stop

the pain can help prevent future attacks as well.

Easing Inflammation

People with gout have increased levels of uric acid, which is a by-product of metabolism, in their bloodstreams. Occasionally, this uric acid will crystallize inside a joint—usually the big toe—where it can cause intensely painful inflammation lasting for hours or even days.

Stopping the inflammation can stop the pain, says Dr. Antonelli. Anti-inflammatory drugs such as ibuprofen (Advil, Motrin IB, Nuprin), available over the counter, often will do the trick. Or your doc-

NATURAL ALTERNATIVES

While medications may lower the level of uric acid in the blood, certain foods do just the opposite. These foods may trigger gout attacks in those who are susceptible. The worst offenders are foods high in purines. Here are 12 menu items *loaded* with purines. If you have gout, you might be better off without them!

Anchovies	Kidney
Bacon	Liver
Consommé	Mussels
Gravies	Sardines
Heart	Sweetbreads
Herring	Turkey

tor may recommend prescription drugs such as indomethacin (Indameth, Indocin) or fenoprofen (Nalfon) instead.

"The earlier you take them, the more effective they are," says Dr. Antonelli. In fact, people who have frequent gout attacks may take anti-inflammatory drugs regularly to prevent problems.

Aspirin also can relieve gout pain. To be effective, however, it must be taken in large doses. At lower doses, aspirin actually may trigger attacks, Dr. Antonelli says. That's why doctors usually treat gout with other anti-inflammatory drugs.

Yet all of these medications can cause side effects, including bleeding, stomach pain and even kidney problems. If side effects are particularly bad, your doctor may give you anti-inflammatory steroids instead. Prescription drugs such as prednisone (Deltasone, Meticorten, Orasone) and dexamethasone (Decadron, Decaject, Dexasone), taken orally or by injection, can stop attacks, usually within a day. Though steroids can cause side effects such as water retention and high blood pressure when taken for long periods of time, they're quite safe for short-term use.

Another effective prescription anti-inflammatory drug is colchicine. Taken orally or by injection within hours of an attack, colchicine is more than 95 percent effective at relieving gout pain. The problem, as Dr. Antonelli delicately puts it, is that colchicine "causes some gastric distress." This can mean nausea, vomiting or out-of-control diarrhea.

AT A GLANCE

FENOPROFEN

Brand name: Nalfon

How taken: Capsule, tablet

Prescription: Yes

	YES	NO
Generic substitutes	✓	
Potentially addicting		✓
May cause drowsiness	✓	
Alcohol discouraged	✓	

Possible drug interactions include: This drug taken in combination with aspirin or anti-clotting drugs may result in an increase in bleeding; taking it with digitalis (a heart medicine) or lithium (used for manic depression) may result in high blood levels of these drugs.

Possible side effects include: Skin rash, headache, stomach cramps, dizziness, indigestion and nausea or vomiting.

DEXAMETHASONE

Brand names: Decadron, Decaject, Dexasone

How taken: Cream, injection, liquid, spray, tablet

Prescription: Yes

	YES	NO
Generic substitutes	✓	
Potentially addicting	✓	
May cause drowsiness		✓
Alcohol discouraged	✓	

Possible drug interactions include: Taking this drug may decrease the effects of diuretics (water pills). This drug taken in combination with oral diabetes drugs and insulin may result in an increase in blood sugar levels; taking it with digitalis (a heart medication) may cause irregular heartbeat.

Possible side effects include: Increased appetite, indigestion, weight gain, increased risk of infection, nervousness and insomnia.

CAUTION: Discontinue this drug 72 hours before vaccination and do not resume it for at least 14 days afterward.

Beyond Symptoms

Although anti-inflammatory drugs can relieve the pain of gout, they don't stop the disease itself. That's why doctors sometimes prescribe drugs that reduce the amount of uric acid in the bloodstream. These drugs rout gout either by slowing the body's production of uric acid or by speeding its excretion through the urine.

A tablet called allopurinol (Lopurin, Zyloprim) works well, says Dr. Antonelli. To be effective, however, it must be taken every day. "If you stop taking it, you may have more attacks," she says.

In fact, once you get gout, subsequent attacks can be triggered whether your uric acid levels go up *or* down. So when you first start taking allopurinol, your doctor may give you several doses of colchicine as well. Once your uric acid levels stabilize, allopurinol alone should be effective.

Another prescription tablet for gout is probenecid (Benemid, Probalan). As with allopurinol, it may be used in conjunction with colchicine for the first few weeks of treatment.

Regardless of the drug you take, it's important to drink lots of water to dilute uric acid in the bloodstream and in the urine, adds Dr. Antonelli. "I tell people to drink six to eight glasses a day in addition to their normal intake—the more the better."

AT A GLANCE

ALLOPURINOL

Brand names: Lopurin, Zyloprim

How taken: Tablet

Prescription: Yes

	YES	NO
Generic substitutes	✓	
Potentially addicting		✓
May cause drowsiness	✓	
Alcohol discouraged	✓	

Possible drug interactions include: Taking this drug may increase the effects of azathioprine (an arthritis drug), mercaptopurine (a leukemia drug) and oral anti-clotting drugs. This drug taken in combination with ampicillin may cause a skin rash.

Possible side effects include: Skin rash or sores, hives, itching and temporary increase in gout attacks.

PROBENECID

Brand names: Benemid, Probalan

How taken: Tablet

Prescription: Yes

	YES	NO
Generic substitutes	✓	
Potentially addicting		✓
May cause drowsiness		✓
Alcohol discouraged	✓	

Possible drug interactions include: The effects of this drug may decrease if taken with aspirin. Taking this drug may increase the effects of indomethacin (an anti-inflammatory drug) and methotrexate (used for psoriasis, cancer and rheumatoid arthritis).

Possible side effects include: Headache, joint pain, redness or swelling, loss of appetite and nausea or vomiting.

503

Heart Rhythm Drugs

Conductors That Keep the Beat

The heart beats, on average, 72 times a minute, 4,320 times an hour and 103,680 times a day. In your entire lifetime, it may beat well beyond 2.5 *billion* times. What's more, it does so with remarkable precision, only occasionally—so the saying goes—missing a beat.

Yet the heart depends on electricity to run correctly. Should the electrical current run too strong or too weak, arrive too soon or too late, the rhythm falters. The term for these arrhythmic beats is, reasonably enough, arrhythmias.

"If you have a few extra beats here and there and they're not causing symptoms, they're usually not a problem," says John F. Setaro, M.D., director of the Cardiovascular Disease Prevention Center at Yale University School of Medicine.

If, on the other hand, the arrhythmias are frequent and causing symptoms—dizziness, for example—then you'll probably need medications. "If the heart seriously goes out of rhythm," says Dr. Setaro, "the circulation can come to a standstill."

An Old Standby

Doctors have known for more than a century that quinine, a compound found in the bark of a South American tree, was active against malaria. By chance, they also discovered that people who had malaria *and* heart rhythm problems improved on both counts after taking the drug.

A modern relative of quinine is quinidine (Cardioquin, Duraquin, Quinaglute Dura-Tabs). Usually taken orally, quinidine often is used to slow dangerously fast heartbeats, a condition called tachycardia, says Dr. Setaro.

Other prescription drugs that can slow runaway heartbeats are procainamide (Procan SR, Promine, Pronestyl) and disopyramide (Norpace). Like quinidine, they usually are taken orally, although procainamide may be injected

AT A GLANCE

QUINIDINE

Brand names: Cardioquin, Dura-quin, Quinaglute Dura-Tabs

How taken: Capsule, tablet

Prescription: Yes

	YES	NO
Generic substitutes	✓	
Potentially addicting		✓
May cause drowsiness		✓
Alcohol discouraged	✓	

Possible drug interactions include: The effects of this drug may increase if taken with antacids. Taking this drug may increase effects of other heart medications, especially digoxin. This drug taken in combination with anti-clotting drugs may increase the risk of bleeding.

Possible side effects include: Dizziness, nausea, vomiting, diarrhea, blurred vision and ringing in the ears.

PROCAINAMIDE

Brand names: Procan SR, Promine, Pronestyl

How taken: Capsule, tablet, injection

Prescription: Yes

	YES	NO
Generic substitutes	✓	
Potentially addicting		✓
May cause drowsiness		✓
Alcohol discouraged	✓	

Possible drug interactions include: The effects of this drug may increase if taken with antacids. Taking this drug may increase the effects of blood pressure medications. This drug taken in combination with pimozide (an antipsychotic medication) may result in irregular heartbeat.

Possible side effects include: Diarrhea and loss of appetite.

when faster action is required.

Each of these medications may cause side effects, including diarrhea, nausea and loss of appetite. They also may cause *pro*arrhythmia, an allergic-type reaction to medication that makes the heart problem worse. Because of the possibility of such a reaction, your doctor will want to keep you under supervision when you begin taking these drugs.

Heart Tonics

Quinidine isn't the only heart rhythm medication derived from nature. Another class of prescription drugs, called digitalis, comes from the leaves of an herb called foxglove.

Digitalis drugs such as digoxin (Lanoxicaps, Lanoxin) and digitoxin (Crystodigin) work by regulating the electrical signals passing through the heart. This can cause it to beat more slowly and with better control, says Paul Walinsky, M.D., professor of medicine at Thomas Jefferson University Hospital in Philadelphia.

Digitalis drugs are very effective at relieving symptoms of heart dis-ease, such as fatigue, shortness of breath and swelling of the legs, says Dr. Walinsky. They also can give people more physical endur-ance so they can get about more normally.

Digitalis drugs aren't a cure for heart disease, however. People who

AT A GLANCE

DIGOXIN

Brand names: Lanoxicaps, Lanoxin

How taken: Capsule, liquid, tablet, injection

Prescription: Yes

	YES	NO
Generic substitutes	✓	
Potentially addicting		✓
May cause drowsiness	✓	
Alcohol discouraged		✓

Possible drug interactions include: The effects of this drug may increase if taken with other heart drugs, steroids, diuretics (water pills), anti-fungal medications and ibuprofen; effects may decrease if taken with fiber supplements, cholesterol-lower-ing drugs such as cholestyramine or anti-diarrheal drugs such as bismuth subsalicylate (Pepto-Bismol). This drug taken in combination with many cold and allergy remedies, asthma drugs, diet pills and antacids may result in irregular heartbeat.

Possible side effects include: De-creased sex drive, fatigue and nausea.

DIGITOXIN

Brand name: Crystodigin

How taken: Tablet

Prescription: Yes

	YES	NO
Generic substitutes	✓	
Potentially addicting		✓
May cause drowsiness	✓	
Alcohol discouraged		✓

Possible drug interactions include: The effects of this drug may increase if taken with other heart drugs, diuretics (water pills), steroids, anti-fungal medications and ibuprofen; effects may decrease if taken with fiber supplements, cholesterol-lowering drugs such as cholestyra-mine or anti-diarrheal drugs such as bismuth subsalicylate (Pepto-Bismol). This drug taken in combina-tion with many cold and allergy remedies, asthma drugs, diet pills and antacids may result in irregular heartbeat.

Possible side effects include: De-creased sex drive, nausea and fatigue.

AT A GLANCE

ACEBUTOLOL

Brand name: Sectral

How taken: Capsule

Prescription: Yes

	YES	NO
Generic substitutes		✓
Potentially addicting		✓
May cause drowsiness	✓	
Alcohol discouraged	✓	

Possible drug interactions include: Taking this drug may decrease the effects of theophylline and other asthma medications and insulin or oral diabetes drugs. This drug taken in combination with blood pressure medications may result in low blood pressure; taking it with monoamine oxidase (MAO) inhibitors (used for depression) or nonprescription nasal decongestant sprays may result in increased blood pressure.

Possible side effects include: Fatigue, insomnia, dizziness and decreased sex drive.

VERAPAMIL

Brand names: Calan, Isoptin, Verelan

How taken: Capsule, injection, tablet

Prescription: Yes

	YES	NO
Generic substitutes	✓	
Potentially addicting		✓
May cause drowsiness		✓
Alcohol discouraged	✓	

Possible drug interactions include: Taking this drug may increase the effects of other heart drugs and certain anti-seizure medications. This drug taken in combination with glaucoma medications such as betaxolol and timolol may result in low blood pressure and slow heart rate.

Possible side effects include: Headache, fatigue, flushing, dizziness and constipation.

take them usually do so for life, often in combination with other drugs. Unfortunately, these medications usually become less effective over time. They also can cause uncomfortable side effects, including fatigue and nausea. Finally, they can be dangerous should potassium levels in your bloodstream decline. To prevent this, your doctor may give you potassium supplements along with your medication.

A Safer Option

Because many heart rhythm drugs cause uncomfortable, even dangerous side effects, your doctor may begin your treatment with medications called beta-adrenergic blocking agents, or beta-blockers. Beta-blockers aren't as effective as some other drugs, but they are usually safer. So for many patients, they are worth a try, says Dr. Setaro.

Prescription oral beta-blockers such as propranolol (Inderal) and acebutolol (Sectral) or injectable forms such as esmolol (Brevibloc) work by reducing the force of electrical signals that stimulate the heart. Beta-blockers are used both to prevent arrhythmias and to stop attacks already in progress.

Even though these medications are not as powerful as, say, the digitalis drugs, "some people do pretty well with beta-blockers," Dr. Setaro says.

Electrical Insulators

A class of drugs called calcium channel blockers also can reduce the force of the heartbeat.

They do this by reducing the amount of calcium passing through special channels in heart-muscle cells. This in turn helps "insulate" the heart from surplus stimulation, which steadies the rhythm.

Calcium channel blockers such as verapamil (Calan, Isoptin, Verelan) and diltiazem (Cardizem) work very well, says Dr. Setaro. "Sometimes the heart can pretty much run away with itself, and very often these drugs are used to slow it down," he says.

During severe episodes of heart rhythm disturbances, calcium blockers may be given by injection to get things under control. More often, they're taken orally to prevent arrhythmias from occurring.

For most people, calcium blockers are extremely safe. When given by injection, however, they may cause additional heart problems. In most cases, lowering the dose will prevent this, says Dr. Setaro.

Immune System Suppressants

More Protection—With Less

We can't see them, but we live in the midst of veritable clouds of bacteria, viruses and parasites. The only reason these teeming creatures don't make us sick more often is that our immune systems are very good at destroying them before they cause trouble.

There are times, however, when you want the immune system to work a little less efficiently. For people having transplant surgery or those with immune system disorders such as rheumatoid arthritis, medications that dampen immunity can speed recovery or even, in some cases, save a life.

The immune system is an extremely vigilant sentinel, but it doesn't always know what's good for you. In the early days of transplants, for example, operations often failed because the immune system, failing to recognize the new organ as a friend, attacked it as an enemy. The result was organ rejection and often death.

By using immune system suppressants, however, doctors can

AT A GLANCE

CYCLOSPORINE

Brand name: Sandimmune

How taken: Liquid, capsule, injection

Prescription: Yes

	YES	NO
Generic substitutes		✓
Potentially addicting		✓
May cause drowsiness		✓
Alcohol discouraged	✓	

Possible drug interactions include: The effects of this drug may increase if taken with sex hormones (estrogen or testosterone), cimetidine (used for ulcers) and some antibiotics, antifungal medications and heart drugs. This drug taken in combination with other medications that suppress the immune system or cancer drugs may increase the risk of infection.

Possible side effects include: Bleeding, tender gums, high blood pressure, nausea, muscle tremors and kidney or liver problems.

CAUTION: Avoid vaccines such as the polio vaccine.

AZATHIOPRINE

Brand name: Imuran

How taken: Tablet, injection

Prescription: Yes

	YES	NO
Generic substitutes	✓	
Potentially addicting		✓
May cause drowsiness		✓
Alcohol discouraged	✓	

Possible drug interactions include: The effects of this drug may increase if taken with some gout medications. This drug taken in combination with other immune system suppressants, cancer drugs or cortisone (a steroid) may increase the risk of infection.

Possible side effects include: Nausea, vomiting, fatigue and loss of appetite.

CAUTION: Avoid vaccines such as the polio vaccine.

AT A GLANCE

METHOTREXATE

Brand names: Mexate, Rheumatrex

How taken: Tablet, injection

Prescription: Yes

	YES	NO
Generic substitutes	✓	
Potentially addicting		✓
May cause drowsiness		✓
Alcohol discouraged	✓	

Possible drug interactions include:
Interactions are unlikely (unless also taking aspirin, ibuprofen or other nonsteroidal anti-inflammatory drugs).

Possible side effects include:
Mouth or lip sores, stomach pain, flushing, nausea and diarrhea.

CAUTION: Avoid vaccines such as the polio vaccine. May be dangerous if taken with aspirin, ibuprofen or other nonsteroidal anti-inflammatory drugs.

cialized immune system cells called T-lymphocytes.

When cyclosporine came into use in the early 1980s, the survival rate of transplanted organs immediately rose by 10 to 15 percent. At the same time, there was a significant decrease in postsurgical complications, says Dr. Elzinga.

"It's made cardiac and liver transplantation very successful, whereas before they were only marginally successful," says Dr. Elzinga. "Cyclosporine really sparked a revolution."

The drug usually is given in high doses several hours to a day before surgery, and then given in smaller amounts for the rest of your life. "People who have had transplants are pretty much committed to lifelong immunosuppression," says Dr. Elzinga. "The dose is tapered over time, but it's never removed completely."

Before there was cyclosporine, doctors usually used the prescription drug azathioprine (Imuran) to prevent rejection. Taken orally or by injection, azathioprine profoundly dampens the immune system. It may be less effective than cyclosporine, however, which is why it's used less often, says Dr. Elzinga.

Other prescription immune system suppressants, taken orally or by injection, include methotrexate (Mexate, Rheumatrex), prednisone (Deltasone, Meticorten, Orasone) and cyclophosphamide (Cytoxan, Neosar). Yet another option, given

now prevent rejection, enabling transplanted organs to survive, says Lawrence Elzinga, M.D., assistant professor of medicine at Oregon Health Sciences University in Portland.

The immune system suppressant most in use today for organ transplants is cyclosporine (Sandimmune). This powerful prescription medication, taken orally or by injection, blocks the activity of spe-

by injection, are specialized cells known as monoclonal antibodies (Orthoclone OKT3). Because these medications act in different ways, they're often combined—for example, cyclosporine plus azathioprine and prednisone—for greater effectiveness.

Saving the Body from Itself

These powerful medications aren't used only in the operating room. Doctors also use them to treat autoimmune disorders, conditions such as psoriasis and rheumatoid arthritis, in which the immune system, rather than protecting the body, begins attacking it instead.

For example, with methotrexate, doctors can virtually eliminate the silvery skin scales of psoriasis, says Alan Menter, M.D., medical director of the Psoriasis Center and chairman of the dermatology division at Baylor University Medical Center in Dallas. "There's no other drug that has as good a record or works as well for psoriasis as methotrexate," says Dr. Menter.

It isn't considered a cure for psoriasis, though. To date there is no cure. But in most cases, he adds, the skin will begin to clear within 30 days of treatment and may be completely clear within three months. But because methotrexate can cause serious side effects—nausea or lung problems, for example—it's usually used only when other psoriasis treatments aren't

effective. Also, the psoriasis eventually does come back.

Methotrexate also works well for rheumatoid arthritis, another immune system disorder. In one study, researchers at Boston's Brigham and Women's Hospital treated 12 people with methotrex-

AT A GLANCE

PREDNISONE

Brand names: Deltasone, Meticorten, Orasone

How taken: Liquid, tablet

Prescription: Yes

	YES	NO
Generic substitutes	✓	
Potentially addicting		✓
May cause drowsiness		✓
Alcohol discouraged	✓	

Possible drug interactions include: The effects of this drug may decrease if taken with antacids, antibiotics or antifungal drugs. Taking this drug may decrease the effects of diuretics (water pills) and digitalis (a heart medication); taking it may increase or decrease the effects of insulin.

Possible side effects include: Stomach upset, acne, bruising, weight gain and insomnia.

CAUTION: See your doctor if you experience unusual bruising or irregular heartbeat. Avoid vaccines such as the polio vaccine.

ate for seven years. In more than 80 percent of the cases, swelling was significantly reduced, and half of the patients reported considerable improvement in joint pain as well.

Cyclosporine also has been used for immune system disorders, including psoriasis, arthritis and inflammatory bowel disease.

Powerful Drugs, Powerful Side Effects

Although doctors are excited about the many possibilities of these drugs, they remain concerned about their many possible side effects.

Cyclosporine, for example, commonly causes nausea, muscle tre-

---

AT A GLANCE

CYCLOPHOSPHAMIDE

Brand names: Cytoxan, Neosar

How taken: Liquid, tablet, injection

Prescription: Yes

	YES	NO
Generic substitutes	✓	
Potentially addicting		✓
May cause drowsiness		✓
Alcohol discouraged		✓

Possible drug interactions include: Taking this drug may increase the effects of antibiotics, antifungal drugs, anti-thyroid medications or drugs for gout. This drug taken in combination with other medications that suppress the immune system may increase the risk of infection.

Possible side effects include: Fatigue, nausea, vomiting, dizziness, loss of appetite, confusion, agitation and darkening of the skin and fingernails.

CAUTION: Avoid vaccines such as the polio vaccine.

MONOCLONAL ANTIBODIES

Brand name: Orthoclone OKT3

How taken: Injection

Prescription: Yes

	YES	NO
Generic substitutes		✓
Potentially addicting		✓
May cause drowsiness		✓
Alcohol discouraged		✓

Possible drug interactions include: This drug taken in combination with cancer drugs or other medications that suppress the immune system may increase the risk of infection.

Possible side effects include: Nausea, headache, chest pain, irregular heartbeat, dizziness and shortness of breath.

CAUTION: Avoid vaccines such as the polio vaccine.

mors and kidney poisoning. Azathioprine, while somewhat safer, also may cause nausea as well as damage to the liver or bone marrow. Even methotrexate, which is relatively safe, may cause liver damage when taken for a long time, says Dr. Menter.

In addition, suppressing the immune system invariably increases the risk of infection, particularly when the drugs are given in high doses, as they are for organ transplant surgery, says Dr. Elzinga. "Infection is more of a problem in the first one to six months following the transplant," he adds. "It's not as much of a problem once they're on the lower doses."

When side effects are severe, changing the dose or changing drugs often will help clear things up. The goal, doctors agree, is to use the medications in the lowest effective doses.

"What we like to do is give people drug holidays, to get them off the drugs for a while," says Dr. Menter. "I think it's important not to push the drugs to the limit."

Incontinence Drugs

Warranties against Wetness

Day after day, the bladder quietly collects urine from the kidneys. Except for an occasional reminder that a trip to the bathroom would be very much appreciated, it usually goes about its job without your even being aware of it.

But for people with urinary incontinence, the bladder isn't so cooperative. It lets go when it should hold on, often with little or no warning. Even sneezing or laughing can open the gates, says Jerry G. Blaivas, M.D., urologist and clinical professor at The New York Hospital–Cornell Medical Center in New York City.

In many cases these people can control incontinence with therapies such as exercise and biofeedback. When natural measures don't work, however, medications may be used. "Any patient who has the concern, awareness and motivation, we can make dry," says Dr. Blaivas.

Many people have a condition known as urge incontinence, in

NATURAL ALTERNATIVES

To help control an unruly bladder, try these simple techniques. **Make frequent pit stops.** Don't wait until your bladder reaches its limit before finding a bathroom. Urinating more frequently can help prevent problems later.

Go regularly. Research indicates you can "train" your body to gain additional control. In one study, nursing-home residents who went to the bathroom at the same times every day had fewer accidents than those who merely waited for nature's call.

Try Kegels. By strengthening your pelvic muscles, these special exercises can help increase your holding power. To identify the muscles involved, tighten the muscles around your anus without tensing the buttocks or abdomen muscles (imagine trying to hold back a bowel movement). Next, try to stop, then restart your urine flow. To do a Kegel: Moving back to front, clench the muscles while counting to four, then relax to four. Repeat for two minutes three times daily for a total of about 40 to 50 Kegels.

which the bladder overreacts to the slightest stimulation, says Deborah Erickson, M.D., assistant professor of surgery in the Division of Urology at Pennsylvania State University College of Medicine in Hershey. For these people, nature's call can come quickly—often too quickly to get to a bathroom in time.

To help keep you dry, your doctor may recommend drugs to calm an "excitable" bladder. Taken orally, prescription medications such as propantheline (Pro-Banthine) and oxybutynin (Ditropan) work by blocking acetylcholine, a chemical that causes the bladder to contract—and overreact.

These drugs can prevent many accidents, but they aren't a cure, says Dr. Erickson. In addition, they may cause side effects, including constipation, a dry mouth and blurred vision. If they don't work for you, your doctor may recommend other medications instead.

Many people have found relief with some medications that are also used to treat depression. Prescription drugs such as imipramine (Janimine, Norfranil, Tofranil) can help make the bladder less sensitive, says Dr. Erickson. But these medications aren't entirely free of problems. If you quit taking them suddenly, you may experience chills, muscle aches and other uncomfortable symptoms. "If you stop taking one of these drugs, you may need to decrease the dose gradually to prevent these side effects," she says.

Other prescription drugs that have been used for incontinence include muscle relaxants such as dicyclomine (Antispas, A-Spas, Bentyl) and flavoxate (Urispas). Usually taken orally, these medications are rarely a doctor's first choice. But for people who can't tolerate other drugs, says Dr. Erickson, "they may be helpful, with fewer side effects."

A second type of incontinence is called stress incontinence. For people with this condition, anything that increases pressure in the abdomen—coughing, sneezing, laughing, even stepping off a curb—can spell trouble.

Stress incontinence occurs most often in women, often following pregnancy or with advancing age, when the pelvic floor muscles have become too weak to support the bladder in the correct position, says Dr. Erickson. It also can occur if the urethral sphincter—the round mus-

---

AT A GLANCE

PROPANTHELINE

Brand name: Pro-Banthine

How taken: Tablet

Prescription: Yes

	YES	NO
Generic substitutes	✓	
Potentially addicting		✓
May cause drowsiness	✓	
Alcohol discouraged		✓

Possible drug interactions include: The effects of this drug may decrease if taken with antacids, diarrhea medicines or some antifungal drugs. Taking this drug may increase the effects of narcotics, antihistamines, antidepressants and sedatives.

Possible side effects include: Dizziness, constipation, blurred vision and dryness of the nose, mouth or throat.

OXYBUTYNIN

Brand name: Ditropan

How taken: Tablet, liquid

Prescription: Yes

	YES	NO
Generic substitutes	✓	
Potentially addicting		✓
May cause drowsiness	✓	
Alcohol discouraged	✓	

Possible drug interactions include: Taking this drug may increase the effects of antihistamines, antidepressants, muscle relaxants, sedatives and bronchodilators (used for asthma).

Possible side effects include: Constipation, blurred vision and dryness of the mouth, nose or throat.

AT A GLANCE

IMIPRAMINE

Brand names: Janimine, Norfranil, Tofranil

How taken: Tablet, capsule, injection

Prescription: Yes

	YES	NO
Generic substitutes	✓	
Potentially addicting		✓
May cause drowsiness	✓	
Alcohol discouraged	✓	

Possible drug interactions include: The effects of this drug may increase if taken with thyroid, anti-spasmodic, ulcer or blood pressure medicines. This drug taken in combination with monoamine oxidase (MAO) inhibitors (used for depression) may result in high blood pressure; taking it with diet pills or decongestants may cause heart problems.

Possible side effects include: Nausea, headache, fatigue, dizziness, increased appetite and a dry mouth.

DICYCLOMINE

Brand names: Antispas, A-Spas, Bentyl

How taken: Tablet, liquid, capsule, injection

Prescription: Yes

	YES	NO
Generic substitutes	✓	
Potentially addicting		✓
May cause drowsiness	✓	
Alcohol discouraged		✓

Possible drug interactions include: The effects of this drug may decrease if taken with antacids, diarrhea medicines and some antifungal drugs. Taking this drug may increase the effects of narcotics, antihistamines, sedatives, some heart rhythm drugs and other anti-spasmodic drugs.

Possible side effects include: Constipation, dizziness, blurred vision and dryness of the mouth, nose or throat.

cle inside the urethra—becomes too weak to reliably prevent leakage.

To increase tension on this all-important muscle, your doctor may recommend a drug called phenyl-propanolamine (Control, Prolamine, Propagest). Taken orally, this over-the-counter and prescription medication (it's the active ingredient in many cold remedies and diet aids) can help keep urine in until you decide to let it out.

Phenylpropanolamine rarely causes serious side effects, although some people may experience nausea, insomnia or a dry mouth. In addition, some people may experience high blood pressure, although it will return to normal levels when they stop taking the drug, says Dr. Erickson.

For some women, particularly those past menopause, the hormone estrogen may be used to control stress incontinence, says Michael Vernon, M.D., director of geriatrics at East Carolina University School of Medicine in Greenville, North Carolina. Prescription medications containing estrogen (Estraval, Premarin), usually taken orally, work by increasing the amount of tissue that surrounds the urethra. This enables the surrounding muscles to get a better "grip" for controlling urination, says Dr. Vernon.

Estrogen also can be combined with phenylpropanolamine for

AT A GLANCE

PHENYLPROPANOLAMINE

Brand names: Control, Prolamine, Propagest

How taken: Tablet, capsule

Prescription: Sometimes, depending on strength

	YES	NO
Generic substitutes	✓	
Potentially addicting		✓
May cause drowsiness		✓
Alcohol discouraged		✓

Possible drug interactions include: This drug taken with digitalis (a heart drug) or stimulant drugs such as caffeine or cold medicines may result in irregular heartbeat; taking it with beta-blockers (heart and blood pressure drugs) or monoamine oxidase (MAO) inhibitors (used for depression) may result in high blood pressure.

Possible side effects include: Nausea, insomnia and dry mouth.

AT A GLANCE

FLAVOXATE

Brand name: Urispas

How taken: Tablet

Prescription: Yes

	YES	NO
Generic substitutes		✓
Potentially addicting		✓
May cause drowsiness	✓	
Alcohol discouraged		✓

Possible drug interactions include: Interactions are unlikely.

Possible side effects include: Blurred vision and dryness of the mouth or throat.

extra effectiveness, he adds.

When taken in low doses, estrogen is generally quite safe, although some women may experience uncomfortable side effects such as bloating or breast pain. Also, some experts worry that long-term use of estrogen may increase the risk of endometrial cancer or breast cancer. Before taking this medication, you should discuss these risks with your doctor.

Inflammatory Bowel Disease Drugs

Strong Relief for Intestinal Pain

It often begins with abdominal pain, weight loss and diarrhea. Then there may be fever or bloody stool. It *feels* like the flu, you tell your doctor, but it won't go away. What kind of bug is this?

Perhaps you don't have a bug at all, but inflammatory bowel disease (IBD). This painful inflammation of the intestinal wall affects approximately 500,000 Americans. It appears to be somewhat hereditary and may somehow be triggered by alterations in the body's immune system, says Samuel Meyers, M.D., an IBD expert and clinical professor of medicine at Mount Sinai School of Medicine of the City University of New York.

Although it's convenient to talk about IBD as though it were one disease, in fact it is two. Ulcerative colitis causes inflammation in the colon, that part of the intestinal tract closest to the "exit door." Crohn's disease can cause inflammation anywhere in the intestinal tract, but its favorite spot is the ileum, which is at the end of the small intestine. The symptoms of the two diseases are somewhat similar, as are the treatments.

Apart from surgery (and not always then), there is no cure for either form of IBD. There are drugs, however, that can help quell the inflammation, ease the pain and discourage both from coming back.

Standard Treatments

For mild to moderate IBD, the drug most commonly prescribed is sulfasalazine (Azulfidine, Azulfidine EN-tabs). Taken orally, the drug is used for flare-ups of both Crohn's disease and ulcerative colitis. For preventing inflammation, however, it works best for colitis, says Dr. Meyers. This is because sulfasalazine works best in an environment rich in bacteria, like the colon.

"The advantage of sulfasalazine is that it's one of the oldest medicines used for IBD, and we always feel secure using something familiar," says Dr. Meyers. Yet it also can cause side effects, including nausea and headache. For this reason, as many as one in five people can't take it.

Sulfasalazine is the grandfather of an entire class of prescription

AT A GLANCE

SULFASALAZINE

Brand names: Azulfidine, Azulfidine EN-tabs

How taken: Liquid, tablet

Prescription: Yes

	YES	NO
Generic substitutes	✓	
Potentially addicting		✓
May cause drowsiness		✓
Alcohol discouraged	✓	

Possible drug interactions include: Taking this drug may increase the effects of diabetes drugs and anti-clotting medications, such as aspirin and warfarin.

Possible side effects include: Dizziness, sore muscles and joints, headache, itching and skin rash.

MESALAMINE

Brand names: Asacol, Rowasa

How taken: Enema, suppository

Prescription: Yes

	YES	NO
Generic substitutes		✓
Potentially addicting		✓
May cause drowsiness		✓
Alcohol discouraged	✓	

Possible drug interactions include: Interactions are unlikely.

Possible side effects include: Stomach cramps, gas, mild headache and nausea.

drugs known as 5-aminosalicylic acids (5-ASAs). The newer 5-ASAs seem to work as well as sulfasalazine without the side effects. Taken orally or rectally, drugs such as mesalamine (Asacol, Rowasa) and olsalazine (Dipentum) work for both types of IBD, says William Ruderman, M.D., chairman of the Department of Gastroenterology at the Cleveland Clinic–Florida in Fort Lauderdale. Unlike sulfasalazine, some of the 5-ASAs are designed to relieve inflammation higher up in the intestinal tract.

Today, sulfasalazine remains a best seller among IBD drugs. But in the future, Dr. Ruderman says, "I think we will see the newer 5-ASA drugs taking over more and more."

The Big Guns

Both sulfasalazine and the other 5-ASAs are less effective when IBD is severe. That's when steroids shine. For stopping inflammation fast, these potent drugs, in use since the 1950s, remain the gold standard, says Dr. Meyers.

For example, prescription drugs

such as prednisone (Deltasone, Orasone, Prednicen-M), beta-methasone (Betatrex, Celestone, Soluspan) and prednisolone (Hydeltrasol, Pediapred) can begin relieving pain and inflammation almost immediately, says Dr. Meyers. These drugs may be taken orally, rectally or by injection.

Another potent inflammation fighter is called adrenocortico-tropic hormone, also known as corticotropin and ACTH (Acthar). This prescription drug, given by injection, works by stimulating the adrenal glands to make more cortisone, a natural steroid. "Instead of giving a steroid, ACTH helps people produce it themselves," explains Dr. Meyers.

AT A GLANCE

PREDNISONE

Brand names: Deltasone, Orasone, Prednicen-M

How taken: Liquid, tablet

Prescription: Yes

	YES	No
Generic substitutes	✓	
Potentially addicting		✓
May cause drowsiness		✓
Alcohol discouraged	✓	

Possible drug interactions include: The effects of this drug may decrease if taken with antacids, antibiotics or antifungal drugs. Taking this drug may decrease the effects of diabetes medications, diuretics (water pills) and digitalis.

Possible side effects include: Increased appetite, weight gain, salt and water retention, loss of potassium and risk of infection.

CAUTION: See your doctor if you experience unusual bruising or irregular hearbeat. Avoid vaccines such as the polio vaccine.

CORTICOTROPIN

Brand names: Acthar

How taken: Injection

Prescription: Yes

	YES	No
Generic substitutes	✓	
Potentially addicting		✓
May cause drowsiness		✓
Alcohol discouraged	✓	

Possible drug interactions include: The effects of this drug may decrease if taken with antacids, griseofulvin (an antifungal medication) and phenylbutazone (used for arthritis).

Possible side effects include: Increased appetite, indigestion, nervousness or restlessness, sleep disturbances and risk of infection.

Although steroids and ACTH are extremely effective, they also can cause serious side effects, such as mood changes, high blood pressure and osteoporosis. For this reason, says Dr. Ruderman, these drugs are used as briefly as possible. As soon as the inflammation is tamed, they're discontinued and, in some cases, replaced with safer drugs.

When steroids don't help and your symptoms are severe, your doctor may recommend a short-term course of immune system–modulating drugs. By altering your immune system—which is thought to play a significant role in IBD—these powerful medications can help suppress inflammation in the intestine as well, says Dr. Ruderman.

Studies have shown that prescription drugs such as mercaptopurine (Purinethol) and azathioprine (Imuran), taken orally or by injection, can help relieve symptoms in 60 to 70 percent of people who have hard-to-treat IBD.

Unfortunately, these drugs, some-

AT A GLANCE

MERCAPTOPURINE

Brand name: Purinethol

How taken: Tablet

Prescription: Yes

	YES	NO
Generic substitutes		✓
Potentially addicting		✓
May cause drowsiness		✓
Alcohol discouraged	✓	

Possible drug interactions include: Taking this drug may decrease or increase the effects of gout medications; taking it may increase the effects of anti-thyroid medications. This drug taken in combination with cyclosporine (an immunosuppressant) or anti-inflammatory steroids may increase the risk of infection.

Possible side effects include: Fatigue, weakness and yellow eyes or skin.

AZATHIOPRINE

Brand name: Imuran

How taken: Injection, tablet

Prescription: Yes

	YES	NO
Generic substitutes	✓	
Potentially addicting		✓
May cause drowsiness		✓
Alcohol discouraged	✓	

Possible drug interactions include: The effects of this drug may increase if taken with gout medications. Taking this drug may decrease the effects of anti-clotting drugs and some muscle relaxants; taking it may increase the effects of anti-inflammatory steroids.

Possible side effects include: Fatigue, cough, fever, lower back pain and difficulty urinating.

times called immunomodulators or immunosuppressants, can be dangerous. Possible side effects include infections, inflammation of the pancreas or even cancer, says Dr. Meyers. These drugs are also slow acting, requiring three or more months to be effective. And when treatment is stopped, symptoms quickly return. "They are used only when people don't respond to other medications and surgery is not appropriate," says Dr. Meyers.

In fact, none of the drugs used to treat IBD is perfect. As a result, people often are treated in "layers." For example, someone with IBD might first be given sulfasalazine or another 5-ASA—the first layer. "If that's not enough, you add on the corticosteroid layer. If that's not enough, you go to surgery or the immunosuppressants," says Dr. Meyers. Then, when you take them *off* the medications, he adds, you peel off the layers, one at a time.

Laxatives

A Helping Hand When Needed

It's one thing to read in the bathroom. But when you're finishing entire chapters of *War and Peace*, you're probably spending way too much time in there.

But you're not alone. Doctors say Americans complain more about constipation than any other gastrointestinal problem and spend approximately $400 million a year trying to relieve it.

Constipation usually can be relieved with natural remedies, such as eating more fiber and getting more exercise. But sometimes nature needs a helping hand, says Edmund Leff, M.D., a colon and rectal specialist with offices in

Phoenix and Scottsdale. "For occasional use, a mild laxative is okay," he says.

Bulk Gets You Going

For most constipation, bulk-forming laxatives are the drugs of choice, says Dr. Leff. These simple preparations, sold over the counter and taken orally, are packed with nondigestible fibers. Like thousands of tiny sponges, these fibers soak up many times their weight in intestinal water. This can make hard stools soften up, prompting easy, regular bowel movements.

There are many bulk-forming laxatives to choose from, including methylcellulose (Citrucel, Cologel), psyllium (Siblin, Perdiem Plain, Syllact) and polycarbophil (Equal-actin, Fibercon, Mitrolan).

These preparations usually begin working within one to three days and may be taken safely for several weeks, says Dr. Leff. They may, however, cause gas and cramping during the first week of treatment, he adds. And because they're so absorbent, it's important to drink plenty of water, at least four to eight glasses every day.

A Soft Touch

When stools are hard and painful to pass, your doctor may recommend stool softeners such as docusate sodium (Colace, Dialose) and docusate calcium (Doxidan, Surfak). Sold over the counter and by prescription, these drugs, usually taken orally, allow fats and fluids to penetrate the stool. This makes the stool larger, softer and easier to eliminate.

A time-honored stool lubricant is mineral oil. Sold over the counter and taken orally, mineral oil helps ease the passage of hard stools. However, it also can block the body's absorption of vitamins A, D, E and K. For this reason many doctors suggest avoiding mineral oil and sticking with softeners instead. If you do take mineral oil, however, be sure to take it during the day and not at night because of its potential to cause pneumonia.

NATURAL ALTERNATIVES

Constipation is preventable! In the majority of cases, doctors say, you can keep things moving by heeding these simple suggestions.

Seek fiber. "Eating a high-fiber diet may be all you need," says Edmund Leff, M.D., a colon and rectal specialist with offices in Phoenix and Scottsdale. Good sources for dietary fiber include whole grains, fruit and vegetables.

Fill your glass. Drink plenty of fluids. By keeping the contents of your colon well lubricated, you can help stools move smoothly along. Have at least four to six (eight-ounce) glasses of water every day.

Heed the call. In today's high-pressure world, it's easy to postpone your basic needs. Over time, this can lead to constipation, says Dr. Leff. To prevent problems, don't procrastinate when nature calls.

Get physical. Exercise. When you move the rest of your body, your bowels will move more easily, too.

Fast Action

When you want a more powerful purging, osmotic laxatives are very effective. Taken orally or rectally, they cause water to rush into the bowel, which results in a rapid bowel movement, says William Ruderman, M.D., chairman of the Department of Gastroenterology at the Cleveland Clinic–Florida in Fort Lauderdale. Taken orally, they work within three hours; rectally, within 15 minutes.

Available over the counter and by prescription, laxatives such as magnesium hydroxide (Phillips' Milk of Magnesia), sodium phosphate (Fleet Phospho-Soda, K-Phos Neutral) and magnesium citrate (Citroma, Citro-Nesia) are very effective and, when used as directed, safe, says Dr. Ruderman.

A drug called glycerin (Fleet Babylax, Sani-Supp) also draws water into the bowel. Sold over the counter or by prescription and taken rectally, glycerin usually will cause a bowel movement within 30 minutes. But because it can irritate the rectum, doctors say it shouldn't be used regularly.

In fact, all of the laxatives that draw water into the bowel should be used with restraint, says Dr. Ruderman. When overused, they can alter the body's normal balance of minerals and fluids. More worrisome is the tendency of some to cause dependence: People who abuse laxatives may find it increasingly difficult to have a bowel movement without them.

CASTOR OIL: ITS TIME HAS PASSED

People have been using castor oil—or at least the plant from which it's derived, *Ricinus communis*—for thousands of years.

But what's traditional, doctors agree, isn't necessarily safe. Castor oil is one of the most powerful stimulant laxatives on the market today, and doctors rarely recommend it, says William Ruderman, M.D., chairman of the Department of Gastroenterology at the Cleveland Clinic–Florida in Fort Lauderdale.

When taken in normal doses, castor oil may cause such a thorough emptying of the bowel that several days may pass before the next bowel movement does. It also can cause dehydration, painful cramping and even damage to the colon wall.

So even though some old-timers still swear by castor oil, it doesn't belong in the modern medicine chest. "It's very potent stuff," says Dr. Ruderman, "and it tastes terrible."

AT A GLANCE

PSYLLIUM

Brand names: Metamucil, Naturacil, Perdiem Plain, Siblin, Syllact

How taken: Granules, powder, wafers, caramels

Prescription: No

	YES	NO
Generic substitutes	✓	
Potentially addicting		✓
May cause drowsiness		✓
Alcohol discouraged		✓

Possible drug interactions include: Interactions are unlikely.

Possible side effects include: Side effects are unlikely.

DOCUSATE SODIUM

Brand names: Colace, Dialose

How taken: Tablet, capsule, liquid, syrup

Prescription: No

	YES	NO
Generic substitutes	✓	
Potentially addicting	✓	
May cause drowsiness		✓
Alcohol discouraged		✓

Possible drug interactions include: Interactions are unlikely.

Possible side effects include: Diarrhea, nausea and cramping.

POLYCARBOPHIL

Brand names: Equalactin, Fibercon, Mitrolan

How taken: Tablet, chewable tablet

Prescription: No

	YES	NO
Generic substitutes	✓	
Potentially addicting		✓
May cause drowsiness		✓
Alcohol discouraged		✓

Possible drug interactions include: Interactions are unlikely.

Possible side effects include: Skin rash, itching and difficulty swallowing.

PHENOLPHTHALEIN

Brand names: Ex-Lax, Medilax

How taken: Chewing gum, tablet, chewable tablet, wafers

Prescription: No

	YES	NO
Generic substitutes		✓
Potentially addicting	✓	
May cause drowsiness		✓
Alcohol discouraged		✓

Possible drug interactions include: Interactions are unlikely.

Possible side effects include: Cramping and potassium loss.

AT A GLANCE

BISACODYL

Brand names: Bisac-Evac, Carter's Little Pills, Dulcolax

How taken: Enema, liquid, suppository, tablet

Prescription: No

	YES	NO
Generic substitutes	✓	
Potentially addicting	✓	
May cause drowsiness	✓	
Alcohol discouraged		✓

Possible drug interactions include: Interactions are unlikely.

Possible side effects include: Cramping and diarrhea.

MAGNESIUM CITRATE

Brand names: Citroma, Citro-Nesia

How taken: Liquid, suppository, tablet

Prescription: No

	YES	NO
Generic substitutes	✓	
Potentially addicting	✓	
May cause drowsiness	✓	
Alcohol discouraged		✓

Possible drug interactions include: Taking this drug may keep antibiotics such as tetracyclines from working.

Possible side effects include: Gas, cramping, diarrhea and increased thirst.

Aggressive Action

The most powerful laxatives of all are called stimulant laxatives. When you *must* have a bowel movement—for example, before undergoing a bowel examination—your doctor may recommend a drug such as phenolphthalein (Ex-Lax, Medilax), bisacodyl (Bisac-Evac, Carter's Little Pills, Dulcolax) or a polyethylene glycol electrolyte solution (Colyte, Golytely).

These prescription and over-the-counter drugs, taken orally or rectally, stimulate secretion of fluid into the bowel. At the same time, they prompt muscular contractions in the bowel wall, which hastens bowel movements.

Indeed, they may hasten things too well. Stimulant laxatives sometimes cause nausea, cramps and explosive diarrhea. In fact, they're too powerful to be used without a doctor's supervision. "I generally avoid them unless absolutely necessary, and then use them only on a short-term basis," explains Dr. Ruderman.

Malaria Drugs

Battling a Tropical Threat

Malaria is among the world's most common infections, and one of the most devastating. Caused by microscopic parasites that usually enter the bloodstream following mosquito bites, malaria causes symptoms such as sweating, high fever and agonizing chills. Worldwide, it strikes approximately 270 million people a year, killing more than 2 million.

Although malaria is rare in the United States, travelers to regions such as central and southern Africa often are exposed to this very dangerous disease. Experts agree that treating malaria—or better yet, preventing it—always should get top priority.

Standard Protection

Although there isn't yet a vaccine that will prevent malaria, there are several medications that can help keep the infection at bay, both in mosquito country and once you get home.

A standard medication used for malaria is the prescription drug chloroquine (Aralen). Usually taken orally, chloroquine is used for both the prevention and treatment of malaria, states Hans Lobel, M.D., head of the malaria surveillance section at the Centers for Disease

---

AT A GLANCE

CHLOROQUINE

Brand name: Aralen
How taken: Tablet, injection
Prescription: Yes

	YES	NO
Generic substitutes	✓	
Potentially addicting		✓
May cause drowsiness	✓	
Alcohol discouraged	✓	

Possible drug interactions include: Interactions are unlikely.

Possible side effects include: Nausea, itching, diarrhea, stomach cramps and blurred vision.

Control and Prevention in Atlanta.

When chloroquine is used to prevent malaria, it usually is taken in a low dose once a week, beginning one week before traveling and continuing for four weeks after you return. When the drug is used for treatment, it usually is taken in high doses and can completely relieve symptoms in a day or two. In these larger amounts the drug may cause headache, itching or an upset stomach. In general, however, it's quite safe, says Dr. Lobel.

Resistance Fighters

How effective a drug is depends on the sensitivity of the parasite," Dr. Lobel says. Some organisms become resistant and simply don't respond to chloroquine. When that happens, other drugs—alone or in combination—may be used instead.

For example, the prescription drug mefloquine (Lariam), taken orally, can be used to treat species of the parasite that aren't affected

---

AT A GLANCE

MEFLOQUINE

Brand name: Lariam
How taken: Tablet
Prescription: Yes

	YES	NO
Generic substitutes		✓
Potentially addicting		✓
May cause drowsiness		✓
Alcohol discouraged	✓	

Possible drug interactions include: This drug taken in combination with heart or blood pressure drugs such as diltiazem, quinidine or verapamil may result in slowed heartbeat; taking it with anti-seizure drugs or with other antimalarial drugs such as quinine or chloroquine may increase the risk of seizures.

Possible side effects include: Nausea, dizziness, headache and difficulty concentrating.

PYRIMETHAMINE and SULFADOXINE

Brand name: Fansidar
How taken: Tablet
Prescription: Yes

	YES	NO
Generic substitutes		✓
Potentially addicting		✓
May cause drowsiness	✓	
Alcohol discouraged	✓	

Possible drug interactions include: This drug taken in combination with anti-thyroid drugs, amphotericin B (an antifungal drug), colchicine (used for gout) or cancer drugs such as methotrexate and interferon may increase the risk of side effects.

Possible side effects include: Nausea, fever, fatigue, diarrhea and swelling or burning of the tongue.

AT A GLANCE

PRIMAQUINE

Brand name: Generic only
How taken: Tablet
Prescription: Yes

	YES	NO
Generic substitutes	✓	
Potentially addicting		✓
May cause drowsiness	✓	
Alcohol discouraged	✓	

Possible drug interactions include: This drug taken in combination with oral diabetes drugs, quinacrine (used for intestinal tract infections), aceto-hydroxamic acid (used for kidney stones), furazolidone (an anti-parasitic drug) and methyldopa (used for high blood pressure) may increase the risk of side effects.

Possible side effects include: Fever, nausea, fatigue, discoloration of urine and pain in the back, leg or stomach.

QUININE

Brand names: Legatrin, Quinamm, Quindan, Quiphile
How taken: Capsule, tablet
Prescription: Sometimes, depending on strength

	YES	NO
Generic substitutes	✓	
Potentially addicting		✓
May cause drowsiness	✓	
Alcohol discouraged	✓	

Possible drug interactions include: This drug taken in combination with mefloquine (another malaria drug) may increase the risk of side effects.

Possible side effects include: Nausea, diarrhea, headache, stomach cramps, blurred vision and ringing in the ears or temporary hearing loss.

by chloroquine. When used to prevent malaria, mefloquine is taken once a week. If you've already been infected, however, a single large dose should do the trick, says Dr. Lobel.

As with chloroquine, mefloquine is quite safe, although it may cause some stomach upset.

Another potent prescription medication is a combination of pyrimethamine plus sulfadoxine (Fansidar). "This is very effective most of the time," says Dr. Lobel.

Unfortunately, the drug may cause dangerous skin reactions. For that reason it's rarely used to prevent disease. "If it's used for treatment, which is only a single dose, then the risk of serious reactions is very small," Dr. Lobel adds.

The prescription drug primaquine is also used for treating malaria. Taken orally, primaquine often is used in combination with chloroquine for added effectiveness. But primaquine may cause anemia when taken by people with certain enzyme deficiencies. As a result, it may be used only when other drugs aren't appropriate or available.

Perhaps the oldest medication for malaria is quinine. Originally extracted from the bark of the cinchona tree, quinine (Legatrin, Quinamm, Quiphile) is commonly used when the malaria-causing parasites are resistant to chloroquine. "Quinine can be used for seven days all by itself, or it can be combined with another drug so you don't have to take it for so long," explains Dr. Lobel.

Quinine generally is quite safe, although it can cause headache, nausea and nervousness. As a result, people taking this drug require careful supervision by their doctors.

Male Hormones

Chemical Jump-Starts

As a boy enters puberty, he undergoes many physical changes. His voice deepens, his genitals develop and he begins getting body hair. At the same time, he becomes taller and more muscular and grows out of his clothes at an astounding rate.

These changes are due to powerful chemicals called male hormones, chiefly testosterone. (Women also produce testosterone, but in smaller amounts.) Produced primarily in the testicles, it gives a man his sex drive and typical male characteristics, such as a beard.

Should a boy have too little male hormone—because of problems with the testicles or pituitary gland, for example—he may have retarded growth or delayed puberty. In men, low levels of testosterone reduce sex drive. To treat these and other conditions, doctors often prescribe low doses of testosterone or other male hormones, powerful synthetic medications that act almost exactly like the body's natural hormones.

Long-Term Replacements

Perhaps the most common use for male hormones is in boys or men who have low testosterone

AT A GLANCE

TESTOSTERONE

Brand names: Andro 100, Delatest, Testein P.A.

How taken: Injection

Prescription: Yes

	YES	NO
Generic substitutes	✓	
Potentially addicting		✓
May cause drowsiness		✓
Alcohol discouraged	✓	

Possible drug interactions include: Taking this drug may increase the effects of insulin or anti-clotting drugs. This drug taken in combination with other steroids or anti-nausea, anti-infective or anti-thyroid drugs, oral contraceptives, heart drugs, gold (used for arthritis) or large doses of acetaminophen may result in liver damage.

Possible side effects include: Acne or oily skin, bloating, hair loss, irregular menstrual periods, increases in body hair and changes in breast size, mood or libido.

FLUOXYMESTERONE

Brand names: Android-F, Halotestin

How taken: Capsule, tablet

Prescription: Yes

	YES	NO
Generic substitutes	✓	
Potentially addicting		✓
May cause drowsiness		✓
Alcohol discouraged	✓	

Possible drug interactions include: Taking this drug may increase the effects of insulin or anti-clotting drugs. This drug taken in combination with other steroids or anti-nausea, anti-infective or anti-thyroid drugs, oral contraceptives, heart drugs, gold (used for arthritis) or large doses of acetaminophen may result in liver damage.

Possible side effects include: Acne or oily skin, bloating, hair loss, irregular menstrual periods, increases in body hair and changes in breast size, mood or libido.

levels, a condition called hypogonadism, says Irma Ullrich, M.D., professor of medicine at West Virginia Medical Center's Health Sciences Center in Morgantown.

Given orally or by injection, prescription medications such as testosterone (Andro 100, Delatest, Testrin P.A.), fluoxymesterone (Android-F, Halotestin) and methyltestosterone (Android-5, Oreton, Virilon) can quickly boost flagging testosterone supplies to acceptable levels, says Dr. Ullrich.

In boys with delayed puberty, the drugs may be used for four to six months to jump-start the body's natural production of testosterone. "They can help hasten the maturation of the pituitary gland,"

AT A GLANCE

METHYLTESTOSTERONE

Brand names: Android-5, Oreton, Virilon

How taken: Tablet, capsule, injection

Prescription: Yes

	YES	NO
Generic substitutes	✓	
Potentially addicting		✓
May cause drowsiness		✓
Alcohol discouraged	✓	

Possible drug interactions include: Taking this drug may increase the effects of insulin or anti-clotting drugs. This drug taken in combination with other steroids or anti-nausea, anti-infective or anti-thyroid drugs, oral contraceptives, heart drugs, gold (used for arthritis) or large doses of acetaminophen may result in liver damage.

Possible side effects include: Acne or oily skin, bloating, hair loss, irregular menstrual periods, increases in body hair and changes in breast size, mood or libido.

NANDROLONE

Brand names: Anabolin, Durabolin, Kabolin

How taken: Injection

Prescription: Yes

	YES	NO
Generic substitutes	✓	
Potentially addicting		✓
May cause drowsiness		✓
Alcohol discouraged	✓	

Possible drug interactions include: Taking this drug may increase the effects of insulin or anti-clotting drugs. This drug taken in combination with other steroids or anti-nausea, anti-infective or anti-thyroid drugs, oral contraceptives, heart drugs, gold (used for arthritis) or large doses of acetaminophen may result in liver damage.

Possible side effects include: Acne or oily skin, bloating, irregular menstrual periods, changes in body hair or hair loss and changes in breast size, mood or libido.

explains Dr. Ullrich. Should a boy be physically incapable of producing testosterone, however, the drugs may need to be taken for life, she says.

Men who produce too little testosterone may show little interest in sex. For these guys, a dose of male hormone can often get the fires burning, says Lila Wallis, M.D., hormone expert and clinical professor of medicine at Cornell University Medical College in New York City.

In some cases, women also may be given male hormones. Taken in low doses, the drugs may be used to help relieve postmenopausal mood problems or flagging sexual desire. But because these drugs can cause male characteristics such as facial hair, their use in women can be tricky, Dr. Wallis says. As a result, they're usually used only when other medications won't work.

Growth Stimulators

Male hormones aren't used only to stimulate (or maintain) sexual maturation. They also can be used to improve the appetite, speed the production of red blood cells and accelerate muscle growth, says Dr. Wallis.

For example, someone who has had major surgery might be given a male hormone drug such as nandrolone (Anabolin, Durabolin, Kabolin) or oxymetholone (Anadrol) to speed the healing process. "They can be used for short periods of time to give patients more energy, increase their appetite and help them gain weight," explains Dr. Wallis.

The same drugs, taken orally or by injection, can stimulate the production of red blood cells, which makes them helpful in treating some types of anemia, says Dr. Ullrich.

While these medications have many important and legitimate uses, they also are commonly *misused* by ambitious athletes looking to add a quick—and illegal—edge to their training. Often taken by injection, male hormones (which also may be called anabolic steroids) can enable athletes to train harder and recover more quickly. Yet the medications are rife with

dangers. Even when used appropriately, they can cause breast enlargement in men and increase the risk for prostate cancer and heart disease. People taking them require close supervision to prevent problems. "These medications are extremely potent and we really don't know all of their long-term effects," warns Dr. Wallis.

AT A GLANCE

OXYMETHOLONE

Brand name: Anadrol
How taken: Tablet
Prescription: Yes

	YES	NO
Generic substitutes		✓
Potentially addicting		✓
May cause drowsiness		✓
Alcohol discouraged	✓	

Possible drug interactions include: Taking this drug may increase the effects of insulin or anti-clotting drugs. This drug taken in combination with other steroids or anti-nausea, anti-infective or anti-thyroid drugs, oral contraceptives, heart drugs, gold (used for arthritis) or large doses of acetaminophen may result in liver damage.

Possible side effects include: Acne or oily skin, bloating, irregular menstrual periods, changes in body hair or hair loss and changes in breast size, mood or libido.

Menstrual-Problem Drugs

Timely Help for Monthly Woes

For many women, the only predictable thing about their periods is that they're unpredictable. The flow may be light one month and heavy the next. Sometimes you know when they're due, and sometimes they hit from the blue.

These month-to-month variations usually are caused by normal fluctuations in your body's chemistry. Sometimes, however, changes in the menstrual cycle are caused by physical problems—like too much of one hormone or too little of another. In that case, your doctor may recommend medication to help put your cycles back on track.

When Periods Stop

Of course, some menstrual irregularities are *meant* to be off-track. Consider, for example, a woman who hasn't had a period for several months. Doctors call this condition amenorrhea. "The most common cause of amenorrhea is pregnancy," says Phillip C. Galle, M.D., an infertility and re-productive specialist in Springfield, Illinois.

But sometimes menstrual periods stop because the body's delicate balance of hormones goes awry. For instance, a woman can produce normal amounts of estrogen but still not ovulate. In this case she may need to take supplemental progesterone, or progestin (Cycrin, Depo-Provera, Medroxyprogesterone). This medication, usually taken orally or by injection, can often promote a more regular bleeding pattern, says Dr. Galle.

More regular menstrual cycles can also be achieved by giving low doses of estrogen along with progesterone. In fact, the two hormones may be given simultaneously in the form of oral contraceptives such as norethindrone and ethinyl estradiol (Brevicon, ModiCon, Ortho-Novum 1/35), says Jacqueline Gutmann, M.D., a fertility specialist at the Philadelphia Fertility Institute and assistant clinical associate at the University of Pennsylvania. "These are ideal for women who want reliable contraception as well as regular periods," she adds.

In general, low-dose hormone therapy is quite safe, although some women may experience side effects such as fatigue or weight gain. When this occurs, making small changes in dosage often will clear things up, says Dr. Galle.

Periods That Cause Pain

Virtually every woman has had painful, crampy periods. Cramps occur when the uterus, in its efforts to expel the lining, undergoes powerful contractions. Cramps that are overly vigorous can be extremely uncomfortable. This condition is called dysmenorrhea and is among the most common problems gynecologists treat.

Perhaps the most effective medications for treating cramps are nonsteroidal anti-inflammatory drugs, or NSAIDs. Prescription medications such as mefenamic acid (Ponstel) and naproxen (Anaprox, Naprosyn) and over-the-counter drugs like aspirin (Anacin, Genuine Bayer Aspirin), ibuprofen (Advil, Motrin IB, Nuprin), and naproxen (Aleve), usually taken orally, work by blocking the production of chemicals called prostaglandins, which cause uterine contractions.

In most cases, these are the only medications that people need to relieve painful cramps, says Roger P. Smith, M.D., chief of the Section of General Obstetrics and Gynecology at the Medical College of Georgia in Augusta. "If the pain doesn't improve significantly from taking a NSAID, then you have to wonder if you have the right diag-

NATURAL ALTERNATIVES

There are several things you can do at home to help prevent menstrual cramps from cramping your style.

Relax in a hot bath. Surrounding yourself with warmth will increase blood flow and relax muscles throughout your body, including those in the pelvic area.

Get turned on. Researchers have found that sex with orgasm causes the uterus to contract vigorously, which can temporarily relieve menstrual cramps. On the other hand, sex without orgasm may make the cramps worse, doctors say.

Get some exercise. Physical activity such as swimming or walking can help take your mind off achy monthly cramps.

Mind your minerals. Be sure to get enough calcium, potassium and magnesium. Women who get adequate amounts of these important minerals appear to be less bothered by cramps than those who don't.

nosis," comments Dr. Smith.

The NSAIDs are safe for occasional use, but they can cause diarrhea, stomach pain or other side effects. To reduce discomfort, always take these medications with food or milk, says Dr. Smith.

For severe cramps that aren't relieved by NSAIDs, your doctor may recommend oral contraceptives as well. Those that contain estrogen and a progestin (Brevicon, Loestrin 1/20, Nordette) are very effective for controlling, or even eliminating, menstrual pain, says Dr. Smith.

A significant drawback to this therapy is that these prescription

---

AT A GLANCE

PROGESTIN

Brand names: Amen, Cycrin, Depo-Provera, Medroxyprogesterone

How taken: Injection, tablet

Prescription: Yes

	YES	NO
Generic substitutes	✓	
Potentially addicting		✓
May cause drowsiness		✓
Alcohol discouraged		✓

Possible drug interactions include: Taking this drug may decrease the effects of insulin.

Possible side effects include: Blood clots, fatigue, weight gain and midcycle bleeding.

CAUTION: May cause birth defects if taken during pregnancy.

NORETHINDRONE and ETHINYL ESTRADIOL

Brand names: Brevicon, ModiCon, Ortho-Novum 1/35

How taken: Tablet

Prescription: Yes

	YES	NO
Generic substitutes		✓
Potentially addicting		✓
May cause drowsiness		✓
Alcohol discouraged		✓

Possible drug interactions include: The effects of this drug may decrease if taken with antibiotics, sedatives, anti-seizure drugs or nonsteroidal anti-inflammatory drugs.

Possible side effects include: Blood clots, acne, midcycle bleeding and weight gain.

CAUTION: Cigarette smokers taking this medication may have an increased risk of dangerous heart and circulation problems, including blood clots.

drugs must be taken 21 days a month to deliver just a few days of benefits. "That's not a good payback unless you need contraception, too," Dr. Smith adds.

Other prescription drugs that can relieve menstrual pain include danazol (Danocrine) and GnRH agonists (Lupron, Lupron Depot, Synarel). Taken orally or by injection, these medications are extremely effective. But they're also likely to cause side effects, including weight gain and irregular periods, says Dr. Smith. As a result, they're usually only used as a last resort, and then only for a short time.

The Monthly Blues

In the days before their menstrual periods, some women experience a condition known as PMS, or premenstrual syndrome. As their hormone levels change, so do their bodies—and sometimes their moods. PMS can cause an incredible array of symptoms, ranging from acne and anxiety to irritability and breast tenderness.

No one is sure what causes PMS, although many experts believe it's related to drops in levels of progesterone. For some women, prescription progesterone, often taken orally or by injection during the week before their period, can help relieve the symptoms.

Another way to steady hormonal swings is with prescription oral contraceptives. Of course, this is only helpful for women who don't want to become pregnant, says Dr. Smith.

Virtually all women can relieve PMS symptoms by taking over-the-counter painkillers, such as acetaminophen (Anacin 3, Halenol, Tylenol) or aspirin. "Taking an over-the-counter drug is a sensible

MEFENAMIC ACID

Brand name: Ponstel

How taken: Capsule

Prescription: Yes

	YES	NO
Generic substitutes	✓	
Potentially addicting		✓
May cause drowsiness	✓	
Alcohol discouraged	✓	

Possible drug interactions include: Taking this drug may increase the effects of lithium (used for manic depression), anti-clotting drugs and oral drugs for diabetes; taking it may decrease the effects of blood pressure medications, including diuretics (water pills).

Possible side effects include: Dizziness, diarrhea, stomach cramps and heartburn.

CAUTION: Do not take for more than seven days at a time, unless recommended by your doctor. Increased side effects and toxicity may result.

AT A GLANCE

NAPROXEN

Brand names: Anaprox, Naprosyn, Aleve

How taken: Liquid, tablet

Prescription: Sometimes, depending on strength

	YES	No
Generic substitutes		✓
Potentially addicting		✓
May cause drowsiness		✓
Alcohol discouraged	✓	

Possible drug interactions include: Taking this drug may increase the effects of anti-clotting drugs; taking it may decrease the effects of blood pressure medications, including diuretics (water pills). This drug taken in combination with dipyridamole (a heart drug), sulfinpyrazone (used for gout), valproic acid (an anti-seizure drug) and other anti-inflammatory drugs, such as aspirin, may increase the risk of bleeding.

Possible side effects include: Dizziness, diarrhea, stomach cramps, heartburn and increased sensitivity to light.

HYDROCHLOROTHIAZIDE

Brand name: Hydro-chlor, HydroDIURIL

How taken: Tablet, liquid

Prescription: Yes

	YES	No
Generic substitutes	✓	
Potentially addicting		✓
May cause drowsiness		✓
Alcohol discouraged	✓	

Possible drug interactions include: Taking this drug may increase the effects of blood pressure drugs, lithium (used for manic depression) and digoxin (a heart drug).

Possible side effects include: Dry mouth, nausea, vomiting and muscle cramps. In rare cases may cause weakness or sensitivity to sunlight.

---

place to start," says Dr. Smith.

For women who don't respond to general treatments such as painkillers, it may be worthwhile to tackle individual symptoms, adds Dr. Gutmann. For example, a mild prescription diuretic such as hydrochlorothiazide (Hydro-chlor, HydroDIURIL), taken orally, can be a big help for bloating.

Migraine Drugs

Loosening the Vise

Headaches come in all types. There are tension headaches, ice cream headaches and Monday morning headaches. But when it comes to sheer pain—head-pounding, bell-clanging, head-in-a-vise pain—migraines are in a class by themselves.

Attacks can be triggered by stress, diet and many other factors. They also tend to run in families, says Roger Cady, M.D., medical director of the Shealy Institute for Comprehensive Health Care in Springfield, Missouri.

Migraines begin when blood vessels mysteriously constrict, reducing the flow of blood within the brain. This may cause dizziness, mood changes and other "pre-migraine"

NATURAL ALTERNATIVES

There are several techniques that may help relieve—or even prevent—migraine pain.

Chill out. Apply an ice pack at the first hint of pain. By constricting blood vessels in your head, this can help reduce the swelling that accompanies migraines.

Try to relax. For most people, emotional factors—too much work, too much tension—can play a role in migraine pain.

Pay attention to what you eat. As many as 30 percent of people who have migraines are sensitive to certain foods. Some common culprits are aged cheeses, processed meats, beer and Chinese food, which may contain the food additive monosodium glutamate (MSG).

Keep a regular schedule. People who alternate late nights with all-day sleepfests are far more likely to have migraines than those who keep regular hours.

AT A GLANCE

ASPIRIN

Brand names: Anacin, Genuine Bayer Aspirin, Empirin

How taken: Tablet, capsule, chewing gum, suppository

Prescription: No

	YES	NO
Generic substitutes	✓	
Potentially addicting		✓
May cause drowsiness		✓
Alcohol discouraged	✓	

Possible drug interactions include: Taking this drug may increase the effects of methotrexate (used for psoriasis, cancer and rheumatoid arthritis) and some oral diabetes drugs; taking it may decrease the effects of probenecid and sulfinpyrazine (used for gout). This drug taken in combination with anti-clotting and pain-killing medications, zidovudine (used to treat AIDS) and some antibiotics and diabetes drugs may increase the risk of bleeding and other side effects.

Possible side effects include: Nausea or vomiting, indigestion and stomach discomfort or cramps.

DICLONFENAC

Brand name: Voltaren

How taken: Tablet

Prescription: Yes

	YES	NO
Generic substitutes		✓
Potentially addicting		✓
May cause drowsiness	✓	
Alcohol discouraged	✓	

Possible drug interactions include: This drug taken in combination with anti-clotting drugs, antibiotics or anti-inflammatory medications may increase the risk of bleeding; taking it with diuretics (water pills), heart medications, gout drugs and antifungal drugs may increase the risk of serious side effects.

Possible side effects include: Skin rash, headache, nausea, vomiting, dizziness or light-headedness, indigestion, diarrhea, stomach cramps or irritation and heartburn.

symptoms. Then, within the next 24 hours, the abnormally narrowed blood vessels will suddenly expand and become inflamed. This expansion is accompanied by pounding pain—the "ache" in headache.

Although there isn't a cure for migraines, there are drugs that can short-circuit—or even prevent—the whole migraine cascade.

Aspirin and Friends

Caught early, some migraines can be chased away with over-the-counter painkillers such as aspirin (Anacin, Genuine Bayer Aspirin, Empirin), acetaminophen (Acephen, Maximum Strength Panadol, Tylenol), ibuprofen (Advil, Motrin IB, Nuprin) or naproxen (Aleve).

"My favorite first-line therapy is to use two Alka-Seltzer and one aspirin at the first hint of a migraine," says Dr. Cady. Alka-Seltzer aids the absorption of aspirin, which in turn blocks pain-causing chemicals called prostaglandins. At the same time, aspirin "thins" the blood, improving blood flow throughout the brain.

If you need something stronger, your doctor may recommend prescription drugs that work much like aspirin does. Medications such as naproxen (Anaprox, Naprosyn), diclofenac (Voltaren) and mefenamic acid (Ponstel), taken orally or by suppository, also block prostaglandins. In one study, 46 people having migraines were given injections of diclofenac. In 88 percent of cases, the pain was completely relieved within 30 minutes.

All of these drugs, however,

AT A GLANCE

ACETAMINOPHEN

Brand names: Acephen, Maximum Strength Panadol, Tylenol

How taken: Capsule, tablet

Prescription: No

	Yes	No
Generic substitutes	✓	
Potentially addicting		✓
May cause drowsiness		✓
Alcohol discouraged	✓	

Possible drug interactions include: This drug taken in combination with zidovudine (used to treat AIDS) may increase the risk of side effects, such as fatigue and weakness.

Possible side effects include: Side effects are unlikely.

ERGOTAMINE

Brand names: Ergomar, Ergostat

How taken: Inhaler, tablet

Prescription: Yes

	Yes	No
Generic substitutes	✓	
Potentially addicting		✓
May cause drowsiness		✓
Alcohol discouraged	✓	

Possible drug interactions include: This drug taken in combination with birth control pills may increase the risk of serious side effects.

Possible side effects include: Nausea, vomiting, diarrhea, dizziness, muscle weakness, swelling of the legs and feet and sensitivity to cold temperatures.

including aspirin, can cause stomach pain, bleeding or even ulcers when taken for long periods. You can help prevent side effects by always taking them with food, says Dr. Cady. If you're still having stomach pain, see your doctor.

More Prescription Power

Although aspirin and related drugs can be very effective for ordinary headaches, they rarely work for migraines. Even if they do, they may take several hours to begin working—an eternity when measured in migraine time. For more specific treatment, your doctor may recommend you take prescription drugs called ergot alkaloids instead.

Originally used in obstetrics to stimulate uterine contractions, the ergots work by quickly narrowing the dilated blood vessels that are causing your pain.

When taken by injection, drugs such as ergotamine (Ergomar, Ergostat) and dihydroergotamine mesylate (D.H.E. 45) may completely relieve a migraine in as little as 15 minutes. They also are effective when taken orally, although they will take longer to kick in, says Seymour Diamond, M.D., executive director of the National Headache Foundation and director of the Diamond Headache Clinic in Chicago.

The ergots have some drawbacks, however. They only work when taken in the early stages of a migraine and can cause nausea, vomiting and muscle weakness, says Dr. Diamond. They may also cause more serious side effects, like blood circulation problems from narrowing of the blood vessels. For these reasons, doctors usually prescribe the smallest possible amounts, then carefully increase the doses if needed.

Because the ergots can be so dangerous, doctors have always had to weigh the benefits against

---

AT A GLANCE

SUMATRIPTAN

Brand names: Imigran, Imitrex

How taken: Injection, tablet

Prescription: Yes

	YES	NO
Generic substitutes		✓
Potentially addicting		✓
May cause drowsiness	✓	
Alcohol discouraged	✓	

Possible drug interactions include: Taking this drug may increase the effects of ergotamine-containing preparations (also used to treat migraines).

Possible side effects include: Nausea, dizziness, feelings of heaviness, pain or tightness in the chest, pain or irritation at the injection site and sensation of warmth or cold, tingling or numbness.

the risks and monitor effects on individual patients.

A prescription drug called suma-triptan (Imigran, Imitrex), usually taken by injection, provides benefits equal or superior to other drugs, without the side effects.

Sumatriptan works by mimicking the brain's naturally occurring chemical called serotonin, which is in short supply in the brain before and during migraines. In studies, between 70 and 90 percent of people given injections of sumatriptan had relief within 60 to 90 minutes, with most saying the treatment was "good" or "excellent."

Best of all, sumatriptan causes few side effects and can be taken at any time during a migraine attack. "It's an excellent drug," says Dr. Diamond.

Head Off Headache Pain

If you have two or more migraines a month and the pain is uncommonly severe, your doctor may recommend you take medications daily to prevent them.

There are several prescription drugs that can head off migraines, the most popular being beta-adrenergic blocking agents, or beta-blockers. Drugs such as propranolol (Inderal), timolol (Blocadren) and nadolol (Corgard), taken orally, prevent the dilation of blood vessels in the brain. They can be very helpful, says Dr. Diamond.

While the beta-blockers are quite safe, they can cause slowing of the heart rate, which may cause fatigue, depression and anxiety. Also, people with asthma may experience increased breathing difficulties when taking these drugs.

For people who can't take beta-blockers, a class of prescription drugs called calcium channel blockers may be helpful. Again, however, drugs such as verapamil (Calan, Isoptin, Verelan) and

AT A GLANCE

PROPRANOLOL

Brand name: Inderal

How taken: Capsule, liquid, tablet

Prescription: Yes

	YES	NO
Generic substitutes	✓	
Potentially addicting		✓
May cause drowsiness	✓	
Alcohol discouraged	✓	

Possible drug interactions include: Taking this drug may decrease the effects of some asthma drugs; taking it may increase the effects of some blood pressure drugs. This drug taken in combination with monoamine oxidase (MAO) inhibitors (used for depression) may result in high blood pressure.

Possible side effects include: Insomnia, dizziness and weakness. May also affect libido and (in men) sexual function.

nifedipine (Adalat, Procardia), taken orally, may cause side effects, including constipation, dizziness and weight gain.

The third choice for preventing migraines is a class of drugs called antidepressants. Taken orally in low doses, drugs such as amitriptyline (Elavil, Emitrip, Endep) and doxepin (Sinequan) can prevent migraine attacks even in people who aren't depressed. But antidepressants commonly cause drowsiness and other side effects. They also can interact with many other drugs. They're usually reserved for the most serious cases, says Dr. Diamond.

Muscle Relaxants

Tension Breakers, Spasm Unmakers

The man bending over with his palm on his lower back—let's call him Bob—obviously is in pain. What Bob needs, you may think, is a muscle relaxant. What he probably really needs is aspirin, says Stanley Yarnell, M.D., medical director of physical medicine and rehabilitation at St. Mary's Hospital in San Francisco.

"Most people with muscle pain need an analgesic or an anti-inflammatory drug, not a muscle relaxant," says Dr. Yarnell. Most muscle relaxants, he explains, are simply too powerful to use for a wrenched back.

Although often used inappropriately in cases such as Bob's, muscle relaxants are effective when used to treat symptoms caused by serious neurological problems such as strokes, spinal cord injuries or brain disorders. By blocking signals from the brain (or acting directly on muscles), these prescription drugs, such as diazepam, baclofen or methocarbamol, can help relieve flexor spasms, a type of involuntary muscle movement or tightness called spasticity.

A Prescription for Rehabilitation

Following a stroke, a person's arm might be so stiff that he can't bend it. Or he can't walk because his legs are stiff and shaky.

NATURAL ALTERNATIVES

If you've played just a little too hard and now you find yourself with extremely tight, sore muscles, here are a few tips from Virginia Graziani, M.D., assistant professor of rehabilitation medicine at Jefferson Medical College of Thomas Jefferson University in Philadelphia.

Put it on ice. Applying cold for 20 to 30 minutes several times a day will help relieve pain and swelling by reducing blood flow to the troubled area. If you don't have cold packs, use ice cubes wrapped in a washcloth or dish towel.

Add heat. After cold has done its work—most doctors recommend that you apply cold for at least a day—soak your muscles in a warm bath or whirlpool. Heat will dilate the blood vessels and help the muscles heal. It feels good, too.

Sleep tight. Sleeping on a firm mattress not only is good for sore muscles, it also can help prevent them from getting sore in the first place. The mattress does some of the work for you by holding up your bones.

Stretch away. Gentle exercise can help relax tight muscles. Of course, by keeping your muscles loose and limber in the first place, you'll greatly reduce your chances of getting hurt in the future. "I usually recommend walking three times a week for half an hour," says Dr. Graziani.

"Some people have spasms that actually make their legs and body jump," says Virginia Graziani, M.D., assistant professor of rehabilitation medicine at Jefferson Medical College of Thomas Jefferson University in Philadelphia. For these and similar cases, muscle relaxants can help.

One of the muscle relaxants of choice in such cases is diazepam, a drug better known as a sedative (Valium, Valrelease). Another drug of choice is baclofen (Lioresal). "I use baclofen now and again to relieve spasticity and muscle tightness in people with multiple sclerosis—it helps them walk more smoothly," says Dr. Yarnell.

Baclofen, taken orally, is sometimes used in conjunction with physical therapy. Once the muscles are relaxed, Dr. Graziani says, a person can proceed with range-of-motion exercises recommended by a therapist.

When muscle tightness and spasms are caused by problems of

the spinal cord, diazepam, taken orally, often along with baclofen, can bring quick relief, says Dr. Graziani. Diazepam not only relaxes the muscles, it helps people fall asleep at night—a time when muscle spasms can be most annoying.

Another muscle relaxant called dantrolene (Dantrium) acts directly on the muscle fibers. Taken orally, it's very effective for relieving all types of spasms and tightness, says Dr. Graziani. The problem with dantrolene is that it has a serious potential to cause liver problems, including fatal hepatitis. It also can cause debilitating muscle weakness. Consequently, this drug usually is used only when others don't work, Dr. Graziani says.

For Bum Backs

Returning for a moment to our poor friend Bob and his bad back: A smart doctor may prescribe a muscle relaxant if Bob is in *serious* pain. For muscle spasms that aren't caused by brain or

---

AT A GLANCE

DIAZEPAM

Brand names: Valium, Valrelease

How taken: Capsule, injection, liquid, tablet

Prescription: Yes

	YES	NO
Generic substitutes	✓	
Potentially addicting	✓	
May cause drowsiness	✓	
Alcohol discouraged	✓	

Possible drug interactions include: Taking this drug may increase the effects of digoxin (a heart drug) and phenytoin (an anti-seizure drug); taking it may decrease the effects of levodopa (used for Parkinson's disease).

Possible side effects include: Lethargy and dizziness.

BACLOFEN

Brand name: Lioresal

How taken: Tablet

Prescription: Yes

	YES	NO
Generic substitutes	✓	
Potentially addicting		✓
May cause drowsiness	✓	
Alcohol discouraged	✓	

Possible drug interactions include: Taking this drug may increase the effects of sedatives and blood pressure drugs; taking it may decrease the effects of diabetes drugs.

Possible side effects include: Dizziness, nausea, constipation and headache.

AT A GLANCE

DANTROLENE

Brand name: Dantrium
How taken: Capsule, injection
Prescription: Yes

	YES	NO
Generic substitutes		✓
Potentially addicting		✓
May cause drowsiness	✓	
Alcohol discouraged	✓	

Possible drug interactions include: Taking this drug may increase the effects of some sedatives.

Possible side effects include: Muscle weakness and rashes.

CHLORZOXAZONE

Brand names: Paraflex, Parafon Forte DSC
How taken: Tablet
Prescription: Yes

	YES	NO
Generic substitutes	✓	
Potentially addicting		✓
May cause drowsiness	✓	
Alcohol discouraged	✓	

Possible drug interactions include: Taking this drug may increase the effects of some sedatives.

Possible side effects include: Urine discoloration.

CYCLOBENZAPRINE

Brand name: Flexeril
How taken: Tablet
Prescription: Yes

	YES	NO
Generic substitutes	✓	
Potentially addicting		✓
May cause drowsiness	✓	
Alcohol discouraged	✓	

Possible drug interactions include: Taking this drug may increase the effects of sedatives and atropine-like drugs (used for asthma). This drug taken in combination with monoamine oxidase (MAO) inhibitors (used for depression) may result in fever, seizures and life-threatening reactions.

Possible side effects include: Dizziness, dry mouth and constipation.

METHOCARBAMOL

Brand names: Carbacot, Delaxin, Robaxin
How taken: Injection, tablet
Prescription: Yes

	YES	NO
Generic substitutes	✓	
Potentially addicting		✓
May cause drowsiness	✓	
Alcohol discouraged	✓	

Possible drug interactions include: Taking this drug may increase the effects of some sedatives.

Possible side effects include: Weakness and urine discoloration.

spinal cord problems—a wrenched back, for example, or a painfully stiff neck—doctors sometimes prescribe muscle relaxants such as carisoprodol (Rela, Soma, Soprodol), chlorzoxazone (Paraflex, Parafon Forte DSC) or cyclobenzaprine (Flexeril). These are most often taken orally, and sometimes they are given in combination with painkillers such as aspirin.

Keep in mind, however, that all muscle relaxants affect the central nervous system to some degree, often causing sleepiness, lethargy and muscle weakness. In addition, many can be addicting. That's why sticking with mild painkillers and anti-inflammatory drugs alone may be preferable, says Dr. Yarnell.

Nausea Drugs

Gravity's Little Helpers

A lesson from Physics 101: What goes up always comes down.

A lesson from Stomach 101: What goes down can all too often come back up again.

The truth is, nausea and vomiting are important mechanisms for removing possibly harmful substances from your body. But there are some conditions, like motion sickness and pregnancy, that can stimulate nausea without conferring any particular benefits. That's when nausea drugs can help.

Taming the Trigger

Despite that feeling of having a whirlpool in your gut, nausea doesn't begin in the stomach but in the brain. More specifically, it begins within a specialized group of cells in the brain that are called, appropriately enough, the vomiting center.

Although some nausea drugs act directly on the stomach, most act on the brain itself, says Charles D. Wood, Ph.D., former professor of pharmacology at Louisiana State University in Shreveport. Which one your doctor recommends depends on what, exactly, is making you sick.

When Movin' It Means Losin' It

According to some NASA studies, "up to 70 percent or more of the untreated crew members will have symptoms of motion sickness," says Dr. Wood. Closer to Earth, taking a car trip, airplane flight or ocean cruise can have some of the same tipping, tilting, downright nauseating effects.

For sensitive travelers, over-the-counter antihistamines such as dimenhydrinate (Dimetabs, Dramamine, Hydrate), diphenhydramine (Benadryl, Valdrene) and meclizine (Bonine) often can help keep nausea at bay—even if the bay is choppy. Usually taken by mouth, these drugs provide protection for up to eight hours, says Dr. Wood.

Stronger still are prescription antihistamines. Drugs such as hydroxyzine (Atarax, Hydroxacen, Vistaril) and meclizine (Antivert, Meni-D), usually taken orally, can be more effective than their over-the-counter counterparts, according to Dr. Wood.

Of course, stronger drugs may cause stronger side effects—for example, increased sweating, dizziness, a dry mouth and blurred vision—as well. In fact, virtually all of the antihistamines recommended to combat nausea may cause some minor discomfort.

If side effects are a problem, tell your doctor. A different drug (or maybe a lower dose) may work just as well—without the discomfort.

NATURAL ALTERNATIVES

Drugs aren't the only way to relieve nausea. Here are some tips from the experts to help you calm your stomach *before* it gets into trouble.

Stick with easy-to-digest meals. Doctors traditionally have recommended soda crackers (like soup crackers) both for travelers and moms-to-be. But eating small amounts of any low-fat, starchy foods—rice, for instance—can help calm the queasies, says Edwin M. Monsell, M.D., Ph.D., head of the Division of Otology and Neurology at Henry Ford Hospital in Detroit. (Some people, however, do best on an empty stomach.)

Distract yourself. Studies have shown that people who keep their minds busy with mental exercises tend to get sick less often than those who sit passively. So sing a song. Recite some poetry. Try to remember Latin verbs. Do anything *except* concentrate on your stomach.

Watch the horizon. If you feel car sickness coming on, take your eyes *off* those telephone poles zipping by and put them *on* stationary objects far off in the distance. This little trick can help keep two of your sense organs—the eyes and inner ears—in happy harmony.

For longer-lasting protection from motion sickness, your doctor may prescribe an adhesive patch containing scopalamine (Transderm Scōp). The patch, when affixed behind the ear, slowly releases the drug into your bloodstream. "It is good for about three days, so you don't have to worry about taking additional pills," says Dr. Wood. As with antihistamines, however, scopalamine may cause a dry mouth, dizziness, drowsiness and other side effects.

Tough Relief

For severe nausea—caused by some cancer treatments, for example—your doctor may pre-

---

AT A GLANCE

DIMENHYDRINATE

Brand names: Dimetabs, Dramamine, Hydrate

How taken: Liquid, capsule, injection, tablet

Prescription: Sometimes, depending on strength

	YES	NO
Generic substitutes	✓	
Potentially addicting		✓
May cause drowsiness	✓	
Alcohol discouraged	✓	

Possible drug interactions include: This drug taken in combination with stomach drugs, some antibiotics and antifungal drugs may increase side effects; taking it with alcohol, painkillers, sleeping pills, antihistamines and anti-seizure drugs may increase its sedative effects.

Possible side effects include: Dry mouth, nose or throat, thickening of mucus, confusion, dizziness and difficult or painful urination.

SCOPALAMINE

Brand name: Transderm Scōp

How taken: Patch, injection

Prescription: Yes

	YES	NO
Generic substitutes	✓	
Potentially addicting		✓
May cause drowsiness	✓	
Alcohol discouraged	✓	

Possible drug interactions include: The effects of this drug may increase if taken with nervous system depressants (such as antihistamines, sedatives, sleeping pills and painkillers), antidepressants and alcohol; its effects may decrease if taken with antacids, antifungal and diarrhea medications.

Possible side effects include: Dry mouth, nose, throat or skin, dizziness, blurred vision, confusion, constipation and increased vulnerability to heatstroke.

CAUTION: Using alcohol or taking nervous system depressants may lead to unconsciousness and possibly death.

AT A GLANCE

PROMAZINE

Brand names: Primazine, Prozine-50, Sparine

How taken: Injection, tablet

Prescription: Yes

	YES	NO
Generic substitutes	✓	
Potentially addicting		✓
May cause drowsiness	✓	
Alcohol discouraged	✓	

Possible drug interactions include: Taking this drug may increase the side effects of many blood pressure drugs. This drug taken in combination with heart drugs may increase the risk of severe low blood pressure; taking it with anti-psychotic drugs, antidepressants, other nausea drugs and nervous system depressants (such as antihistamines, sedatives, sleeping pills and painkillers) may increase the risk of serious side effects.

Possible side effects include: Constipation, decreased sweating, dizziness, nasal congestion and dryness of the mouth.

METOCLOPRAMIDE

Brand names: Clopra, Octamide, Reglan

How taken: Injection, liquid, tablet

Prescription: Yes

	YES	NO
Generic substitutes	✓	
Potentially addicting		✓
May cause drowsiness	✓	
Alcohol discouraged	✓	

Possible drug interactions include: Taking this drug may increase the side effects of nervous system depressants (such as antihistamines, sedatives, sleeping pills or painkillers).

Possible side effects include: Dizziness, restlessness and, if taken in high doses, diarrhea.

scribe powerful drugs, taken orally or by injection, like promazine (Primazine, Prozine-50, Sparine), fluphenazine (Permitil, Prolixin) or metoclopramide (Clopra, Octamide, Reglan).

Another option for severe nausea is dronabinol (Marinol), which contains some of the active ingredients found in marijuana. Because it can cause mood changes, it's usually used only when other drugs don't work.

It's important to remember that all nausea drugs are better at preventing problems than eliminating them, says Dr. Wood. If you wait until you're already sick before taking them, you may be too late. As a rule, doctors say, you should take your medication half an hour to an hour before you actually need it.

Pregnancy Problems

More than half of all pregnant women experience morning sickness—and not just in the morning, either.

Most women can calm their stomachs without medication: by sipping ginger ale, for example, or avoiding heavy meals and snacking lightly throughout the day. "But when nausea is severe, we don't shy away from drugs," says Kathleen Kuhlman, M.D., a maternal and fetal medicine specialist at Thomas Jefferson University Hospital in Philadelphia.

Prescription drugs such as prochlorperazine (Compazine, Contrazine) and chlorpromazine (Thorazine, Thor-Prom), taken

---

AT A GLANCE

DRONABINOL

Brand name: Marinol

How taken: Capsule

Prescription: Yes

	YES	NO
Generic substitutes		✓
Potentially addicting	✓	
May cause drowsiness	✓	
Alcohol discouraged	✓	

Possible drug interactions include: The sedative effects of this drug may increase if taken with nervous system depressants (such as antihistamines, sedatives, sleeping pills or pain-killers).

Possible side effects include: Dizziness, confusion and poor coordination.

MECLIZINE

Brand names: Antivert, Bonine, Meni-D

How taken: Capsule, tablet

Prescription: Sometimes, depending on strength

	YES	NO
Generic substitutes	✓	
Potentially addicting		✓
May cause drowsiness	✓	
Alcohol discouraged	✓	

Possible drug interactions include: Taking this drug may increase the side effects of alcohol and nervous system depressants such as antihistamines, sleeping pills, prescription pain medications and muscle relaxants, sedatives and narcotics.

Possible side effects include: Dry mouth and drowsiness.

orally, rectally or by injection, can help relieve morning sickness while causing few side effects, she says. A drug called doxylamine (Unisom Nighttime Sleep Aid), sold over the counter, can help in two ways, she adds. "It's used as a sleeping med-ication, but some people find that Unisom, taken once a night, will also decrease the nausea of pregnancy."

If you are pregnant, however, you shouldn't take *any* drugs without the consent of your doctor.

Osteoporosis Drugs

The Bone Boosters

We tend to think of bones as being dry and life-less, but in fact, they are very much alive, consisting of nerves, blood vessels and layers of tough material. The most important component in this complex structure is calcium. It is calcium that gives bones their strength and hardness. Take away calcium and your bones become subject to warping and cracking.

This is exactly what often happens in people with osteoporosis, a bone-thinning disease that causes bones to lose calcium more quickly than it can be replaced. Often linked to the hormonal changes of menopause, the disease usually strikes women over the age of 50 and can result in a 30 to 50 percent loss of bone mass over the course of a lifetime. Not surprisingly, there are approximately 1.5 million osteoporosis-related bone fractures every year.

It's not possible to make bones young again, but with appropriate lifestyle changes and medications you can stem bone loss, possibly reducing bone fractures by as much as 60 percent, says Stanley Wallach, M.D., director of endo-crinology and co-director of the metabolic bone disease center at the Hospital for Joint Diseases in New York City.

Bone Up with Calcium

The human body contains more than 35 ounces of calcium, most of which is stored in the bones. The calcium isn't locked away, however, but is constantly being broken down, used else-

NATURAL ALTERNATIVES

Doctors agree that preventing osteoporosis is a lot easier than treating it once it occurs. To keep your bones strong:

Fill up on calcium. For most people, this means boning up with dairy products: low-fat milk, yogurt and cheeses.

Add some D. For your bones to harden, they need vitamin D, which is produced in the skin following exposure to sunlight. It's a good idea to spend at least five to ten minutes a day in the sun (without using sunscreen on your face and hands), three times a week. Or, if you can't tolerate the sun, you can drink fortified milk (which contains vitamin D) or take a multivitamin containing 200 to 400 international units of this important nutrient. Because vitamin D is toxic in large doses, vitamin D capsules are not recommended.

Get moving. Studies have shown that regular weight-bearing exercise—such as walking, aerobics or lifting weights—can help increase bone mass.

Be careful about your habits. Drinking excessive alcohol can interfere with bone production. In addition, smoking cigarettes may contribute to bone loss.

where by the body and then replaced in the bone. If the amount used exceeds the amount stored, then serious bone loss can result.

Most people think of calcium as just a mineral supplement. If you're at risk for osteoporosis, however, it's also an effective medicine—one you may need to take every day.

The National Institutes of Health have recommended that women consume at least 1,000 milligrams of calcium (BioCal, Os-Cal 500, Caltrate 600) a day to prevent bone loss. For women past menopause, when bone loss is greatest, 1,500 milligrams is recommended, says Edward G. Lufkin, M.D., associate professor of medicine at the Mayo Clinic in Rochester, Minnesota. "We do recommend that every woman routinely take calcium supplements after menopause," says Dr. Lufkin. "Calcium supplements are very effective for reducing bone loss."

Although calcium is generally safe when taken in these doses, a few people may experience constipation, headache or other side effects. If this happens to you, stop taking it and see your doctor.

In addition to supplements, don't be surprised if your doctor advises you to boost the calcium intake in your diet. Foods that are particularly rich in this important mineral include milk, yogurt and other dairy products. Combining a good diet with calcium supplements, says Dr. Wallach, can help put your bones in the safety zone.

Hormone Helpers

The hormone estrogen plays an important part in bone production. But after menopause, a woman's decreasing estrogen supply causes a corresponding loss in bone mass. In fact, bone loss is greatest in the 3 to 6 years following menopause, although the process may continue for 20 years more.

Bone loss can be stopped with prescription estrogen supplements (Estraderm, Ogen, Premarin), says Dr. Wallach. Estrogen can reduce

---

AT A GLANCE

CALCIUM

Brand names: BioCal, Caltrate 600, Os-Cal 500

How taken: Capsule, liquid, tablet

Prescription: Sometimes, depending on strength

	YES	NO
Generic substitutes	✓	
Potentially addicting		✓
May cause drowsiness		✓
Alcohol discouraged	✓	

Possible drug interactions include: Taking this drug may decrease the effects of etidronate (used for some bone disorders), cellulose sodium phosphate (used for kidney stones), magnesium sulfate (a laxative) or tetracycline (an antibiotic). This drug taken in combination with heart drugs such as digoxin may increase the risk of irregular heartbeat.

Possible side effects include: Constipation and headache.

ESTROGEN

Brand names: Premarin, Estraderm, Ogen

How taken: Tablet, patch

Prescription: Yes

	YES	NO
Generic substitutes	✓	
Potentially addicting		✓
May cause drowsiness		✓
Alcohol discouraged		✓

Possible drug interactions include: Taking this drug may decrease the effects of tricyclic antidepressants or bromocriptine (used to treat infertility and menstrual problems). This drug taken in combination with many drugs, including acetaminophen, oral contraceptives and gold (used for arthritis) may result in liver damage.

Possible side effects include: Nausea, weight gain or fluid retention and breast tenderness or pain.

CAUTION: Estrogen should not be taken during pregnancy.

AT A GLANCE

CALCITONIN

Brand names: Cibacalcin, Calcimar, Miacalcin

How taken: Injection, nasal spray

Prescription: Yes

	YES	NO
Generic substitutes		✓
Potentially addicting		✓
May cause drowsiness		✓
Alcohol discouraged		✓

Possible drug interactions include: Interactions are unlikely.

Possible side effects include: Nausea, diarrhea, loss of appetite, flushing and stomach pain.

Strength by Injection

When osteoporosis is advanced, however, estrogen may be less effective. In addition, there are some women who can't take estrogen. In either case, a prescription drug called calcitonin (Cibacalcin, Calcimar, Miacalcin) can be used instead. Calcitonin works by decreasing the number of cells that dissolve bone tissue.

"It will stabilize bone mass in at least 70 percent of cases, and, in some cases, it will help increase bone mass," says Dr. Wallach. Additionally, calcitonin can help relieve pain (such as back pain) caused by osteoporosis-related deterioration of the vertebrae, he adds.

Yet calcitonin has drawbacks as well. Although a nasal form of the drug is available, calcitonin is also given by injection three times a week in some cases, or even twice a day. Also, some people become resistant to its effects after several months of treatment.

Emerging Treatments

There are several promising new approaches that researchers say may be used not only to prevent osteoporosis but also to treat it.

They are most excited about a medication called etidronate (Didronel). Studies have shown that this drug can cause an increase in spinal bone density and decrease the fractures of spinal ver-

osteoporosis-related fractures by as much as 50 percent. Estrogen does more than just stop bone loss, adds Dr. Lufkin. "The ultimate effect of estrogen is a slight *increase* in bone density," he says.

The medication isn't without side effects, however. Some women may experience weight gain, bloating or breast pain. There also is concern that when estrogen is taken for long periods of time, the risk of endometrial or breast cancer may increase. But for most women, says Dr. Lufkin, "we continue to believe that estrogen is the treatment of choice both for preventing and treating osteoporosis."

tebrae, a common symptom of osteoporosis.

Etidronate has been approved by the Food and Drug Administration for treating Paget's disease (another type of bone disease), but its use in treating osteoporosis still is experimental, says Dr. Lufkin.

Another drug on the experimental front is sodium fluoride. Used to help prevent cavities in children, this same medication, taken in higher doses, can help boost bone mass. Taken orally, sodium fluoride has been found to increase bone density by as much as 8 percent a year in the lumbar spine and by 4 percent in the upper leg.

"A lot of physicians are using it because one, it's oral and two, it's cheaper than other medications," according to Dr. Wallach. It's still a powerful drug, however, and it should be taken only under special circumstances and with a doctor's supervision.

Painkillers

Providers of Deep Relief

The sheer variety of pain is little less than astounding. There are migraines and tension headaches . . . PMS and menstrual cramps . . . back strain and muscle sprain. The list goes on and on.

Fortunately, the list of remedies is also a long one. There are literally dozens of medications for pain, says Richard M. Linchitz, M.D., medical director of the Pain Alleviation Center in Long Island, New York. These drugs range from common over-the-counter alternatives such as aspirin and acetaminophen to powerful prescription choices such as morphine.

Commonly Used, Uncommonly Potent

In your neighborhood pharmacy or grocery store you'll see shelf after shelf of painkillers. What do they contain? In many cases the active ingredient is aspirin, one of the most popular painkillers on the market today.

We've been using aspirin for almost a century, although a chemical relative, salicin, has been extracted from white willow bark for thousands of years. Usually taken orally, aspirin (Anacin, Genuine Bayer Aspirin, Empirin) quickly blocks the production of prostaglandins, chemicals in your body that cause pain and inflammation.

Aspirin may be inexpensive and readily available, but don't underestimate its abilities. It's an extremely powerful drug, says Dr. Linchitz.

Aspirin can help relieve virtually all types of pain but is most effective at combating pain caused by inflammation—from a joint injury, for example, or during an arthritis flare-up. "If you have a problem with inflammation, there's no question that aspirin can be very effective," says Dr. Linchitz.

Yet aspirin can cause potentially serious side effects, such as stomach pain and internal bleeding, which can make long-term use somewhat dangerous. Aspirin never should be taken in large doses without a doctor's supervision, says Dr. Linchitz. To reduce temporary discomfort, try taking aspirin with food. Or try buffered or coated forms of the drug (Bufferin, Bayer Enteric Aspirin, Bayer Plus), which are easier on the stomach.

Aspirin Substitutes

Next to the bottles of aspirin in your neighborhood pharmacy, you'll probably find three

NATURAL ALTERNATIVES

There are many things you can do to ease aches and pains without opening the medicine chest. Here are some recommendations from top pain experts.

Boost your body's natural painkillers. These body chemicals, called endorphins, flood your bloodstream whenever you do vigorous exercise, be it walking, swimming or soccer.

Put pain on ice. After a sudden injury—twisting an ankle, for example—blood and other fluids pour into the injured tissues. By icing the injury either with an ice pack or ice cubes wrapped in a small towel, you can help constrict blood vessels and numb nerve endings. This helps stop the swelling and relieves the pain, experts say.

Add some soothing heat. The easiest way to apply heat to sore muscles and joints is to recline in a warm, steamy bath. Or try applying a heating pad or hot-water bottle to the sore spots.

Meditate your pain away. Begin by lying on your back with your eyes closed. Take a deep breath and hold it for six seconds while tensing all your muscles. Now breathe out and let your body go limp. Breathe deeply for about half a minute. Repeat until your pain slips away.

AT A GLANCE

ASPIRIN

Brand names: Anacin, Genuine Bayer Aspirin, Empirin

How taken: Tablet, capsule, chewing gum, suppository

Prescription: No

	YES	NO
Generic substitutes	✓	
Potentially addicting		✓
May cause drowsiness		✓
Alcohol discouraged	✓	

Possible drug interactions include: Taking this drug may increase the effects of methotrexate (used for psoriasis, cancer and rheumatoid arthritis) and some oral diabetes drugs. This drug taken in combination with anti-clotting drugs may increase the risk of bleeding.

Possible side effects include: Nausea, indigestion and stomach cramps. Long-term use may cause internal bleeding.

ACETAMINOPHEN

Brand names: Actamin, Datril Extra-Strength, Maximum Strength Panadol, Tylenol

How taken: Tablet, capsule, liquid

Prescription: No

	YES	NO
Generic substitutes	✓	
Potentially addicting		✓
May cause drowsiness		✓
Alcohol discouraged	✓	

Possible drug interactions include: This drug taken in combination with zidovudine (used to treat AIDS) may increase the risk of side effects, such as fatigue and weakness.

Possible side effects include: Side effects are unlikely.

other painkillers—acetaminophen, ibuprofen and naproxen.

Acetaminophen (Actamin, Datril Extra-Strength, Tylenol), taken orally and sold without prescription, is an effective pain reliever. For children with fever, it's the pain reliever of choice because aspirin can trigger a rare neurological disorder known as Reye's syndrome.

On the other hand, acetaminophen has little effect on inflammation, says Dr. Linchitz. If you twisted your ankle and need anti-inflammatory relief, it may not be the drug for you.

Ibuprofen, on the other hand, which is sold over the counter and by prescription, is an excellent inflammation fighter. Like aspirin, ibuprofen (Advil, Motrin, Nuprin), taken orally, blocks the synthesis of prostaglandins. It can help relieve pain and swelling throughout the body, says Peter Staats, M.D., assistant in the Division of Pain Medicine, Department of Anesthesiology and Critical Care Medicine at Johns Hopkins University School of Medicine in Baltimore.

"Ibuprofen and aspirin can both cause bleeding problems. However, the side effects of aspirin can last for 10 to 14 days, while the bleeding problems caused by ibuprofen are much more short-lived. Due to its inhibition of prostaglandin synthesis, ibuprofen has been found to be very effective in the treatment of menstrual cramps." Taken regularly, however, it, too, may cause stomach upset. The discomfort can be reduced by taking the drug with meals, says Dr. Staats.

Naproxen (Aleve), like aspirin and ibuprofen, can help relieve pain and inflammation. Unfortunately, it can also cause stomach upset and bleeding, particularly if taken with alcohol or anti-clotting drugs.

Prescription Strength

When over-the-counter painkillers don't do the trick, your doctor may prescribe medications called nonsteroidal anti-inflammatory drugs, or NSAIDs.

Aspirin, ibuprofen and naproxen also are NSAIDs. Some of their pre-

HELP IS IN YOUR HANDS

In the past, when people in the hospital needed drugs for pain, they had to ask for them. This meant calling a nurse (and waiting); making the request (and waiting); finally getting the drug (and waiting for it to start working). The only thing that *wasn't* waiting was the pain— and it was getting worse.

Today there's a new form of pain relief called patient-controlled analgesia, or PCA. This system lets the patient decide how much medication he or she needs. Then it delivers it.

Here's how PCA works. A patient in the hospital is connected intravenously to a computerized pump. When he is ready for pain medication, all he has to do is push a button. This signals the computer to release small amounts of painkiller into the bloodstream.

The advantage of PCA is that patients can get the jump on pain before it gets a head start. Studies have shown that people using this system have less pain—and use *less* medication—than those who get their medication from doctors and nurses, says Richard M. Linchitz, M.D., medical director of the Pain Alleviation Center in Long Island, New York. "It's much easier to prevent pain than to control it once it's started," he says.

AT A GLANCE

IBUPROFEN

Brand names: Advil, Haltran, Motrin, Nuprin

How taken: Capsule, tablet, liquid

Prescription: Sometimes, depending on strength

	YES	NO
Generic substitutes	✓	
Potentially addicting		✓
May cause drowsiness	✓	
Alcohol discouraged		✓

Possible drug interactions include: This drug taken in combination with anti-clotting and other anti-inflammatory medications may increase the risk of bleeding.

Possible side effects include: Nausea, diarrhea, dizziness, mild stomach cramps, fluid retention (weight gain) and discoloration of urine.

CAUTION: Do not take if you are allergic to aspirin.

MEPERIDINE

Brand names: Demerol, Pethadol

How taken: Liquid, tablet, injection

Prescription: Yes

	YES	NO
Generic substitutes	✓	
Potentially addicting	✓	
May cause drowsiness	✓	
Alcohol discouraged	✓	

Possible drug interactions include: Taking this drug may increase the effects of sedatives and the side effects of some antidepressant drugs.

Possible side effects include: Nausea, dizziness and constipation.

CAUTION: Particularly dangerous if combined with monoamine oxidase (MAO) inhibitors (used for depression).

scription brethren include fenoprofen (Nalfon), indomethacin (Indameth, Indocin) and naproxen (Anaprox, Naprosyn). These powerful drugs, usually taken orally, can be taken at lower doses than aspirin. They provide equal or superior pain relief with fewer side effects, says Dr. Linchitz.

Still, all of the NSAIDs should be taken with food to help prevent stomach upset. And don't be surprised if one drug causes more side effects—or less relief—than another. Everyone reacts differently to different NSAIDs. Your doctor may prescribe several medications before finding one that works best for you.

High-Octane Help

For severe pain—after surgery, for example—your doctor may give you narcotics. These powerful prescription drugs, usually taken orally or by injection, include meperidine (Demerol, Pethadol) and morphine (Astramorph, Roxanol). These narcotics act directly on the central nervous system, often relieving pain within minutes.

For certain types of pain, like a sudden injury, narcotics often are considered the gold standard among painkillers. Yet they have some powerful problems as well. They often cause nausea, dizziness and consti-

---

AT A GLANCE

CODEINE

Brand names: Generic only

How taken: Liquid, tablet

Prescription: Yes

	YES	NO
Generic substitutes	✓	
Potentially addicting	✓	
May cause drowsiness	✓	
Alcohol discouraged	✓	

Possible drug interactions include: Taking this drug may increase the effects of sedatives and the side effects of some antidepressant drugs.

Possible side effects include: Dizziness, nausea and vomiting.

AMITRIPTYLINE

Brand names: Elavil, Emitrip, Endep

How taken: Tablet, liquid, injection

Prescription: Yes

	YES	NO
Generic substitutes	✓	
Potentially addicting		✓
May cause drowsiness	✓	
Alcohol discouraged	✓	

Possible drug interactions include: Taking this drug may increase the effects of sedatives and blood pressure drugs and serious side effects of cimetidine (an ulcer drug); taking it may decrease the effects of guanethidine (a blood pressure drug). This drug taken in combination with phenylephrine (a decongestant) may increase the risk of serious effects on the heart; taking it with or within two weeks of taking monoamine oxidase (MAO) inhibitors (used for depression) may cause severe side effects.

Possible side effects include: Headache, nausea, dry mouth, difficulty urinating, increased appetite and weight gain.

pation. They become less effective over time, so people require greater and greater doses. There's also the possibility of addiction.

But, says Dr. Linchitz, people who take narcotics for pain very rarely become hooked. In one study, Boston researchers followed 12,000 surgical patients who had received morphine for postoperative pain. Only 4 of them later became addicted. In fact, the euphoria associated with narcotics—the high—isn't likely to occur when the drugs are taken for pain, says Dr. Linchitz.

Still, except for cancer patients, who often need long-term pain relief, strong narcotics are usually too powerful and potentially dangerous to be used for long periods of time. Less effective narcotics such as codeine or propoxyphene (Darvon), used occasionally, even over longer periods, are usually not a problem.

Long-Term Help

Some prescription drugs normally used in psychiatry can be used to relieve pain, too. These drugs, called tricyclic antidepressants, work by affecting brain chemicals that control the perception of pain, says Dr. Linchitz. You don't have to be depressed for the drugs to be effective, he adds.

Antidepressants such as amitriptyline (Elavil, Emitrip, Endep), doxepin (Adapin, Sinequan) and clomipramine (Anafranil), usually taken orally, have been used to treat headache, arthritis pain and neuropathy, a type of nerve pain often caused by diabetes.

Unfortunately, antidepressants don't bring quick relief. "It's not pop a pill, get some relief," says Dr. Staats. They may take days or weeks to become effective.

But once they do kick in, these drugs may be even more effective than narcotics for the treatment of nerve injury pain such as that caused by diabetes, says Dr. Staats. And because they don't cause tolerance or addiction, "they can be very effective for chronic pain," says Dr. Linchitz. Indeed, people who take antidepressants for chronic pain may take them every day for months or years at a time.

Antidepressants aren't without side effects. They can cause dizziness, a dry mouth and difficulty urinating, to name a few. "But in most cases, they're taken in such low doses that side effects aren't serious," says Dr. Staats.

Parasite Drugs

Exit Visas for Pests

When travelers set out for far-flung vacation spots, they usually look forward to collecting fond memories. All too often, however, they return home with something they didn't anticipate—an illness caused by *Giardia*, hookworm or some other parasite.

Parasitic diseases are rare in the United States. But they are fairly common in other parts of the world, particularly in regions where sanitation is poor, says Kenneth Dardick, M.D., director of health for Mansfield, Connecticut, and author of *Foreign Travel and Immunization Guide*.

Depending on the species involved, parasitic infections can cause fever, diarrhea, liver damage, or—in many cases—no symptoms at all. But in all cases, Dr. Dardick says, they can be eliminated with anti-parasitic drugs.

Waterborne Trouble

One of the most common parasitic infections is giardiasis. Caused by a microscopic organism (*Giardia lamblia*) that attaches to the wall of the small intestine, giardiasis can cause cramps, diarrhea and other intestinal upsets or, if left untreated, serious weight loss.

Prescription drugs for giardiasis include metronidazole (Flagyl, Metizol, Protostat), furazolidone (Furoxone) and quinacrine (Atabrine, Mepacrine). When metronidazole is taken in high doses, it can cause queasiness and leave a metallic taste in the mouth. "All of these drugs can cause side effects," says Dr. Dardick. "But in any case, they sure beat giardia."

Amebiasis is yet another common intestinal infection caused by a parasite (*Entamoeba histolytica*) that often inhabits unsanitary water. The organisms hatch in the small intestine and multiply in the bowel. Many people with amebiasis don't have symptoms, although it may cause diarrhea, constipation or, in more serious cases, liver pain or intestinal bleeding.

When amebiasis is mild, it often is treated with prescription drugs such as metronidazole, iodoquinol (Diquinol, Yodoxin) or paromomycin (Humatin). Taken orally, these medications relieve symptoms within a day or two and completely eradicate the organism within two weeks.

In more severe cases, the infection may be treated with several prescription drugs, usually given in stages, says Dr. Dardick. For example, metronidazole might be taken for ten days, followed by iodoquinol, followed by paromomycin. "When it gets into the liver, amebiasis can be quite serious, and the

---

AT A GLANCE

METRONIDAZOLE

Brand names: Flagyl, Metizol, Metric 21, Protostat

How taken: Tablet, injection

Prescription: Yes

	YES	NO
Generic substitutes	✓	
Potentially addicting		✓
May cause drowsiness		✓
Alcohol discouraged	✓	

Possible drug interactions include: This drug taken in combination with disulfiram (used to discourage drinking alcohol) may increase the risk of side effects; taking it with anti-clotting drugs may increase the risk of bleeding.

Possible side effects include: Nausea, diarrhea, dizziness, headache and stomach cramps.

QUINACRINE

Brand names: Atabrine, Mepacrine

How taken: Tablet

Prescription: Yes

	YES	NO
Generic substitutes		✓
Potentially addicting		✓
May cause drowsiness		✓
Alcohol discouraged	✓	

Possible drug interactions include: This drug taken in combination with primaquine (a malaria drug) may increase the risk of side effects.

Possible side effects include: Nausea, dizziness, headache, diarrhea, stomach cramps and discoloration of the skin or urine.

AT A GLANCE

PYRANTEL

Brand names: Antiminth, Pin-X, Reese's Pinworm Medicine

How taken: Liquid

Prescription: Sometimes, depending on strength

	YES	NO
Generic substitutes	✓	
Potentially addicting		✓
May cause drowsiness	✓	
Alcohol discouraged		✓

Possible drug interactions include: The effects of this drug may decrease if taken with piperazine (another worming medication).

Possible side effects include: Dizziness, cramps, diarrhea, headache, loss of appetite, nausea or sleeping problems.

treatment quite difficult," he says.

Again, these medications are quite safe. As with many antibiotic or antiparasitic-type drugs, however, they do alter the body's natural bacterial flora and may cause side effects such as diarrhea or yeast infections.

Pests That Worm Their Way In

Although many infections are caused by microscopic pests, in some cases the culprits are quite a bit larger. Hookworms, for example, can be half an inch long. That's nothing compared to the tapeworm, which can stretch inside the intestine to *60 feet* in length!

Like other parasites, worms often are transmitted in food or water, although in some cases they enter the bloodstream through intact skin, says Peter Schantz, V.M.D., Ph.D., epidemiologist of the parasitic diseases division at the Centers for Disease Control and Prevention in Atlanta.

Depending on the species, worm infections can cause symptoms that range from rashes and cramps to serious blood loss and anemia. In most cases, however, they are easily treated with antihelminthic, or "worming," agents.

Pinworms, for example, which can cause irritation of the skin around the anus, can be eliminated with over-the-counter medications such as pyrantel (Antiminth, Pin-X, Reese's Pinworm Medicine) or prescription drugs such as mebendazole (Vermox). Usually taken orally for one to three days, these drugs are extremely effective, says Dr. Schantz.

Other antiworm medications are available. Treatment depends on various factors, including the type of parasite and so forth.

Doctors say it's best to take antiworm medications with meals to improve their absorption. Although side effects—nausea or headache, for example—are common, they clear up when you stop taking the drugs, says Dr. Schantz.

AT A GLANCE

MEBENDAZOLE

Brand name: Vermox

How taken: Tablet

Prescription: Yes

	YES	NO
Generic substitutes		✓
Potentially addicting		✓
May cause drowsiness	✓	
Alcohol discouraged		✓

Possible drug interactions include: Interactions are unlikely.

Possible side effects include: Nausea, diarrhea and stomach cramps.

IODOQUINOL

Brand names: Diquinol, Yodoxin

How taken: Tablet

Prescription: Yes

	YES	NO
Generic substitutes	✓	
Potentially addicting		✓
May cause drowsiness		✓
Alcohol discouraged	✓	

Possible drug interactions include: Interactions are unlikely.

Possible side effects include: Nausea, diarrhea and stomach pain.

Parkinson's Disease Drugs

Chemical Balancers for the Brain

Deep inside a healthy brain, an exquisite dance occurs. Two chemicals, dopamine and acetylcholine, work together, the "push" of one precisely balancing the "pull" of the other.

Deep inside the brain of someone with Parkinson's disease, however, the nerve cells that produce dopamine die off, leaving way too much acetylcholine. The chemicals lose their rhythm, causing the symptoms that characterize Parkinson's: uncontrollable shaking and "frozen" muscles that refuse to cooperate.

There isn't a cure for Parkinson's disease yet. There are, however, medications that can help restore chemical balance.

Early Treatments

Basically, medications used to treat Parkinson's disease work in one of three ways. They either increase the amounts or effects of dopamine, decrease those of acetylcholine or increase one while decreasing the other.

Some of the oldest drugs for this condition act on the acetylcholine side of the equation. These prescription drugs, taken orally, include benztropine (Cogentin), ethopropazine (Parsidol) and trihexyphenidyl (Artane, Trihexane, Trihexy).

In the early stages of Parkinson's, these drugs can be very effective at bringing the body's chemistry back into balance, says Curt Freed, M.D., professor of medicine and pharmacology at the University of Colorado

---

AT A GLANCE

BENZTROPINE

Brand name: Cogentin

How taken: Tablet, injection

Prescription: Yes

	YES	NO
Generic substitutes	✓	
Potentially addicting		✓
May cause drowsiness	✓	
Alcohol discouraged	✓	

Possible drug interactions include: The effects of this drug may decrease if taken with antacids. Taking this drug may increase the effects of some antidepressants and anticholinergics (used for stomach cramps).

Possible side effects include: Nausea, blurred vision, constipation, difficulty urinating and dryness of the nose, mouth or throat.

LEVODOPA

Brand names: Dopar, Larodopa

How taken: Tablet, capsule

Prescription: Yes

	YES	NO
Generic substitutes	✓	
Potentially addicting		✓
May cause drowsiness	✓	
Alcohol discouraged		✓

Possible drug interactions include: This drug taken in combination with monoamine oxidase (MAO) inhibitors (used for depression) may result in increased blood pressure.

Possible side effects include: Depression, anxiety, confusion, constipation, jerky movements and changes in the color of sweat and urine.

AT A GLANCE

LEVODOPA–CARBIDOPA	YES	NO
Brand name: Sinemet		
How taken: Tablet		
Prescription: Yes		
Generic substitutes	✓	
Potentially addicting		✓
May cause drowsiness	✓	
Alcohol discouraged		✓

Possible drug interactions include: This drug taken in combination with monoamine oxidase (MAO) inhibitors (used for depression) may result in increased blood pressure.

Possible side effects include: Nausea, jerky movements, depression, nervousness and confusion.

SELEGILINE	YES	NO
Brand name: Eldepryl, SD Deprenyl		
How taken: Tablet		
Prescription: Yes		
Generic substitutes		✓
Potentially addicting		✓
May cause drowsiness	✓	
Alcohol discouraged	✓	

Possible drug interactions include: This drug taken in combination with fluoxetine (used to treat depression) or meperidine (a painkiller) may increase the risk of serious side effects.

Possible side effects include: Nausea, stomach pain, a dry mouth and difficulty sleeping.

Health Science Center in Denver. Unfortunately, they become less effective as the condition progresses. Also, these drugs often cause side effects, including constipation, blurred vision and dryness of the mouth, nose and throat. For these reasons, doctors usually tackle the dopamine side of the equation instead.

Dopamine Replacements

In the past, doctors tried to replace dopamine simply by injecting *more* dopamine. It was a good idea that didn't work. As the doctors discovered, dopamine can't travel from the bloodstream where it's injected into the brain where it's needed.

A prescription drug called levodopa, on the other hand, slips very easily into the brain. Once it arrives, it's metabolized into dopamine. Taken orally, levodopa (Dopar, Larodopa) may reduce or even eliminate symptoms for years at a time.

Unfortunately, it also can cause serious side effects, including nausea, vomiting and involuntary muscle contractions called dyskinesias.

To get the benefits of levodopa

without the side effects, it's often packaged with a drug called carbidopa. This levodopa-carbidopa combination (Sinemet), sold by prescription, is taken orally. "You can take ten times less, and it has fewer side effects than levodopa alone," says Dr. Freed. "It's a very clever drug combination."

Clever, but not perfect. Some people just don't improve with levodopa, alone or in combination. Among those who do respond, the improvements often are temporary. Symptoms generally return within five to ten years.

Chemical Enhancers

There are also medications that can help keep problems at bay by making the brain more responsive to natural dopamine and to levodopa. One dopamine "enhancer" is a prescription drug called selegiline (SD Deprenyl, Eldepryl). In the

---

AT A GLANCE

AMANTADINE

Brand names: Symadine, Symmetrel

How taken: Capsule, liquid

Prescription: Yes

	YES	NO
Generic substitutes	✓	
Potentially addicting		✓
May cause drowsiness	✓	
Alcohol discouraged	✓	

Possible drug interactions include: Taking this drug may increase the effects of anticholinergics (used for stomach cramps) and pemdine (used for hyperactivity).

Possible side effects include: Nausea, headache, dizziness and insomnia.

CAUTION: May be dangerous when taken by people with epilepsy or certain heart problems.

PERGOLIDE

Brand name: Permax

How taken: Tablet

Prescription: Yes

	YES	NO
Generic substitutes		✓
Potentially addicting		✓
May cause drowsiness	✓	
Alcohol discouraged	✓	

Possible drug interactions include: The effects of this drug may decrease if taken with drugs used to treat mental illness, such as haloperidol. Taking this drug may increase the effects of blood pressure drugs.

Possible side effects include: Nausea, stomach pain, low back pain and weakness.

early stages of the disease, it can ward off symptoms for months or years at a time.

In one study, 44 percent of people not taking selegiline had to be put on levodopa within one year to control their symptoms. Among those taking selegiline, only 25 percent needed the additional medication. Selegiline also may be combined with levodopa to make it more effective, says Dr. Freed.

Another helpful medication is amantadine (Symadine, Symmetrel). Taken orally, this prescription drug makes the brain more responsive to dopamine. "It's usually used in combination with levodopa," says Dr. Freed.

Other prescription drugs that can boost the effects of dopamine include bromocriptine (Parlodel) and pergolide (Permax). Again, these drugs usually are used to augment the effects of levodopa, not to replace it, explains Dr. Freed.

Pituitary Drugs

Adjustments for Hormonal Stability

The pituitary gland is a pea-size bundle of tissue tucked away at the base of the brain. Despite its small size, this gland is responsible for producing many important hormones, including those needed for growth and fertility. In fact, this little wonder has so many responsibilities that it has been referred to as the body's master gland.

When the pituitary gland malfunctions—this usually means producing too much of one hormone or too little of another—the effects can be wide-ranging. In most cases, however, pituitary problems can be readily relieved with medications that help restore your body's natural chemical balance.

Necessary Replacements

One of the key functions of the pituitary gland is to produce a hormone that enables children to grow. When levels of this hormone are low—a condition doctors call hypopituitarism—children stop growing and the onset

AT A GLANCE

SOMATREM

Brand name: Protropin

How taken: Injection

Prescription: Yes

	Yes	No
Generic substitutes		✓
Potentially addicting		✓
May cause drowsiness		✓
Alcohol discouraged		✓

Possible drug interactions include:
The effects of this drug may decrease if taken with cortisone medicines (used for inflammation).

Possible side effects include:
Side effects are unlikely.

SOMATROPIN

Brand name: Humatrope

How taken: Injection

Prescription: Yes

	YES	NO
Generic substitutes		✓
Potentially addicting		✓
May cause drowsiness		✓
Alcohol discouraged		✓

Possible drug interactions include:
The effects of this drug may decrease if taken with hydrocortisone (used for inflammation).

Possible side effects include:
Side effects are unlikely.

of puberty can be delayed, says Kay McFarland, M.D., an endocrinologist and professor of medicine at the University of South Carolina School of Medicine in Columbia.

In most cases, just replacing the missing growth hormone will help jump-start growth and development. Prescription medications such as somatrem (Protropin) and somatropin (Humatrope) are virtually identical to the body's natural growth hormone, says Dr. McFarland. Given by injection, they can enable children to shoot up an extra two inches within the first year of treatment. After that, growth rates gradually decline as the bones approach their full adult size.

Because these medications simply replace what should have been in the body in the first place, side effects are rare, says Dr. McFarland. There is one serious drawback, however: One year's treatment may cost as much as $20,000.

Another product of the pituitary gland is known as antidiuretic hormone, or ADH. This hormone, also known as vasopressin, is what enables the kidneys to store water. When ADH levels are low—causing a rare condition known as diabetes insipidus—the kidneys lose some of their holding power. As a result, people need to urinate frequently. At the same time, they're always thirsty because the body is trying to replace missing fluids.

In most cases, this condition can be treated by replacing the missing

ADH with man-made hormones, says Dr. McFarland. Prescription medications such as vasopressin (Pitressin), given by injection, or lypressin (Diapid), a nasal spray, will quickly restore normal kidney function. Although side effects such as headache or stomach cramps may occur, they generally disappear as the body adjusts to the medication.

It isn't always necessary to replace the missing hormone, adds Dr. McFarland. Taken orally, prescription drugs such as clofibrate (Abitrate, Atromid-S) or chlorpropamide (Diabinese, Glucamide) can stimulate the gland to produce more ADH on its own, usually without serious side effects.

Too Much of a Good Thing

Some people, instead of producing low amounts of pituitary hormones, produce too much.

AT A GLANCE

VASOPRESSIN

Brand name: Pitressin

How taken: Injection

Prescription: Yes

	YES	NO
Generic substitutes	✓	
Potentially addicting		✓
May cause drowsiness	✓	
Alcohol discouraged		✓

Possible drug interactions include: The effects of this drug may increase if taken with steroids, anti-seizure drugs, diabetes drugs, tetracycline antibiotics and antidepressants; effects may decrease if taken with lithium (used for manic depression), anti-clotting drugs or norepinephrine (a blood pressure drug).

Possible side effects include: Cramps, nausea and pain at the injection site.

CLOFIBRATE

Brand names: Abitrate, Atromid-S

How taken: Capsule

Prescription: Yes

	YES	NO
Generic substitutes	✓	
Potentially addicting		✓
May cause drowsiness	✓	
Alcohol discouraged	✓	

Possible drug interactions include: Taking this drug may increase the effects of anti-clotting drugs.

Possible side effects include: Rash, nausea, gas and diarrhea.

Depending on the hormones, this can lead to problems ranging from excessive growth to infertility or menstrual problems, says Joshua Hoffman, M.D., an internist and assistant clinical professor of medicine at the University of California, Davis, Medical Center in Sacramento.

When the pituitary gland secretes too much of a hormone called prolactin, for example, it can lead to infertility, menstrual irregularity or galactorrhea, a condition in which milk is produced even in the absence of childbirth. In men, excess prolactin can lead to impotence and reduced libido, says Dr. Hoffman.

In many cases, surgery to remove pituitary tumors that often cause this condition may be needed. Sometimes, however, prolactin levels can be decreased with medica-

AT A GLANCE

BROMOCRIPTINE

Brand name: Parlodel

How taken: Tablet, capsule

Prescription: Yes

	YES	NO
Generic substitutes		✓
Potentially addicting		✓
May cause drowsiness	✓	
Alcohol discouraged	✓	

Possible drug interactions include: The effects of this drug may decrease if taken with female hormone drugs (birth control pills) or with phenothiazines (used to treat nervous disorders). This drug taken in combination with ergot alkaloids like dihydroergotamine (used for migraines) may result in severe high blood pressure.

Possible side effects include: Fatigue, confusion, cramps, dizziness, headache, nausea and a dry mouth.

PERGOLIDE

Brand name: Permax

How taken: Tablet

Prescription: Yes

	YES	NO
Generic substitutes		✓
Potentially addicting		✓
May cause drowsiness	✓	
Alcohol discouraged	✓	

Possible drug interactions include: The effects of this drug may decrease if taken with sedatives and certain other medications used to treat nervous, mental and emotional disorders.

Possible side effects include: Dry mouth, nausea, dizziness, chest pain, constipation, diarrhea and low back pain.

tions alone. Prescription drugs such as bromocriptine (Parlodel) and pergolide (Permax), taken orally, often can stem prolactin production by more than 90 percent.

With both of these medications, however, side effects such as nausea or dizziness can be a problem. "This is why we start treatment slowly," says Dr. Hoffman. By starting treatment with small amounts of medication, then gradually increasing the dose over time, much of the discomfort can be reduced or eliminated, he says.

Occasionally, the pituitary gland, rather than producing too little growth hormone, produces too much. If this condition develops in childhood, it can lead to gigantism, in which a child can grow to an astounding size. If left untreated, it can also develop into a condition called acromegaly, which can result in massive skull bones and enlargement of the hands, feet and internal organs.

Taken orally or by injection, prescription medications such as bromocriptine or octreotide (Sandostatin) can be used to treat the gland. For most people, however, the medications aren't particularly effective, according to Dr. McFarland. "They're usually used only when other methods fail, or to shrink the gland prior to surgery," she says.

Psoriasis Drugs

Skin-Deep Relief

Your skin is a marvelous organ. Weighing approximately nine pounds, it's washable, stretchable and waterproof. It even mends itself.

One reason skin is so durable is that it's constantly renewing itself. Old cells die and new cells form at roughly the same pace. In people with psoriasis, however, new cells pop up at vastly accelerated rates.

Within days, the skin can accumulate layer upon layer of flaky, scaly, unsightly and sometimes itchy cells.

Psoriasis usually occurs in patches—on the scalp, for example, or the chest or elbows. But in severe cases, it can cover the entire body, says Mark G. Lebwohl, M.D., professor of dermatology and director of the Division of Clinical Dermatology at Mount Sinai School of Medicine in New York City.

Doctors aren't sure what causes psoriasis. It often runs in families, and outbreaks may be triggered by cuts, infections or flaws in the immune system. The condition also tends to become worse in cold weather.

This doesn't mean that you need to pack up and move to Mexico, although some sufferers do find relief in sunny climes. In most cases psoriasis can be controlled with medicated lotions and creams.

In other cases more powerful drugs may come to the rescue.

Surface Relief

For most people with psoriasis, the best medicine may be a steroid cream or ointment, says Guy Webster, M.D., Ph.D., assistant professor of dermatology at Jefferson Medical College of Thomas Jefferson University in Philadelphia.

Steroid preparations are sold over the counter and by prescrip-

---

AT A GLANCE

HYDROCORTISONE

Brand names: Allercort, Cortaid, Lemoderm

How taken: Cream, liquid, lotion, ointment, spray

Prescription: Sometimes, depending on strength

	YES	NO
Generic substitutes	✓	
Potentially addicting		✓
May cause drowsiness		✓
Alcohol discouraged		✓

Possible drug interactions include: Interactions are unlikely.

Possible side effects include: Mild stinging of the skin.

FLUOCINOLONE

Brand names: Bio-Syn, Flurosyn, Synemol

How taken: Cream, ointment, liquid, spray

Prescription: Yes

	YES	NO
Generic substitutes	✓	
Potentially addicting		✓
May cause drowsiness		✓
Alcohol discouraged		✓

Possible drug interactions include: Interactions are unlikely.

Possible side effects include: Mild stinging of the skin.

CAUTION: May cause thinning of the skin when used for long periods of time.

AT A GLANCE

COAL TAR

Brand names: Doak Tar Lotion, Tegrin Skin Cream, Zetar Emulsion

How taken: Soap, lotion, cream, ointment, bath oil, shampoo

Prescription: Sometimes, depending on strength

	YES	No
Generic substitutes	✓	
Potentially addicting		✓
May cause drowsiness		✓
Alcohol discouraged		✓

Possible drug interactions include: This drug used in combination with other psoriasis drugs or antibiotics such as tetracycline may result in skin sensitivity.

Possible side effects include: Skin irritation, stinging or temporary discoloration of blonde, bleached or tinted hair (if used on scalp).

CAUTION: Do not use if you plan to spend time in the sun.

ANTHRALIN

Brand names: Anthra-Derm, Drithocreme, Lasan

How taken: Cream, ointment

Prescription: Yes

	YES	No
Generic substitutes		✓
Potentially addicting		✓
May cause drowsiness		✓
Alcohol discouraged		✓

Possible drug interactions include: This drug used in combination with other psoriasis drugs or antibiotics such as tetracycline may result in increased skin sensitivity.

Possible side effects include: Skin irritation or staining.

tion. Drugs such as hydrocortisone (Allercort, Cortaid, Lemoderm) and betamethasone (Alphatrex, Dermabet) may relieve outbreaks, making the redness and scales disappear within days, says Dr. Webster.

As a rule, psoriasis that occurs in delicate areas—near the genitals, for example—is best treated with mild steroid creams such as hydro-cortisone. For hard-to-treat cases that occur on tougher areas of the body, such as on the elbows or knees, high-power prescription creams such as fluocinolone (Bio-Syn, Flurosyn, Synemol) may do a better job.

The problem with steroid creams, particularly the more potent varieties, is that they can cause skin damage with long-term

AT A GLANCE

METHOXSALEN

Brand names: 8-MOP, Oxsoralen Lotion, Oxsoralen-Ultra

How taken: Capsule, lotion

Prescription: Yes

	YES	NO
Generic substitutes		✓
Potentially addicting		✓
May cause drowsiness		✓
Alcohol discouraged		✓

Possible drug interactions include: This drug taken in combination with other psoriasis drugs or drugs that make the skin photosensitive may result in increased skin sensitivity.

Possible side effects include: Nausea and skin itching or irritation.

CAUTION: May contribute to serious sunburns and premature aging of the skin. May increase the risk for cataracts and skin cancer.

METHOTREXATE

Brand names: Folex, Mexate, Rheumatrex

How taken: Injection, tablet

Prescription: Yes

	YES	NO
Generic substitutes	✓	
Potentially addicting		✓
May cause drowsiness		✓
Alcohol discouraged	✓	

Possible drug interactions include: Taking this drug may decrease the effects of digoxin (a heart drug) and phenytoin (used to treat seizures).

Possible side effects include: Cramps, fatigue, fever, diarrhea, difficulty urinating, sores on the lips or in the mouth or throat, an increased risk of infection and skin sensitivity to sunlight.

CAUTION: Avoid vaccines such as the polio vaccine. May be dangerous if taken with aspirin, ibuprofen or other nonsteroidal anti-inflammatory drugs.

use. They also can be expensive, especially when psoriasis covers large areas.

Less expensive and often as effective are medications containing coal tar, which really *is* made from coal. Sold over the counter and by prescription, coal tars (Doak Tar Lotion, Tegrin Skin Cream, Zetar Emulsion) very quickly remove surplus skin cells and slow the rate at which new cells are formed. Some coal tars are applied directly to the skin as lotions or creams. Others are mixed in shampoos or poured into bathwater.

Because coal tars are cheaper than steroids, they're occasionally recommended for people with widespread problems, Dr. Lebwohl says. Still, no one enjoys using them, he adds. "They're black, they smell, and they stain everything," he explains.

Some of the same complaints may be leveled at creams and lotions containing anthralin (Anthra-Derm, Drithocreme, Lasan). Like coal tar, this prescription medication can stain everything from bed sheets to bathtub porcelain. It's rarely used in this country, although British doctors often prefer it to other treatments. "I guess British patients are tougher," comments Dr. Lebwohl.

It may seem as though the remedies for psoriasis are worse than the disease. But in fact, almost anything that's greasy—even petroleum jelly or mineral oil—can help. "If you keep the skin greasy, the psoriasis often goes away," says Dr. Webster.

From the Inside Out

When external creams and ointments don't make psoriasis go away, your doctor may recommend oral drugs that can tackle the problem from the inside.

Perhaps the most effective remedy is one called PUVA, which stands for psoralen plus ultraviolet-A. Psoralens are a class of prescription drugs that include methoxsalen (8-MOP, Oxsoralen Lotion, Oxsoralen-Ultra). Psoralens make the skin—and the psoriasis—extremely sensitive to ultraviolet light. More than 90 percent of people treated with PUVA will be completely clear of psoriasis for weeks or months at a time.

PUVA has many drawbacks, however. It's inconvenient, often requiring more than 30 treatments to be effective. It also can increase the risk for skin cancer. Cancers caused by PUVA, however, rarely spread and are easily removed, adds Dr. Lebwohl. "Most people consider it worth the risk," he says.

Other powerful prescription drugs that can help clear psoriasis include methotrexate (Folex, Mexate, Rheumatrex), etretinate (Tegison) and cyclosporine (Sandimmune). All of these oral drugs can be effective, but they're also rife with side effects, sometimes causing lung, liver or kidney damage. They're used only when safer treatments don't work, says Dr. Webster.

Sedatives

Prescriptions for Stress

Deadlines loom. Money is tight. Traffic is bumper-to-bumper. That's modern life. It's not surprising that sedatives are among the most commonly prescribed drugs in America.

Sedatives, also called tranquilizers or anxiolytics, can help relieve virtually all types of stress, says Matthew A. Menza, M.D., assistant professor of psychiatry and neurology and director of the Consultation Psychiatry Service at Robert Wood Johnson University Hospital in New Brunswick, New Jersey. And when used conscientiously under a doctor's supervision, they can be effective *and* safe.

Sedatives sometimes are used for problems such as chronic anxiety. More often, they're used for temporary relief of the kind of short-term stress that might accompany, say, a death in the family.

Historically, the first sedative was alcohol. This was followed by the

NATURAL ALTERNATIVES

Too much stress in your life? Sedatives may help, but long before you start with them, try these simple, natural stress relievers, suggests Matthew A. Menza, M.D., assistant professor of psychiatry and neurology and director of the Consultation Psychiatry Service at Robert Wood Johnson University Hospital in New Brunswick, New Jersey.

Get moving. Exercise allows you to blow off steam. It also stimulates the release of endorphins, soothing chemicals inside the body that help relieve pain and anxiety.

Try something new. Stress-reduction techniques such as yoga, meditation or biofeedback can work wonders. So can taking a stroll in the woods, listening to soothing music or playing with the dog.

Take a break. Time off from work—whether a single afternoon or an entire week—may literally be what the doctor ordered.

Switch to decaf. When you're already anxious, the last thing you need is caffeine.

AT A GLANCE

FLURAZEPAM

Brand names: Dalmane, Durapam
How taken: Capsule
Prescription: Yes

	YES	NO
Generic substitutes	✓	
Potentially addicting	✓	
May cause drowsiness	✓	
Alcohol discouraged	✓	

Possible drug interactions include: Taking this drug may increase the effects of antihistamines, muscle relaxants, digoxin (a heart drug) and certain drugs used for seizures; taking it may decrease the effects of levodopa (used for Parkinson's disease).

Possible side effects include: Lethargy and unsteadiness.

DIAZEPAM

Brand names: T-Quil, Valium, Vazepam
How taken: Capsule, injection, liquid, suppository, tablet
Prescription: Yes

	YES	NO
Generic substitutes	✓	
Potentially addicting	✓	
May cause drowsiness	✓	
Alcohol discouraged	✓	

Possible drug interactions include: Taking this drug may increase the effects of antihistamines, muscle relaxants, digoxin (a heart drug) and certain drugs used for seizures; taking it may decrease the effects of levodopa (used for Parkinson's disease).

Possible side effects include: Lethargy and unsteadiness.

barbiturates, powerful drugs that were (and are) too dangerous for regular use as sedatives. Today, a class of drugs called benzodiazepines, such as alprazolam, diazepam and lorazepam, are the sedatives of choice. "They cause less dependence and are much safer than the barbiturates," Dr. Menza says.

Interference in the Brain

More than 2,000 different benzodiazepines have been produced in the laboratory, and more than a dozen of these are commercially available. Despite some slight differences, all work in essentially the same way: By damping electrical activity in the brain, they help control stressful emotions in your life.

To relieve temporary stress, your doctor may prescribe benzodiazepines such as temazepam (Razepam, Restoril) or flurazepam (Dalmane, Durapam). Taken orally—usually for no more than two to three weeks—these drugs work very quickly to relieve anxiety, says Dr. Menza.

For problems like panic attacks, high-potency prescription benzodiazepines such as lorazepam (Alzapam, Ativan) or clonazepam (Klonopin) can be very helpful. Typically, you might take one of these drugs for several months, says Theodore A. Stern, M.D., associate professor of psychiatry at Harvard Medical School. Then, when the "symptom cycle" is broken, you may not need them anymore.

In deciding which of these drugs to prescribe, your doctor may consider how long they remain active in the body. For example, a drug such as diazepam (T-Quil, Valium, Vazepam) can cause prolonged sedation, making it a poor choice for someone—a heavy equipment operator, for example—who must be alert in the morning.

In this instance, the drug of choice might be alprazolam (Xanax). It goes to work quickly and is not especially sedating. Also, much of it is eliminated from the body within 12 hours. This means you can take it at night and count

---

AT A GLANCE

ALPRAZOLAM

Brand name: Xanax

How taken: Tablet

Prescription: Yes

	YES	NO
Generic substitutes		✓
Potentially addicting	✓	
May cause drowsiness	✓	
Alcohol discouraged	✓	

Possible drug interactions include: The effects of this drug may decrease if taken with theophylline (an asthma drug). Taking this drug may increase the effects of digoxin (a heart drug); taking it may decrease the effects of levodopa (used for Parkinson's disease).

Possible side effects include: Lightheadedness.

BUSPIRONE

Brand name: BuSpar

How taken: Tablet

Prescription: Yes

	YES	NO
Generic substitutes		✓
Potentially addicting		✓
May cause drowsiness	✓	
Alcohol discouraged		✓

Possible drug interactions include: This drug taken in combination with monoamine oxidase (MAO) inhibitors (used for depression) may result in severe high blood pressure.

Possible side effects include: Mild fatigue.

582

AT A GLANCE

NADOLOL

Brand name: Corgard

How taken: Tablet

Prescription: Yes

	YES	NO
Generic substitutes		✓
Potentially addicting		✓
May cause drowsiness	✓	
Alcohol discouraged	✓	

Possible drug interactions include: Taking this drug may increase the effects of blood pressure medications such as reserpine and verapamil; taking it may decrease the effects of theophylline (an asthma drug). This drug taken in combination with monoamine oxidase (MAO) inhibitors (used for depression) may result in severe high blood pressure.

Possible side effects include: Lethargy, fatigue, slow heart rate and cold feet or hands.

PROPRANOLOL

Brand names: Inderal, Ipran

How taken: Capsule, injection, liquid, tablet

Prescription: Yes

	YES	NO
Generic substitutes	✓	
Potentially addicting		✓
May cause drowsiness	✓	
Alcohol discouraged	✓	

Possible drug interactions include: Taking this drug may increase the effects of blood pressure medications such as reserpine and verapamil; taking it may decrease the effects of theophylline (an asthma drug). This drug taken in combination with monoamine oxidase (MAO) inhibitors (used for depression) may result in severe high blood pressure.

Possible side effects include: Lethargy, fatigue, slow heart rate and cold feet or hands.

on being fully alert the next day.

Unfortunately, the benzodiazepines can cause side effects such as unwanted drowsiness and impaired memory. "Anytime you use a drug that affects the brain you can get a variety of symptoms," says Dr. Stern. To reduce side effects—and to reduce the risk of addiction—your doctor may prescribe these drugs for only a few weeks at a time. This will allow him to keep a close eye on your progress—and your problems.

Alternative Actions

Aside from the benzodiazepines, there are several other types of drugs that can help relieve anxiety. One is the prescription drug buspirone (BuSpar), which is a sedative in a class by itself. It tends to cause fewer side effects than the benzo-diazepines. Also, it's less likely to lead to addiction, Dr. Stern says.

Another class of prescription drugs targets the *symptoms* of anxiety. These drugs, which are called beta-blockers (short for beta-adren-ergic blocking agents), are used for many ailments, including heart conditions.

Drugs such as nadolol (Corgard) and propranolol (Inderal, Ipran) taken orally or by injection, work by blocking the action of a stimulating chemical in the body called norepinephrine. This in turn reduces the force and speed of your heartbeat and prevents blood vessels surrounding the brain from dilating.

An advantage of beta-blockers, says Dr. Stern, is that they can relieve symptoms of anxiety without causing unwanted sedation.

When taken to treat performance anxiety, for example, they can prevent the hands from shaking and the heart from beating rapidly. This helps to relieve stage fright without decreasing mental alertness—or the quality of a performance.

Still, beta-blockers are powerful drugs. "They may have fewer central nervous system side effects, but they have many more profound effects on the rest of the body," according to Dr. Stern. Possible side effects include dizziness (due to low blood pressure) and breathing difficulties.

It's important to remember that sedatives aren't a cure for anxiety, Dr. Menza says. So if stress is a constant and serious problem in your life, you may want to consider psychological counseling. With good help, you may rarely need the drugs at all.

Seizure Drugs

Convulsion Stoppers

Although electricity has changed our lives for the better, it can be a terrible force when it's out of control.

Nowhere is this more apparent than inside the brain. The same electrical signals that enable us to sing a song or think a thought are also capable of erupting into electrical surges. These surges may cause the body to jerk and twitch or the mind to temporarily go

AT A GLANCE

PHENYTOIN

Brand names: Dilantin, Diphenylan

How taken: Capsule, injection, liquid, tablet

Prescription: Yes

	YES	NO
Generic substitutes	✓	
Potentially addicting		✓
May cause drowsiness	✓	
Alcohol discouraged		✓

Possible drug interactions include: Taking this drug may decrease the effects of anti-inflammatory steroids, cyclosporine (an immunosuppressant), doxycycline (an antibiotic) and levodopa (used for Parkinson's disease); taking it may increase the effects of chloramphenicol (an antibiotic) and cimetidine (an ulcer drug) and increase or decrease the effects of oral anti-clotting drugs.

Possible side effects include: Bleeding, tender or enlarged gums, mild fatigue, skin rashes and excessive growth of body hair.

CARBAMAZEPINE

Brand names: Epitol, Tegretol

How taken: Liquid, tablet

Prescription: Yes

	YES	NO
Generic substitutes	✓	
Potentially addicting		✓
May cause drowsiness	✓	
Alcohol discouraged		✓

Possible drug interactions include: Blood levels of this drug may rise if taken with erythromycin (an antibiotic). Taking this drug may increase the effects of sedatives; taking it may decrease the effects of doxycycline (an antibiotic) and warfarin (an anti-clotting drug).

Possible side effects include: Constipation, dry mouth or throat and urination difficulties.

CAUTION: May be dangerous when taken with lithium (used for manic depression) or monoamine oxidase (MAO) inhibitors (used for depression).

blank. Doctors call this an epileptic seizure.

Not all seizures require treatment, says Ronald P. Lesser, M.D., associate professor of neurology and neurosurgery and director of the Epilepsy Center at Johns Hopkins University School of Medicine in Baltimore. But when they occur frequently, because of epilepsy or other brain disorders, you may need anti-seizure drugs.

Cutting the Power

Anti-seizure drugs work by controlling the signals in certain parts of the brain. The most

AT A GLANCE

VALPROIC ACID

Brand names: Dalpro, Depakene, Myproic Acid
How taken: Capsule, liquid, tablet
Prescription: Yes

	YES	NO
Generic substitutes	✓	
Potentially addicting		✓
May cause drowsiness	✓	
Alcohol discouraged	✓	

Possible drug interactions include: Taking this drug may increase the effects of anti-clotting drugs and antidepressants and may increase the risk of bleeding.

Possible side effects include: Lethargy, weight changes and temporary hair loss.

ETHOSUXIMIDE

Brand name: Zarontin
How taken: Liquid, tablet
Prescription: Yes

	YES	NO
Generic substitutes		✓
Potentially addicting		✓
May cause drowsiness	✓	
Alcohol discouraged		✓

Possible drug interactions include: Taking this drug may increase the effects of phenytoin (another anti-seizure drug).

Possible side effects include: Lethargy and fatigue.

widely used of these drugs are phenytoin (Dilantin, Diphenylan), carbamazepine (Epitol, Tegretol) and valproic acid (Dalpro, Depakene, Myproic Acid). These prescription drugs can prevent many types of seizures, including the dramatic *grand mal* convulsions characteristic of some types of epilepsy.

For the milder attacks known as *petit mal* seizures, also characteristic of some forms of epilepsy, doctors often prescribe a drug called ethosuximide (Zarontin) or valproic acid.

Perhaps the oldest of the anti-seizure drugs is phenobarbital (Barbita, Luminal, Solfoton). Phenobarbital is relatively safe and effective for long-term control of various kinds of seizures, says Theodore A. Stern, M.D., associate professor of psychiatry at Harvard Medical School. Unfortunately, phenobarbital tends to cause more sedation and attention difficulties than other anti-seizure drugs, such as the prescription drugs primidone (Myidone, Mysoline) and clonazepam (Klonopin).

To stop attacks already in progress, your doctor first may use a kind of drug known as a benzodiazepine. Two benzodiazepines used for this purpose are lorazepam (Ativan) and diazepam (Valium). Generally, these drugs (used to fight anxiety) are given by injection to get into the body more quickly and stop the seizure, says Dr. Lesser.

Common Problems

The perfect anti-seizure drug would prevent seizures without affecting normal brain function. Unfortunately, such a drug doesn't exist. Each of the anti-seizure drugs may cause problems, including lethargy, memory loss and poor concentration and coordination. In addition, phenytoin may cause an annoying increase in body hair or growth of the gums, while carbamazepine may cause upset stomach and blurred or double vision, and valproic acid can cause upset stomach, weight changes and temporary hair loss.

To keep side effects to a minimum, your doctor may prescribe a very low dose, then gradually increase it. The goal, says Dr.

AT A GLANCE

PHENOBARBITAL

Brand names: Barbita, Luminal, Solfoton

How taken: Capsule, liquid, tablet, injection

Prescription: Yes

	YES	NO
Generic substitutes	✓	
Potentially addicting	✓	
May cause drowsiness	✓	
Alcohol discouraged	✓	

Possible drug interactions include: Taking this drug may decrease the effects of anti-clotting drugs, beta-blockers (used for high blood pressure and heart problems), anti-inflammatory steroids, doxycycline (an antibiotic), griseofulvin (an anti-fungal drug), theophylline (used for asthma) and some oral contraceptives.

Possible side effects include: Weakness, reduced concentration and sluggishness.

PRIMIDONE

Brand names: Myidone, Mysoline

How taken: Liquid, tablet

Prescription: Yes

	YES	NO
Generic substitutes	✓	
Potentially addicting	✓	
May cause drowsiness	✓	
Alcohol discouraged	✓	

Possible drug interactions include: Taking this drug may decrease the effects of anti-clotting drugs, beta-blockers (used for high blood pressure and heart problems), anti-inflammatory steroids, doxycycline (an antibiotic), griseofulvin (an anti-fungal drug), theophylline (used for asthma) and some oral contraceptives.

Possible side effects include: Impaired concentration and sluggishness.

Lesser, is to find the right balance between controlling seizures and causing side effects. It may take several months before your doctor finds the drug (and the dose) that's right for you.

If you experience uncomfortable side effects, let your doctor know. The two of you can work on finding the right drug and the right dose. People who abruptly stop treatment may have more seizures, often within a day or two.

Generic versions of anti-seizure drugs don't necessarily enter the body the same way as the brand-name drugs. Because of this, some people may get too high or too low a level of medicine in the body if the medicine they get is made by a different company from one month to the next. It is important to check this with your doctor.

The good news is that as many as two-thirds of people with epilepsy eventually will stop having seizures. Says Dr. Lesser, "When patients have been seizure-free for five years, they can consider going off their medication."

Sleeping Pills

Rest for Midnight Ramblers

Whoever said time flies never tossed and turned as the midnight hours s-l-o-w-l-y passed. Insomnia is worse than frustrating, however. It also can leave you feeling tired and unable to function well.

There are many reasons people can't fall asleep, the most common being temporary stress and anxiety. It's estimated that about 17 percent of the population often has trouble sleeping, says Peter Hauri, Ph.D., director of the insomnia program at the Mayo Clinic in Rochester, Minnesota. If you find yourself one night staring into quiet darkness, a sleeping pill may help you get to sleep when nothing else you do seems to help.

Sleep in a Bottle

Traditionally, people unable to sleep often reached not for a pill but a potion. Today, of course, alcohol's dangers are well known. So, too, are the dangers of sleeping pills. Doctors agree those drugs, which can lead to addiction, are not meant for long-term use.

But when occasional daytime

NATURAL ALTERNATIVES

Insomnia has many causes—psychological stress, for one—that can't be cured with drugs. So before your doctor writes a prescription, he may ask you to try some other things first. For example:

Knock off the napping. If you sleep two hours every day after work, you'll probably have sleep trouble later on. So try to stay awake until bedtime.

Don't watch the clock. Better yet, don't even have a visible clock in the bedroom. Set the alarm for the time you want to get up, then hide the clock in your top dresser drawer. You should be relaxing, not checking the time every three minutes.

Cut the caffeine. Drinking caffeinated beverages such as coffee or cola late in the day often is a guarantee that you'll burn the midnight oil.

Don't work in bed. If you treat your bed like a second office, a place to pay bills, make business calls and wrestle with taxes, it may treat you like an employee—an employee who doesn't need his rest.

Quit trying so hard. Sometimes sleep is elusive, and there's nothing you can do about it. Instead of getting frustrated (and even *more* awake), try reading a magazine. Drink some milk. Then, when you're really sleepy, go to bed again.

worries cause you nighttime stress, your doctor may recommend drugs called benzodiazepines. "For short-term use, they are very effective sleeping agents," says Matthew A. Menza, M.D., assistant professor of psychiatry and neurology and director of the Consultation Psychiatry Service at Robert Wood Johnson University Hospital in New Brunswick, New Jersey.

There are now more than a half-dozen benzodiazepine medications on the market. Essentially, they work by reducing the activity of the brain, which helps you fall asleep more readily. Just as important,

they help you *stay* asleep.

Though all of these drugs are similar, they differ in how quickly they go to work and how long they remain active in the body. For example, prescription drugs like zolpidem (Ambien) or an older one called triazolam (Halcion) go to work very quickly, but half of the dosage is eliminated within two to five hours. This might make them drugs of choice for someone who typically has difficulties with falling asleep or wakes up at 3:00 in the morning and only needs a few more hours' extra sleep. They also might be prescribed for someone who must be fully alert in the morning, such as a school bus driver, says Dr. Hauri. But be sure you take these medications only as prescribed. Overdosing or using them with alcohol might lead to trouble, including temporary amnesia. You may recall the controversy that arose over Halcion several years ago, with scattered reports of memory loss in people who mixed the drug with alcohol.

For people who have a problem with falling asleep when they first go to bed and also with waking up too much during the night, other drugs may be preferable. These late-night tossers and turners might be given a longer-lasting prescription drug such as estazolam (ProSom) or temazepam (Razepam, Restoril). Taken orally, these medications will help them sleep all through the night. The drugs

---

AT A GLANCE

TRIAZOLAM

Brand name: Halcion

How taken: Tablet

Prescription: Yes

	YES	NO
Generic substitutes		✓
Potentially addicting	✓	
May cause drowsiness	✓	
Alcohol discouraged	✓	

Possible drug interactions include: Taking this drug may increase the effects of sedatives, digoxin (used for heart problems) and phenytoin (used for seizures); taking it may decrease the effects of levodopa (used for Parkinson's disease).

Possible side effects include: Headache, lethargy, nausea and vomiting, nervousness and unsteadiness.

CAUTION: Use with alcohol may cause temporary amnesia.

TEMAZEPAM

Brand names: Razepam, Restoril

How taken: Capsule, tablet

Prescription: Yes

	YES	NO
Generic substitutes	✓	
Potentially addicting	✓	
May cause drowsiness	✓	
Alcohol discouraged	✓	

Possible drug interactions include: Taking this drug may increase the effects of digoxin (a heart drug) and phenytoin (an anti-seizure drug); taking it may decrease the effects of levodopa (used for Parkinson's disease).

Possible side effects include: Dizziness, slurred speech and unsteadiness.

AT A GLANCE

FLURAZEPAM

Brand names: Dalmane, Durapam

How taken: Capsule

Prescription: Yes

	YES	NO
Generic substitutes	✓	
Potentially addicting	✓	
May cause drowsiness	✓	
Alcohol discouraged	✓	

Possible drug interactions include: Taking this drug may increase the effects of digoxin (a heart drug) and phenytoin (used for seizures); taking it may decrease the effects of lev-odopa (used for Parkinson's disease).

Possible side effects include: Lethargy and unsteadiness.

HYDROXYZINE

Brand names: Atarax, Vistaril

How taken: Capsule, liquid, tablet

Prescription: Sometimes, depending on strength

	YES	NO
Generic substitutes	✓	
Potentially addicting		✓
May cause drowsiness	✓	
Alcohol discouraged	✓	

Possible drug interactions include: Taking this drug may increase the effects of other sedatives; taking it may decrease the effects of oral anti-clotting drugs.

Possible side effects include: Dryness of the mouth, nose or throat.

---

remain active for about eight hours.

Then there are the prescription drugs flurazepam (Dalmane, Durapam) and quazepam (Doral), which can remain active for over 24 hours, making a person sleepy and relaxed both night and day, Dr. Hauri says. It not only helps people fall asleep but also can relieve daytime anxiety in certain cases.

Although all of the benzodiazepine drugs are effective for the short run, they may cause side effects, including daytime drowsiness. Some of them also can cause rebound insomnia—long bouts of wakefulness that occur when you stop taking the drug. Potential addiction is also a problem. If you use these drugs no more than once a week, however, you won't be taking any big risks, and you will not become addicted.

Other Sleep Aids

Though the benzodiazepines are doctors' drugs of choice for treatment of short-term insomnia, there are other medications that can be helpful as well.

AT A GLANCE

DIPHENHYDRAMINE

Brand names: Benadryl, Sleep-Eze 3, Sominex Formula 2

How taken: Capsule, liquid, tablet

Prescription: Sometimes, depending on strength

	YES	NO
Generic substitutes	✓	
Potentially addicting		✓
May cause drowsiness	✓	
Alcohol discouraged	✓	

Possible drug interactions include: Taking this drug may increase the effects of sedatives and atropine (an anti-spasmodic drug).

Possible side effects include: Weakness, constipation and a dry nose, mouth or throat.

CAUTION: Do not take if you have bronchitis, pneumonia or active bronchial asthma.

CHLORAL HYDRATE

Brand names: Aquachloral Supprettes, Noctec

How taken: Capsule, liquid, suppository

Prescription: Yes

	YES	NO
Generic substitutes	✓	
Potentially addicting	✓	
May cause drowsiness	✓	
Alcohol discouraged	✓	

Possible drug interactions include: Taking this drug may increase the effects of oral anti-clotting drugs and nervous system depressants like antihistamines.

Possible side effects include: Lightheadedness, nausea, stomach pain, vomiting and weakness.

For example, some researchers suggest prescription antihistamines such as hydroxyzine (Atarax, Vistaril). Taken orally, they can make you drowsy by acting on the central nervous system. (Of course, they help relieve hay fever symptoms as well.) Other prescription and over-the-counter antihistamines, usually taken orally, include diphenhydramine (Benadryl, Sleep-Eze 3, Sominex Formula 2), dimenhydrinate (Calm X, Dimetabs, Dramamine) and doxylamine (Unisom Nighttime Sleep Aid).

Since these drugs are available over the counter and are generally quite safe, they're certainly worth a try. For people with serious insomnia, however, they aren't likely to be very effective, doctors agree.

In low doses, prescription antidepressant drugs such as amitriptyline (Amitril, Elavil, Endep) or trazadone (Desyrel) also can relieve insomnia. In fact, they're often helpful even in people who aren't depressed, says Dr. Menza.

Although these drugs can help and are generally considered safe, they may cause side effects, including dry mouth and occasionally, blurred vision. They're rarely the doctors' first choice, says Dr. Hauri.

In an altogether different class of drugs, a prescription medication called chloral hydrate (Aquachloral Supprettes, Noctec), usually taken orally, can be very effective. It's unlikely to cause addiction and is safe for long-term use. Says Dr. Menza, "It's a perfectly reasonable alternative to the benzodiazepines."

Last, Dr. Hauri reports that in at least one study, simple aspirin was shown to be an effective sleep aid. For occasional restless nights, he recommends two aspirin at bedtime, taken with at least a full glass of water.

Smoking-Cessation Drugs

Gateways to Freedom

Smoking is the single most preventable cause of early death and sickness in the United States. Many stores, restaurants and office buildings have instituted no-smoking zones. Some have even banned it.

So why not stop? Nearly two-thirds of smokers would like to, but can't. "Tobacco is a very powerful, addictive substance," says Douglas E. Jorenby, Ph.D., coordinator of clinical activities at the Center for Tobacco Research and Intervention at the University of Wisconsin Medical School in Madison. "In a given year, about 90 percent of people who attempt to quit smoking will fail," he says.

To help improve the odds, many physicians recommend using stop-smoking drugs. The active ingredient in all of these medications is nicotine, the very same chemical that makes tobacco so addictive. Used for anywhere from 4 to 12 weeks, nicotine gum or nicotine patches can help people make the healthy transition to a smoke-free life by easing withdrawal symptoms.

Patch Up Your Willpower

The most popular stop-smoking medications are sold in patch form. Saturated with nicotine, these prescription patches (Habitrol, Nicoderm, Nicotrol) are affixed to the skin, often on the shoulder. They gradually release nicotine into the bloodstream, simulating the physical effects of smoking.

Stop-smoking patches contain varying amounts of nicotine. A heavy smoker, for example, might use a patch that delivers 22 milligrams of nicotine—the equivalent of about 15 cigarettes. A lighter smoker might do better with a 7-, 11- or 14-milligram patch.

The patches typically are left in place for 24 hours, although one newer patch, Nicotrol, is worn only during the day.

Various studies have shown that nicotine patches can help people quit in about 22 to 42 percent of cases, about double the rate of those using placebo, or dummy, patches. The drugs are most effective, however, when used in combi-

---

AT A GLANCE

NICOTINE PATCH

Brand name: Habitrol, Nicoderm, Nicotrol

How taken: Patch

Prescription: Yes

	YES	NO
Generic substitutes		✓
Potentially addicting	✓	
May cause drowsiness		✓
Alcohol discouraged		✓

Possible drug interactions include: Taking this drug may increase the effects of propranolol (used for high blood pressure).

Possible side effects include: Headache, rapid heartbeat and itching or burning at the application site.

CAUTION: Continuing to smoke while using this drug may cause nausea, diarrhea and other symptoms of nicotine overdose.

NICOTINE GUM

Brand name: Nicorette

How taken: Chewing gum

Prescription: Yes

	YES	NO
Generic substitutes		✓
Potentially addicting	✓	
May cause drowsiness		✓
Alcohol discouraged		✓

Possible drug interactions include: Taking this drug may increase the effects of propranolol (used for high blood pressure).

Possible side effects include: Headache, belching, rapid heartbeat and tender mouth or throat.

CAUTION: Continuing to smoke while using this drug may cause nausea, diarrhea and other symptoms of nicotine overdose.

nation with counseling or other types of stop-smoking programs, says Dr. Jorenby.

The medications are safe, although some people may experience burning or itching where the patch affixes to the skin. The drugs also can cause insomnia, diarrhea or restlessness. When that occurs, lowering the dose should help.

In addition, Dr. Jorenby says, the patches are meant to replace smoking. If you're using a patch, you should not smoke. Doing both could cause nausea, diarrhea, heartbeat irregularities and other symptoms of nicotine overdose, he warns.

Chew Out Smoking

Many smokers have quit with the help of chewing gum. Sold by prescription, nicotine gum (Nicorette), like the patches, delivers steady amounts of nicotine into the bloodstream and is probably just as effective. Although the gum has an unpleasant taste, it has the advantage of enabling smokers to keep their jaws busy while they learn to live without cigarettes. "The gum, when it's used properly, is a very effective aid to smoking cessation," says Dr. Jorenby.

But the gum must be used properly to be effective. Nicotine isn't absorbed through the stomach, so chomping away—the way you chew regular gum—won't work. Instead, you should chew the gum just a few times until the nicotine is released (you'll feel a tingling sensation in your mouth). Then "park" the gum between your gums and the cheek, where the nicotine can be absorbed. After a few minutes, the tingling sensation will begin to fade. Chew the gum to release more nicotine, then put it in back in position.

Also, you shouldn't drink coffee, cola or citrus drinks with nicotine gum. These liquids will temporarily make the inside of your mouth too acidic for the nicotine to be absorbed, says Dr. Jorenby.

As with the patches, he adds, chewing nicotine gum should be just part of a program. "When quitters are given additional support such as counseling, even more of them tend to be successful."

Stimulants

The Fatigue Fighters

Normally, our energy levels ebb and flow in predictable rhythms. Soon after we wake up, for example, our gears just naturally slip into high. At day's end, we get progressively more tired until we finally say good night and turn out the light.

There are times, however, when your energy levels seem to be permanently low. For people with fatigue, or those who just need a little extra pep for a short time, medications called stimulants can be used.

High-Power Relief

When doctors talk about stimulants, they're usually referring to powerful prescription drugs such as amphetamine (Biphetamine), dextroamphetamine (Dexedrine, Dexedrine Spansule, Oxydess II), methamphetamine (Desoxyn) or methylphenidate (Ritalin, Ritalin-SR). Taken orally, these medications cause stimulating chemicals to be released in the brain, giving an energy boost and increased alertness.

Stimulants are used to treat narcolepsy, a serious sleep disorder that causes fatigue and frequent "sleep attacks"—episodes of extreme sleepiness, says E. Don Nelson, Pharm.D., professor of clinical pharmacology at the University of Cincinnati College of Medicine.

With stimulants, people with narcolepsy can stay more alert and live a reasonably active life. The drugs are not a cure, however. People with narcolepsy often need medication for life. "Take the drug away, they'll go to sleep again," says Dr. Nelson.

The same drugs may be given to children with a condition called attention deficit disorder, in which they are unable to sit still or pay attention in class. Prescription medications such as dextroamphetamine and methylphenidate

NATURAL ALTERNATIVES

Many fatigue problems are easily fixed by getting the right amount of sleep and relaxation. Beyond your 40 winks, you might also try the following.

Get up and go. Studies have found that exercising can help boost energy levels and keep them high for up to two hours. Be sure, however, to take things slowly at first. Otherwise you'll have more pain than gain.

Stay trim. People who are overweight usually have extra tissue in the neck and throat. When combined with poor muscle tone, this can cause the airways to partially shut down at night, possibly causing snoring, frequent awakenings and, by the next day, fatigue.

Eat sensibly. If you're overweight, cutting some calories is good; cutting too many, however, can leave you feeling hungry—and fatigued. So rather than embarking on crash diets, talk to your doctor about a sensible weight-loss plan.

Stay motivated. One of the most formidable energy drains is depression. One way to beat negative feelings, experts say, is to stay involved. Take piano lessons. Join a social club. Volunteer your talents at a local hospital or charity. It doesn't really matter what you do—as long as it excites you to do it!

enable the children to focus on the tasks at hand. "Stimulants increase their ability to concentrate," Dr. Nelson says.

A Safer Stimulant

Although most stimulants are sold only with a prescription, one powerful medication is found not only in pharmacies but in restaurants, home kitchens and soda machines. We know it as caffeine, the powerful pick-me-up in coffee, tea, colas and other foods and drinks.

You don't have to raid the pantry to take caffeine, however. It's also the active ingredient in many over-the-counter stimulants (Caffedrine, NōDōz, Vivarin). Taken orally, these medications contain anywhere from 100 to 250 milligrams of caffeine. (A cup of drip coffee, by contrast, may contain 40 to 180 milligrams.)

The caffeine tablets are commonly used by people who don't want coffee or soda but who would still like some extra pep—students studying for exams, for example, or an accountant burning the midnight oil at income tax time.

Is it safe to take caffeine to give yourself a little boost? In most cases, says Dr. Nelson, the answer is yes. But there are some exceptions. People with heart problems or high cholesterol probably shouldn't take the drug without a doctor's supervision. And for some people, caffeine can cause side effects such as headache, diarrhea and insomnia.

Weight Loss in a Pill

Sometimes stimulants are used not to perk you up but to slim you down. Taken orally, prescrip-

---

AT A GLANCE

DEXTROAMPHETAMINE

Brand names: Dexedrine, Dexedrine Spansule, Oxydess II

How taken: Tablet, capsule

Prescription: Yes

	YES	NO
Generic substitutes	✓	
Potentially addicting	✓	
May cause drowsiness		✓
Alcohol discouraged	✓	

Possible drug interactions include: This drug taken in combination with antihistamines, asthma drugs and other stimulants may result in excessive stimulation; taking it with beta-blockers (used for heart problems) or monoamine oxidase (MAO) inhibitors (used for depression) may result in high blood pressure.

Possible side effects include: Restlessness, irritability, insomnia and irregular heartbeat.

CAUTION: Taking this drug for long periods of time can lead to addiction.

METHYLPHENIDATE

Brand names: Ritalin, Ritalin-SR

How taken: Tablet

Prescription: Yes

	YES	NO
Generic substitutes	✓	
Potentially addicting	✓	
May cause drowsiness	✓	
Alcohol discouraged	✓	

Possible drug interactions include: Taking this drug may decrease the effects of blood pressure medications.

Possible side effects include: Restlessness, insomnia, fast heartbeat and loss of appetite.

tion drugs such as amphetamines, phentermine (Adipex-P, Phentercot) and fenfluramine (Pondimin) and a prescription and over-the-counter drug such as phenylpropanolamine (Dex-A-Diet, Dexatrim) have been found to promote weight loss at a rate of about half a pound a week. They do this by suppressing the appetite.

But the use of stimulants as diet pills is an area of considerable controversy. The potential side effects from stimulants—which can range from shaking and insomnia to hallucinations and addiction—can be more dangerous than the extra

AT A GLANCE

CAFFEINE

Brand names: Caffedrine, NōDōz, Vivarin

How taken: Tablet, capsule

Prescription: No

	YES	NO
Generic substitutes	✓	
Potentially addicting	✓	
May cause drowsiness		✓
Alcohol discouraged	✓	

Possible drug interactions include: This drug taken in combination with antihistamines, asthma drugs and beverages that contain caffeine may result in excessive stimulation.

Possible side effects include: Dizziness, rapid heartbeat and insomnia.

FENFLURAMINE

Brand name: Pondimin

How taken: Tablet

Prescription: Yes

	YES	NO
Generic substitutes		✓
Potentially addicting	✓	
May cause drowsiness	✓	
Alcohol discouraged	✓	

Possible drug interactions include: Taking this drug may increase the sedative effects of antihistamines, sedatives, barbiturates and muscle relaxants.

Possible side effects include: Restlessness and irritability, followed by fatigue.

PHENTERMINE

Brand names: Adipex-P, Phentercot

How taken: Tablet, capsule

Prescription: Yes

	YES	NO
Generic substitutes	✓	
Potentially addicting	✓	
May cause drowsiness		✓
Alcohol discouraged	✓	

Possible drug interactions include: Taking this drug may decrease the effects of blood pressure drugs.

Possible side effects include: Restlessness, irritability, insomnia and high blood pressure.

pounds. For the average person, experts say, physical activity and careful dieting is usually a much better approach to weight loss. "No one prefers dope to a good diet and exercise," cautions Dr. Nelson. "The drugs should be used only in people who are extremely overweight, and only as an adjunct to other treatments."

Sun Protectors

Guard against Damaged Skin

Every summer, many devoted sun worshipers take to the great outdoors in search of warmth, relaxation and the perfect tan. What they often get is a lot of damaged skin.

Sunburn, the most painful proof of the sun's devastating power, can do more than ruin your weekend. It also can increase your risk for

NATURAL ALTERNATIVES

Unless you're a relative of Dracula, you probably don't want to avoid the sun altogether. Here are some tips for enjoying your outdoor activities without incurring the wrath of Ol' Sol.

Watch the clock. About 95 percent of the sun's skin-damaging rays hit the Earth between the hours of 10:00 A.M. and 3:00 P.M. (11:00 A.M. and 4:00 P.M. daylight saving time).

Dress defensively. Wear protective clothing when you are out in the sun. Hats, tightly woven fabrics and long sleeves help keep the sun's rays at bay.

Beware of reflective surfaces. It's always the same sun up above, but circumstances on Earth can affect how much sun your skin soaks up. Light-colored surfaces tend to reflect sunlight, so be particularly wary about the time you spend on sand, snow and concrete.

Vacation on a northern seaboard. Be aware that the sun's destructive rays are most powerful at high altitudes (where the air is thinner) and southern latitudes (closer to the equator).

malignant melanoma, which is a life-threatening form of skin cancer. Even tanning can cause permanent damage to the skin, including wrinkles, age spots or cancers, says Frederick Urbach, M.D., professor emeritus of dermatology, at Temple University School of Medicine in Philadelphia.

Although there are a number of medications that can help ease sunburn sting, nothing will reverse damage that has already occurred. That's why it's so important to shut out the rays before they get in.

Ray Bans

When you were a kid, you probably thought that lifeguards were born with brightly colored noses. In fact, what they were doing was protecting themselves with sunblocks. Available over the counter in white or vibrant yellows, greens and pinks, sunblock creams and ointments that contain zinc oxide (Sundown Sport) or titanium dioxide (IT Screen Natural, Neutrogena Chemical-Free Sunblocker) reflect up to 99 percent of incoming light.

For long-term protection, sunblocks are extremely effective, says Dr. Urbach. They aren't without problems, however. For one thing, they aren't invisible, and many people don't want to turn their faces into modern art projects. Also, anything that keeps the sun out may also keep other things—heat and sweat, for example—in. To keep the

AT A GLANCE

PADIMATE O

Brand names: ChapStick Lip Balm, Hawaiian Tropic Dark Tanning Oil with Sunscreen, PreSun Moisturizing Sunscreen

How taken: Balm, lotion, cream, spray

Prescription: No

	YES	NO
Generic substitutes	✓	
Potentially addicting		✓
May cause drowsiness		✓
Alcohol discouraged		✓

Possible drug interactions include: Interactions are unlikely.

Possible side effects include: Dry skin, rash and stinging around the eyelids.

PARA-AMINOBENZOIC ACID (PABA)

Brand name: Solar Lotion 15

How taken: Lotion

Prescription: No

	YES	NO
Generic substitutes	✓	
Potentially addicting		✓
May cause drowsiness		✓
Alcohol discouraged		✓

Possible drug interactions include: Interactions are unlikely.

Possible side effects include: Rash, dry skin and temporary yellow stains on clothing.

discomfort to a minimum, people usually apply sunblocks only to small areas, such as the nose or tips of the ears.

Screen Out Trouble

Unlike sunblocks, medications called sunscreens don't reflect sunlight but chemically absorb the sun's rays, rendering them harmless to the skin underneath.

Every sunscreen is given a sun protection factor, or SPF, says Richard F. Wagner Jr., M.D., professor of dermatology at the University of Texas Medical Branch at Galveston. The higher the number, the greater the protection—but only up to a point. Although some products have SPFs of 20 or even 30, experts agree that they offer little more protection—usually at a higher cost—than a product with an SPF of 15. "For most people, a sunscreen with an SPF of 15 is more than adequate," says Dr. Wagner.

All sunscreens contain one or more ingredients that block a type of sunlight known as ultraviolet B (UV-B), which causes sunburn. Some active ingredients are padimate O (ChapStick Lip Balm, Hawaiian Tropic Dark Tanning Oil with Sunscreen, PreSun Moisturizing Sunscreen) and its chemical cousin para-aminobenzoic acid, or PABA (Solar Lotion 15). These sun-

---

A TAN IN A BOTTLE

Although people are becoming increasingly wary of getting too much sun, not everyone wants to forsake that perfect tan. Rather than getting bronzed by reclining on a beach towel, however, they're opening a bottle instead.

With an over-the-counter chemical called dihydroxyacetone, you really can "tan" without the sun, says Richard F. Wagner, Jr., M.D., professor of dermatology at the University of Texas Medical Branch at Galveston. Usually considered a cosmetic rather than a drug, this chemical binds to amino acids in the skin, rendering them a reddish brown. After several applications, the color may last for several weeks until old skin cells are replaced by new ones.

"It is safe, although the tan doesn't always look like a natural tan," says Dr. Wagner. For best results, tanning lotions should be applied very quickly in a thin layer. Keep in mind that some parts of the body—the elbows and knees, for example—darken more readily than others. If you aren't careful, he warns, you may easily wind up with a splotchy, unconvincing tan.

screens should be applied to the skin 30 minutes to an hour before going outdoors. They are very effective, says Dr. Urbach, although products containing PABA may cause temporary yellow stains on clothing.

Occasionally one of these products also may cause your eyelids to sting or lead to dry skin or a rash. If this happens to you, try a sunscreen with a different active ingredient. There are several to choose from, including cinnamates (Bain de Soleil All Day, Bullfrog, Coppertone Sunscreen Lotion) or oxybenzone (Hawaiian Tropic 15 plus Sunblock, Sundown Sunscreen). Even these may cause reactions, however. "I tell my patients to apply some to a test area—such as the inside of the wrist where the skin is thin—and see if there's a problem," says Dr. Wagner.

In the past, doctors worried primarily about UV-B rays. They now know, however, that another type of ray, called UV-A, also can damage the skin. That's why some sunscreens now include both UV-B and UV-A protection.

One medication used to block UV-A is called Parsol 1789 (another name for a ten-syllable mouthful called butyl methoxydibenzoylmethane). Usually combined with UV-B blockers (Photoplex, Shade UVAGUARD), this medication works extremely well, says Dr. Wagner. "Basically, what we're talking about are *complete* sunblocks," he says.

AT A GLANCE

CINNAMATES

Brand names: Bain de Soleil All Day, Bullfrog, Coppertone Sunscreen Lotion

How taken: Lotion

Prescription: No

	YES	NO
Generic substitutes	✓	
Potentially addicting		✓
May cause drowsiness		✓
Alcohol discouraged		✓

Possible drug interactions include: Interactions are unlikely.

Possible side effects include: Side effects are unlikely.

BUTYL METHOXYDIBENZOYL-METHANE (PARSOL 1789)

Brand names: Photoplex, Shade UVAGUARD

How taken: Lotion

Prescription: No

	YES	NO
Generic substitutes		✓
Potentially addicting		✓
May cause drowsiness		✓
Alcohol discouraged		✓

Possible drug interactions include: Interactions are unlikely.

Possible side effects include: Rash and itching.

AT A GLANCE

BENZOCAINE		
Brand names: Lanacane, Solarcaine		
How taken: Cream, ointment, spray		
Prescription: No		
	YES	NO
Generic substitutes	✓	
Potentially addicting		✓
May cause drowsiness		✓
Alcohol discouraged		✓
Possible drug interactions include: Interactions are unlikely.		
Possible side effects include: Rash, itching, blisters and hives.		

TETRACAINE		
Brand name: Pontocaine		
How taken: Cream		
Prescription: No		
	YES	NO
Generic substitutes		✓
Potentially addicting		✓
May cause drowsiness		✓
Alcohol discouraged		✓
Possible drug interactions include: Interactions are unlikely.		
Possible side effects include: Rash, itching, blisters and hives.		

Easing Burns

You bought a good sunscreen, packed it a day early and promised to use it every day. Yet here you are on the beach in sunny Cancun, while your sunscreen sits forgotten in the hotel a mile away. Now you're as red as a boiled lobster. What can you do?

For minor burns, there are a number of over-the-counter anesthetic sprays and creams that can give quick relief. Medications containing benzocaine (Lanacane, Solarcaine), lidocaine (Ahhh Sunburn Therapy, Bactine Spray) or tetracaine (Pontocaine) can ease sunburn pain almost immediately.

These medications typically relieve pain for anywhere from 15 to 45 minutes. "They do give you immediate relief," Dr. Wagner says. "They don't do anything for the underlying problem, however. The sunburn has to heal itself."

For most people, topical anesthetics aren't likely to cause serious side effects and can be safely used several times a day. Occasionally, however, they may cause rash, itching or even blisters. It's a lot easier, doctors agree, to prevent sunburn than to relieve the pain later.

Thyroid Drugs

Mechanics for Metabolic Tune-Ups

If your body were an automobile, thyroid hormones would be the gas. Produced by a butterfly-shaped gland at the top of the windpipe, these hormones fuel your metabolism. When thyroid levels are low, your "engine" falters. If they surge, it runs too fast.

The two most common thyroid conditions are Graves' disease, in which the thyroid usually produces too much hormone, and Hashimoto's disease, in which it typically produces too little. In the early stages, symptoms caused by too much thyroid hormone—fast heartbeat or gradual weight loss, for example—often are subtle and not too serious. If left untreated, however, thyroid disease can be life-threatening. Fortunately, with medications, many thyroid conditions can be controlled, often within a few weeks.

Too Much of a Good Thing

Graves' disease is an autoimmune disorder, but beyond that, doctors aren't sure what causes it. People with this condition often experience tremors, weight loss, nervousness, heavy sweating, increased appetite, protruding eyes and other uncomfortable, sometimes dangerous, symptoms, says Kay McFarland, M.D., an endocrinologist and professor of medicine at the University of South Carolina School of Medicine in Columbia.

In most cases people with overactive thyroids have radiation therapy to destroy the gland, after which they take replacement thyroid hormones, says Dr. McFarland. Medication and surgery are other options. Prescription drugs such as propylthiouracil and methimazole (Tapazole) put the brakes on thyroid production. Taken orally, they begin relieving symptoms within one to six weeks.

These medications are fairly safe, although they occasionally will cause headache, dizziness, drowsiness or (rarely) an itchy rash. More serious is the risk of agranulocytosis, a dangerous

AT A GLANCE

PROPYLTHIOURACIL

Brand name: Generic only
How taken: Tablet
Prescription: Yes

	YES	NO
Generic substitutes	✓	
Potentially addicting		✓
May cause drowsiness	✓	
Alcohol discouraged		✓

Possible drug interactions include:
Taking this drug may increase the effects of anti-clotting drugs.

Possible side effects include:
Fever, headache, dizziness, joint pain and skin rash.

METHIMAZOLE

Brand name: Tapazole
How taken: Tablet
Prescription: Yes

	YES	NO
Generic substitutes		✓
Potentially addicting		✓
May cause drowsiness	✓	
Alcohol discouraged		✓

Possible drug interactions include:
Taking this drug may increase the effects of anti-clotting drugs.

Possible side effects include:
Headache, fever, dizziness, joint pain and skin rash.

breakdown in the body's immune system. Fortunately, this condition is quite rare, and most people who are treated with these medications won't have serious side effects, says Dr. McFarland.

In the past, doctors often treated Graves' disease with a prescription drug called strong iodine solution or Lugal's solution, a concentrated form of the same mineral found in seafood and iodized salt. Taken orally, this medication very quickly suppresses thyroid production, often relieving symptoms within a day.

The problem with strong iodine solution is that it usually stops working after two to three weeks, Dr. McFarland says. In addition, the drug can cause sneezing, irritation of the eyes and an unpleasant taste in the mouth. Today, it's rarely used except to relieve symptoms prior to surgery or radiation treatments, or for quick relief should thyroid levels suddenly surge.

Several other drugs also may be used to suppress thyroid production. These include lithium (Eskalith, Lithane, Lithobid), iopanoic acid (Telepaque) and ipodate (Bilivist, Oragrafin Calcium, Oragrafin Sodium). "These are all second-line drugs," says Doris Bartuska, M.D., an endocrinologist and professor of medicine at the Medical College of Pennsylvania in Philadelphia. "We use them only when someone has a problem with one of the other drugs."

Note that when taken along with

x-ray dye drugs, iopanoic acid may interfere with certain kinds of x-rays.

Restoring Balance

Just as having too much thyroid hormone speeds the engine, having too little is like running on empty. This condition, called hypothyroidism, makes people weak and tired. It also may cause the thyroid gland to visibly enlarge, causing a lump in the throat called a goiter, says Joshua Hoffman, M.D., an internist and assistant clinical professor of medicine at the University of California, Davis, Medical Center in Sacramento.

Although hypothyroidism can be quite serious, many people don't even know they have a problem for months or even years. "The symptoms usually occur so gradually that people just think that's the way they're supposed to feel," says Dr. Hoffman.

In most cases, this condition is easily reversed with hormone drugs. Prescription medications such as levothyroxine (Levoid, Levoxine, Synthroid) or liothyronine (Cytomel, Triostat), taken orally, are virtually identical to the body's natural thyroid hormone. This means that they can quickly relieve symptoms while causing few side effects. Doctors like them because they're easily absorbed from the gastrointestinal tract, making them easy to control.

While these drugs are made from

AT A GLANCE

STRONG IODINE SOLUTION

Brand name: Generic only
How taken: Liquid
Prescription: Yes

	YES	NO
Generic substitutes	✓	
Potentially addicting		✓
May cause drowsiness	✓	
Alcohol discouraged		✓

Possible drug interactions include: The effects of this drug may increase if taken with other antithyroid drugs.

Possible side effects include: Hives, sneezing, eye irritation, joint pain, confusion, headache, stomach upset and an unpleasant taste in the mouth.

IOPANOIC ACID

Brand name: Telepaque
How taken: Tablet
Prescription: Yes

	YES	NO
Generic substitutes		✓
Potentially addicting		✓
May cause drowsiness		✓
Alcohol discouraged		✓

Possible drug interactions include: Interactions are unlikely.

Possible side effects include: Itching, nausea, vomiting, stinging urination, cramping and diarrhea.

scratch in the laboratory, older thyroid medications derived from animal glands are also available. Although quite effective, these drugs are less predictable than their synthetic counterparts. As a result, they're rarely used today because "they really don't have anything to recommend them," says Dr. Hoffman.

Although thyroid hormone medications—both natural and synthetic—rarely cause serious side effects, they may cause sweating, chest pain, nervousness or other uncomfortable symptoms, says Dr. McFarland. To help prevent this, doctors usually prescribe them in small amounts, gradually increasing the dose as the weeks go by. In most cases just changing the dose—and giving the body time to adjust—will make the side effects disappear.

AT A GLANCE

LEVOTHYROXINE

Brand names: Levoid, Levothroid, Levoxine, Synthroid

How taken: Tablet, injection

Prescription: Yes

	YES	NO
Generic substitutes	✓	
Potentially addicting		✓
May cause drowsiness		✓
Alcohol discouraged		✓

Possible drug interactions include: Taking this drug may increase the effects of anti-clotting drugs; taking it may decrease the effects of diabetes drugs.

Possible side effects include: Side effects are unlikely.

LIOTHYRONINE

Brand names: Cytomel, Triostat

How taken: Tablet, injection

Prescription: Yes

	YES	NO
Generic substitutes	✓	
Potentially addicting		✓
May cause drowsiness		✓
Alcohol discouraged		✓

Possible drug interactions include: Taking this drug may increase the effects of tricyclic antidepressants, digitalis (a heart medication) and anti-clotting drugs.

Possible side effects include: Side effects are unlikely.

Tuberculosis Drugs

New Weapons for an Old Scourge

We often think of tuberculosis (TB) as an "old-fashioned" condition, common a century ago but rarely seen today. Until the early 1940s, however, TB—a bacterial infection that begins in the lungs and causes fever, cough and other flulike symptoms—was the fourth leading cause of death in the United States. Even today, it strikes approximately 25,000 people a year in this country, and the numbers are on the rise, particularly among drug abusers, the homeless and people with AIDS, whose weakened immune systems can't fend off the disease.

Most cases of TB can be controlled with antibiotics, but sometimes this age-old adversary just scoffs at modern treatments and drags on for months or years at a time. When that happens, many different drugs may be needed to keep it under control.

Emerging Trouble

When antibiotics were introduced about 50 years ago, germs were taken by surprise. Diseases such as TB were easy to control—so easy, in fact, that many experts predicted that one day they would be eliminated entirely.

But germs, as scientists now know, can get used to anything, including antibiotics. "What we're seeing recently are outbreaks of TB that are resistant to multiple drugs," says Sam Dooley, M.D., assistant director for science in the Division of Tuberculosis Elimination at the Centers for Disease Control and Prevention in Atlanta.

In treating TB, he explains, it's important that every single germ be destroyed. "The minimum course of therapy is *six months*," Dr. Dooley says. "It requires an absolute minimum of two drugs,

609

although our current recommendation is four drugs—that's a lot of medications to take for a long time."

Tough Treatments

The drug used most often for battling TB is a prescription antibiotic called isoniazid (Laniazid, Nydrazid, Tubizid). Taken orally or by injection, this powerful medication is usually taken daily for at least two months.

About 5 percent of people taking isoniazid will experience side effects. These include a rash, fever or, more rarely, a painful type of nerve inflammation. As a result, the drug usually is given in combination with pyridoxine (vitamin B_6), which helps prevent the inflammation.

Another helpful antibiotic is

AT A GLANCE

ISONIAZID

Brand names: Laniazid, Nydrazid, Tubizid

How taken: Injection, liquid, tablet

Prescription: Yes

	YES	NO
Generic substitutes	✓	
Potentially addicting		✓
May cause drowsiness		✓
Alcohol discouraged	✓	

Possible drug interactions include: The effects of this drug may decrease if taken with anti-inflammatory steroids. Taking this drug may increase the effects of anti-seizure drugs.

Possible side effects include: Diarrhea, nausea, fever, stomach pain, fatigue, unsteadiness, rash and discoloration of the skin, eyes or urine.

RIFAMPIN

Brand names: Rifadin, Rimactane

How taken: Capsule, injection

Prescription: Yes

	YES	NO
Generic substitutes		✓
Potentially addicting		✓
May cause drowsiness	✓	
Alcohol discouraged	✓	

Possible drug interactions include: Taking this drug may decrease the effects of anti-seizure drugs, anti-clotting drugs, beta-blockers (used for high blood pressure), anti-inflammatory steroids, digitoxin (used for heart problems) and oral contraceptives.

Possible side effects include: Diarrhea, fever, nausea, rash, stomach cramps and discoloration of the skin, stool or urine.

AT A GLANCE

ETHAMBUTOL

Brand name: Myambutol

How taken: Tablet

Prescription: Yes

	YES	NO
Generic substitutes		✓
Potentially addicting		✓
May cause drowsiness		✓
Alcohol discouraged		✓

Possible drug interactions include: The effects of this drug may decrease if taken with antacids containing aluminum.

Possible side effects include: Increased blood levels of uric acid.

PYRAZINAMIDE

Brand name: Generic only

How taken: Tablet

Prescription: Yes

	YES	NO
Generic substitutes	✓	
Potentially addicting		✓
May cause drowsiness		✓
Alcohol discouraged	✓	

Possible drug interactions include: Taking this drug may decrease the effects of gout drugs.

Possible side effects include: Increased blood levels of uric acid and joint pain.

rifampin (Rifadin, Rimactane). It's usually taken once a day, although some doctors will prescribe larger doses to be taken twice a week. It rarely causes serious side effects, although some people may experience a rash or flulike symptoms such as fever or nausea.

For added effectiveness, isoniazid, pyridoxine and rifampin can be used in combination. When these drugs are taken together, experts say, a germ's chances for survival are reduced to about 1 in 100 billion. That's powerful medicine!

There are several additional prescription drugs that may be added to this barrage. Medications such as ethambutol (Myambutol), streptomycin or pyrazinamide are very effective. All are quite safe, although pyrazinamide in high doses occasionally may lead to liver problems. Should this occur, other antibiotics can be substituted, says Dr. Dooley.

Ulcer Medications

Fire Extinguishers

We sometimes think of the stomach as being sensitive but, in fact, the stomach is one tough organ. Following a meal, the stomach kneads and grinds food and fluids. At the same time, it secretes powerful acids and enzymes that break down the food even further.

Consider this: On the pH scale, a scientific measure of acidity, stomach acid is stronger than pure lemon juice and just slightly less potent than battery acid! Consider it a miracle that the same stuff that helps digests a piece of steak doesn't digest you in the process.

Sometimes, however, that's exactly what happens. When it does, ulcer drugs can be a big help.

Into the Breech

Normally, the stomach and duodenum—the part of the small intestine that attaches to the stomach—are protected by a number of mechanisms. Sometimes, however—for reasons that are not always clear—the protective mech-

anisms fail and the lining of the stomach or duodenum breaks down. When it does, stomach acid and digestive enzymes begin to gnaw at unprotected tissue. The result can be pain, inflammation and, sometimes, an ulcer.

Occasionally an ulcer will disappear or heal on its own. But in many cases, especially when accompanied by pain, ulcers can be best treated with prescription ulcer medications, says William Ruderman, M.D., chairman of the Department of Gastroenterology at the Cleveland Clinic–Florida in Fort Lauderdale. Some ulcer drugs help augment the body's own protective mechanisms. Others eradicate harmful bacteria. But the most popular ulcer medications are those that actually stem the flow of corrosive acid, says Dr. Ruderman.

Turning Off the Acid Tap

The drugs of choice for treating most ulcers are H_2-receptor antagonists, or H_2-blockers for short. Sold by prescription and usually taken orally one to four times a day, these drugs help block the effects of a body chemical called histamine, which in turn helps reduce the amount of acid in the stomach.

There are four different H_2-blockers your doctor can choose. They are cimetidine (Apo-Cimetidine, Peptol, Tagamet), ranitidine (Zantac), famotidine (Pepcid) and nizatidine (Axid). As a group, these drugs are very effective. They reduce stomach acid secretions by 50 to 80 percent, healing about 75 percent of duode-

nal ulcers in four weeks and 85 to 90 percent after eight weeks, says Dr. Ruderman.

Stomach ulcers, on the other hand, may be more difficult to treat. Healing stomach ulcers may require a full 12 weeks of treatment because the acid concentrations are so much higher. In the long run, however, the success rates are still very good, he adds.

The four different H_2-blockers have much in common. "They've all been given to a few hundred million people by now. They're all very safe and the side effects are

---

NATURAL ALTERNATIVES

With modern drugs, healing ulcers is easy. What's not so easy is preventing them from coming back. Still, there are ways to improve your odds. For example:

Check your medicines. Tell your doctor if you're taking aspirin or other nonsteroidal anti-inflammatory drugs. You may be three times more likely to have ulcers. Indeed, among people with rheumatoid arthritis—who often take large doses of these drugs—the risk for serious ulcers may be increased *ninefold*. Ask your doctor about medications that can counteract their effects.

Toss the cigarettes. Smokers are twice as likely as nonsmokers to develop ulcers, doctors say. And once smokers get ulcers, they heal more slowly and are more likely to have recurrences than nonsmokers.

Go easy on the alcohol. In experiments, alcohol put directly into the stomach causes bleeding and ulcers. It's still not clear how the occasional drink, imbibed in the usual way, affects ulcers. Still, if you do drink, doctors say, it only makes sense to do so in moderation.

Watch the hot stuff. As with alcohol, black and red pepper may cause bleeding. Yet some studies have shown that people who indulge in spicy foods have no problems at all. This is one instance when you must let your stomach—and any resulting discomfort—be your guide.

AT A GLANCE

CIMETIDINE

Brand names: Apo-Cimetidine, Novocimetidine, Peptol, Tagamet

How taken: Tablet, liquid, injection

Prescription: Yes

	YES	NO
Generic substitutes		✓
Potentially addicting		✓
May cause drowsiness		✓
Alcohol discouraged	✓	

Possible drug interactions include: Taking this drug may increase the effects of anti-clotting drugs, sedatives, phenytoin (an anti-seizure drug), propranolol (used for heart and blood pressure problems) and theophylline (an asthma drug).

Possible side effects include: Side effects are unlikely.

RANITIDINE

Brand name: Zantac

How taken: Liquid, injection, tablet

Prescription: Yes

	YES	NO
Generic substitutes		✓
Potentially addicting		✓
May cause drowsiness		✓
Alcohol discouraged	✓	

Possible drug interactions include: Taking this drug may increase the effects of anti-clotting drugs.

Possible side effects include: Side effects are unlikely.

usually minimal," according to Dr. Ruderman.

Potent Alternatives

Although the H$_2$-blockers are the drugs of choice for most types of ulcers, there are times when more powerful drugs are needed. A class of drugs called proton-pump inhibitors—the proton pump is a chemical process in individual cells—can reduce acid secretions by more than 95 percent.

For example, a prescription drug called omeprazole (Prilosec), taken orally once a day, may be prescribed for people with serious duodenal ulcers or reflux esophagitis, the painful splashing of acid into the esophagus. Omeprazole is much more potent in terms of acid suppression than the H$_2$-blockers, says Dr. Ruderman.

But the drug also is expensive, costing more than $1 a day. It's also new, so doctors aren't entirely comfortable with it, as they aren't sure what the long-term side effects may be. As a result, omeprazole usually is prescribed only when H₂-blockers don't work.

Reducing acid is just one way to heal ulcers. A prescription drug called misoprostol (Cytotec) can suppress acid production but may also augment the natural defenses of the stomach. Taken orally four times a day, misoprostol usually is used to prevent ulcers in people who are taking large doses of aspirin or other nonsteroidal anti-inflammatory drugs, which are harsh irritants to the stomach lining. For healing ulcers that already have formed, however, misoprostol appears to be less effective than either omeprazole or the H₂-blockers.

Paste-on Protection

Another way to heal ulcers is to protect them. A prescription drug called sucralfate (Carafate), taken orally, coats ulcers with a tough chemical blanket, which acts like an internal adhesive

---

AT A GLANCE

FAMOTIDINE

Brand name: Pepcid

How taken: Tablet, liquid, injection

Prescription: Yes

	YES	NO
Generic substitutes		✓
Potentially addicting		✓
May cause drowsiness		✓
Alcohol discouraged	✓	

Possible drug interactions include: Interactions are unlikely.

Possible side effects include: Side effects are unlikely.

OMEPRAZOLE

Brand name: Prilosec

How taken: Capsule

Prescription: Yes

	YES	NO
Generic substitutes		✓
Potentially addicting		✓
May cause drowsiness		✓
Alcohol discouraged	✓	

Possible drug interactions include: Taking this drug may increase the effects of phenytoin (an anti-seizure drug), anti-clotting drugs and diazepam (a sedative).

Possible side effects include: Diarrhea and stomach upset.

MISOPROSTOL

Brand name: Cytotec
How taken: Tablet
Prescription: Yes

	YES	NO
Generic substitutes		✓
Potentially addicting		✓
May cause drowsiness		✓
Alcohol discouraged	✓	

Possible drug interactions include:
This drug taken in combination with antacids containing magnesium may result in diarrhea.

Possible side effects include:
Diarrhea and abdominal pain.

CAUTION: May cause miscarriage when taken by pregnant women.

SUCRALFATE

Brand name: Carafate
How taken: Tablet, liquid
Prescription: Yes

	YES	NO
Generic substitutes		✓
Potentially addicting		✓
May cause drowsiness	✓	
Alcohol discouraged	✓	

Possible drug interactions include:
Taking this drug may decrease the effects of phenytoin (an anti-seizure drug), anti-clotting drugs, tetracycline (an antibiotic) and cimetidine (another ulcer drug).

Possible side effects include:
Constipation.

strip. By covering the ulcer, it keeps acids and pepsin, a digestive enzyme, away until the tender tissue heals.

Sucralfate usually is prescribed for duodenal ulcers, and studies show it can heal 60 to 90 percent of cases within six weeks. It's also used to prevent "stress ulcers," a dangerous condition that often threatens critically ill hospital patients.

"Sucralfate's main calling card is that it's not absorbed, so it's extremely safe," says Richard McCallum, M.D., professor of medicine and chief of the Division of Gastroenterology, Hepatology and Nutrition at the University of Virginia Health Sciences Center in Charlottesville.

On the other hand, sucralfate has to be taken up to four times a day and may cause some constipation. Many doctors use it only when other drugs aren't effective.

Stopping the Source

Over the years, doctors have fingered dozens of ulcer suspects, including stress, coffee and spicy foods. Undoubtedly, these and many other factors can make ulcers flare. But the real culprit is almost always a common bacteria called *Helicobacter pylori*, says Dr. McCallum. "Aside from those ulcers caused by nonsteroidal anti-inflammatory drugs, virtually every duodenal ulcer in this country can be linked to the presence of *H. pylori*," he says.

This may explain why so many ulcers, even those that have been successfully targeted with ulcer medications, eventually come back. The *ulcer* was healed, but the underlying *problem*—the bacteria—remained.

In one study, researchers at Baylor College of Medicine in Houston treated 109 ulcer patients either with the H_2-blocker ranitidine alone or ranitidine plus "triple therapy"—bismuth subsalicylate (Pepto-Bismol) combined with two antibiotics for two weeks. Then they kept track of the patients' progress for up to two more years.

Among those in the ranitidine group, more than 50 percent experienced recurrent ulcers within 12 weeks of completion of therapy. Among those receiving triple therapy, only four people (less than 5 percent) had relapses—either because the bacteria were not fully killed off initially or because of the use of nonsteroidal anti-inflammatory drugs (not part of the original therapy).

Despite some compelling evidence, there still is disagreement about whether people should be treated, at least initially, with antibiotics or traditional ulcer drugs such as H_2-blockers. Some doctors argue that the possible benefits of antibiotic therapy may be overshadowed both by the inconvenience (the drugs are taken several times a day for two weeks) and possible side effects, such as diarrhea.

Other doctors are now using antibiotics as first-line treatment. "If people have ulcers and you eradicate the *H. pylori*, then 90 to 95 percent of them will have a cure for up to two years," says Dr. McCallum.

Vaccines

Infection Protection

Few battles have been so successful as those against infectious diseases. Consider polio. In 1952, polio struck more than 20,000 Americans. Today it's been virtually eradicated in the United States. Diphtheria? In 1921, it struck more than 200,000 Americans. In 1990: 4. Equally impressive were the reductions in the incidence of mumps, measles, rubella and many other infectious diseases.

What accounts for these dramatic changes? The answer can be summed up in one word: vaccines.

Fighting Disease with Disease

As early as the 1700s, scientists suspected that giving people mild forms of a disease—for example, by exposing them to tissue infected with smallpox—might reduce their risk of getting the full-fledged version later.

These early "vaccines" were crude, but the underlying principle was sound: You can prevent a disease by first getting a disease: that is, by getting just enough of it to "teach" your immune system what to look for—and attack—in the future. This is called immunity.

Modern vaccines are essentially "imitations" of nature's germs—*minus* their ability to cause disease, says Louisa Chapman, M.D., a medical epidemiologist with the Centers for Disease Control and Prevention in Atlanta. Your im-

---

AT A GLANCE

DTP VACCINE (diphtheria, tetanus and pertussis)

Brand names: DTwP, Tri-Immunol

How taken: Injection

Prescription: Yes

Possible drug interactions include: Interactions are unlikely.

Possible side effects include: Mild fever, irritability and soreness or swelling at the injection site.

When to vaccinate: Immunization is recommended for children at 2, 4, 6 and 18 months, and again at five years. Children seven years of age and older should get a combined tetanus and diphtheria vaccine. Adults should get booster shots of this vaccine every ten years.

POLIOVIRUS VACCINE LIVE ORAL (OPV)

Brand names: Orimune, Poliovax

How taken: Liquid

Prescription: Yes

Possible drug interactions include: The effects of this drug may decrease if taken with cancer drugs, x-rays or high doses of steroids.

Possible side effects include: Side effects are unlikely.

When to vaccinate: Immunization is recommended for children at 2, 4 and 18 months, and again at five years.

CAUTION: Live polio vaccine is not recommended for children who have low resistance to serious infections or who live with other persons who do.

AT A GLANCE

HAEMOPHILUS B POLYSACCHA-RIDE VACCINE

Brand names: Hib TITER, Pedvax, Pro HIBIT

How taken: Injection

Prescription: Yes

Possible drug interactions include: Interactions are unlikely.

Possible side effects include: Diarrhea, mild fever, irritability, lack of appetite and redness or soreness at the injection site.

When to vaccinate: Children should be immunized between their second and fifth birthday. For children attending day-care centers or for those with chronic illnesses such as Hodgkin's disease, immunizations should be given between 18 months and two years.

MMR VACCINE (measles, mumps and rubella)

Brand name: Generic only

How taken: Injection

Prescription: Yes

Possible drug interactions include: Interactions are unlikely.

Possible side effects include: Fever, rash and stinging at the injection site.

When to vaccinate: Immunization is recommended for children at 15 months and for those born after 1957 who have not been previously vaccinated.

CAUTION: Birth defects may result if women become pregnant within three months after receiving this vaccine.

mune system can't tell the difference between a vaccine and a real germ, so it produces antibodies just the same. You get protection without getting sick the first time.

Childhood Protection

By the time you reach adulthood, you've been exposed to—and developed immunity to—many common germs. You don't bother them, they don't bother you. But kids and germs don't have this benevolent relationship.

That's why experts recommend that all children be vaccinated against the Big 8 childhood diseases: Measles, mumps, rubella, diphtheria, tetanus, pertussis, polio and *Haemophilus influenzae* type b, or Hib, a serious infection that can lead to meningitis.

The first vaccination most kids get is called DTP (DTwP, Tri-Immunol). Given by injection, DTP is really three vaccines—diphtheria, tetanus and pertussis—in one.

The vaccine often causes fever and can make kids extremely

AT A GLANCE

HEPATITIS B VACCINE

Brand names: Engerix-B, Recombivax HB

How taken: Injection

Prescription: Yes

Possible drug interactions include: Interactions are unlikely.

Possible side effects include: Soreness at the injection site.

When to vaccinate: Immunization is recommended for everyone, at any age.

INFLUENZA VACCINE

Brand names: Flu-Imune, Fluogen

How taken: Injection

Prescription: Yes

Possible drug interactions include: Interactions are unlikely.

Possible side effects include: Redness, soreness or a hard lump at the injection site.

When to vaccinate: Immunization is recommended for everyone, except infants under the age of six months.

CAUTION: This vaccine is not recommended for those allergic to eggs.

cranky for a day or two. The fevers are generally mild, however, and giving your child acetaminophen can help keep the temperature down. Experts recommend that you give your child one dose at the time of the vaccination and another every four to six hours over the next two to three days.

At the same time as the DTP shot, kids are often given a polio vaccine as well. Taken orally on several occasions, the OPV vaccine actually contains a live polio virus (it's been made very weak so it won't cause disease). The vaccine is very effective, protecting the vast majority of children against this terrible disease, in most cases for life.

There also is an injectable form of the vaccine, which may be used in some adults and children with serious illnesses such as cancer. But in most cases, the oral drug is the preferred form.

Other important vaccines include those for *Haemophilus influenzae* type b (Hib TITER, Pedvax HIB, Pro HIBIT) and the combination MMR (measles, mumps and rubella) vaccine. In addition, the American Academy of Pediatrics has recommended that all children be immunized against hepatitis B as well. Although hepatitis B isn't a children's disease, experts hope that, with early vaccinations, it may someday be eradicated for good.

Fears and Misconceptions

The U.S. Public Health Service would like to see all of the nation's two-year-olds fully immunized. Currently, however, fewer than 63 percent of infants receive all their shots. In some areas, the number is as low as 10 percent.

Why don't all kids get their shots? In some cases, parents feel they can't afford the vaccines. Or perhaps they don't have a regular doctor they can turn to for advice. Some parents worry that vaccinations may actually harm their children.

There have been some cases in which people taking the polio vaccine, or someone in close contact with a person recently immunized, did become infected. This is rare. In fact, experts estimate that the risk is about 1 in every 6.5 million doses.

Some parents worry that the DTP vaccine may cause dangerous convulsions or other neurological conditions. Again, this is rare. In one study, researchers at Vanderbilt University in Tennessee kept tabs on nearly 40,000 kids who received more than 100,000 DTP vaccinations. They concluded that the immunizations only rarely, if ever, cause serious neurological problems.

Shots for Adults

Children get the lion's share of vaccinations, but adults also need protection. The tetanus vaccine, for example, which is routinely given to infants, isn't effective forever. Adults must get booster shots once every ten years to prevent this terrible disease.

Then there's influenza. Every year, as many as one in four Americans are afflicted with the sniffles, muscle aches and general blahs that accompany this seasonal misery, better known as the flu.

For most people, the flu is annoying but nothing to worry about. For the elderly, however, or those with underlying illnesses, a bout with flu can be very serious, sometimes deadly. That's why experts recommend that anyone with a weakened immune system receive an annual flu vaccination. In fact, many doctors advise all of their patients over 65 as well as younger people with health problems to receive the vaccination, says Dr. Chapman.

You have to get a flu shot every year because the viruses themselves are constantly changing. "Every year the viruses that are circulating may be first cousins or even distant cousins to the ones circulating the year before," she says.

It takes about two weeks after getting the shot for your body to develop full immunity, Dr. Chapman adds. So if you wait until the bug is already in your neighborhood before getting immunized, it may be too late.

The height of the vaccination season is from mid-October to mid-November, says Dr. Chapman. But, she adds, "People who are at high risk should get the vaccine as soon as it's available in September."

Index

Boldface references indicate boxed text.

A

Abitrate (clofibrate), 462, 573
Accutane (isotretinoin), 359–60, **359**
Acebutolol, **370**, 371, 452, 508
ACE inhibitors, 451
Acephen. *See* Acetaminophen
Acetaminophen, 35, 407
  for colds, **466**, 467
  for menstrual problems, 537
  for migraines, 541, **541**
  for pain relief, 559, **559**
Acetazolamide, 491
Acetic acid, 483, **485**
Acetylcholine, 567
Acid indigestion. *See* Heartburn
Acidophilus, 121–23
  key facts summarized, **122**
  sweet, **70**
  in yogurt, 108–9
Acne
  drug treatment, 356–60
    natural alternatives, **356**
  zinc for, 246
Acquired immune deficiency
    syndrome. *See* AIDS
Acromegaly, 575
Actamin. *See* Acetaminophen
ACTH, 520–21, **521**
Acthar (corticotropin), 520–21, **521**
Actidose-Aqua (activated charcoal), 399, **399**
Actifed with Codeine, 470–71, **471**
Actigall (ursodiol), 498–99, **499**
Activated charcoal, 399, **399**

Acyclovir, 423–24, **423**, 425, 487
Adalat (nifedipine), 450, 544
Adapin. *See* Doxepin
Addictions, 126
ADH, 572–73
Adipex-P (phentermine), 599–600, **599**
Adolescents, riboflavin deficiency in, 231
Adrenalin (epinephrine), 433, **435**
Adrenocorticotropic hormone, 520–21, **521**
Adrucil (fluorouracil), **455**
Advil. *See* Ibuprofen
AeroBid (flunisolide), 437
Aerolate (theophylline), 435, **436**
Afrin Nasal Spray (oxymetazoline), **473**
Afrinol Repetabs. *See* Pseudoephedrine
Aging
  cherries and, 48
  vitamin B$_6$ and, 129
  vitamin B$_{12}$ and, **132**, 133
Ahhh Sunburn Therapy (lidocaine), 604
AIDS
  drug treatment, 356–60, 363, 427
  hyssop for, 312
  St.-John's-wort for, 329–31
Airplane ear, **483**
Akarpine (pilocarpine), **490**, 491
AK-Dex (dexamethasone), 409–10, **409**
Alamag (aluminum and magnesium), **375**, 377
Alaria, 94
Albuterol, 433, **435**
Alcohol, 116, 157
Alcoholism, 240
Aldactone (spironolactone), 449

I

M

N

P